CONCEPTS IN COMMUNITY HEALTH

Prof. (Dr.) Sujata K. Das

ALLIED HEALTH PRESS

Concepts in Community Health

Author: **Prof. (Dr.) Sujata K. Das**

Allied Health Press
4164 Lakeshore Road
Burlington ON L7L 1A4
Canada
www.alliedhealthpress.com
Email: orders@arclereducation.com

ISBN: 978-1-77956-252-4

ABOUT THE AUTHOR

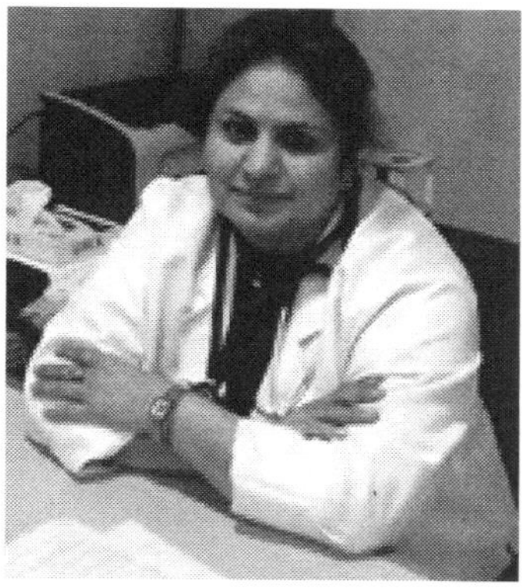

Prof (Dr) Sujata K. Dass, M.B.B.S, D.N.B, Ph.D. (Medicine) is a distinguished neuro-physician and academician, currently serving as an Attending Consultant in the Department of Neurology, B.L. Kapur Hospital, a renowned super-specialty medical institution in the New Delhi. Her illustrious career in medicine and research spans over three decades, characterized by her profound contributions to neurology and her unwavering commitment to medical education.

Dr. Dass began her educational journey at Flushing High School in New York, USA, and completed her High School Diploma thereafter she joined Queens College of the City University of New York as an undergrad student. With a passion for medicine, she pursued her MBBS degree at King George Medical College, Lucknow, U.P., India. Her academic prowess and dedication to medicine were evident early on, setting the stage for a remarkable career. Dr Dass worked under the supervision of Dr M.S. Bains, M.D. as a Visiting Fellow in cardio-thoracic surgery at Memorial Sloan Kettering Cancer Research Center, New York, USA. Dr. Dass furthered her medical training by obtaining a D.N.B. (Family Medicine) and conducted significant research on hematological changes in malaria. Her quest for knowledge and excellence led her back to New York, where she completed her Ph.D. (Medicine) at the Department of Obstetrics & Gynecology, The New York Hospital-Cornell University Medical Center under the mentorship of Prof. Brij B. Saxena. Her groundbreaking work on Sn-Proto and Sn-Mesoporphyrin and the chemoprevention of neonatal jaundice culminated in the award of her D.Sc. (Medicine).

Dr. Sujata Dass joined as the BR Ambedkar Chair Professor in July 2002 in the Institute of Biomedical Sciences, Faculty of Medicine, Bundelkhand University, Jhansi. Her tenure was marked by her dedication to advancing medical research and education. She also served as UGC National Research Award (Professor) at V.P. Chest Institute, University of Delhi. Throughout her career, Dr. Dass has received numerous awards and accolades on a global level. Notable among these are the UGC Research Award, the Fast Track Young Scientist Award from the Department of Science and Technology (DST), and the Women's Award of Highest Honour from Soka University, Japan. She has also received numerous research grants from DST, DBT and ICMR, UGC etc. These awards and grants underscore her exceptional contributions to medical science and research.

Dr. Dass is a respected member of various scientific and administrative bodies like Planning Board (IGNOU), Executive Council - Bhagat Phool Singh Mahila Vishwavidhlaya, Haryana (2008-2011) where she continues to influence the medical community with her insights and expertise. Her commitment to guiding and mentoring students in their master's and doctoral thesis highlights her dedication to nurturing the next generation of medical professionals. Dr. Dass remains a beacon of excellence and a role model for aspiring medical professionals worldwide.

Word Roots, Prefixes, and Suffixes by Chapter

Chapter 1 Introduction to Community Health

Anti-: Against or opposed to (e.g., antibiotic - against life).

Pre-: Before (e.g., prevention - action taken before illness occurs).

Sub-: Under or below (e.g., subclinical - below the level of clinical symptoms).

Pro-: In favor of or supporting (e.g., promote - to support or advance).

-ology: Study of (e.g., sociology - the study of society).

-ic: Pertaining to (e.g., specific - relating to a particular case).

-tion: Action or process (e.g., prevention - the process of preventing).

-al: Pertaining to (e.g., personal - relating to the individual).

Chapter 2 Infectious Disease Epidemiology

Epi-: Means "upon" or "over" (e.g., epidemic - a widespread occurrence of an infectious disease).

Pre-: Means "before" (e.g., prevalence - the proportion of a population found to have a condition before a certain point in time).

Sub-: Means "under" or "below" (e.g., subclinical - a stage of disease not showing obvious symptoms).

Anti-: Means "against" (e.g., antiviral - targeting or inhibiting viruses).

-ology: Refers to the study of (e.g., epidemiology - the study of how diseases spread and affect populations).

-itis: Indicates inflammation (e.g., hepatitis - inflammation of the liver).

-sis: Refers to a process or condition (e.g., diagnosis - the identification of a disease).

-gen: Means "producing" or "causing" (e.g., pathogen - an organism that causes disease).

-emic: Refers to a condition related to blood or a disease affecting a particular group (e.g., epidemic - a widespread occurrence of an infectious disease).

Chapter 3 Enhancing Community and Public Health through Nutritional Strategies

Pre-: Before (e.g., Primary Prevention)

Non-: Not (e.g., Non-Communicable Diseases)

Sub-: Under or below (e.g., Subclinical, not directly mentioned but related)

-ology: Study of (e.g., Epidemiology)

-ic: Related to (e.g., Nutritional, Chronic)

-ist: Specialist or expert (e.g., Nutritionist)

-ion: Process or action (e.g., Promotion)

-al: Pertaining to (e.g., Nutritional, Chronic)

Chapter 4 Empowering Women's Health: Understanding, Care, and Wellness Across the Lifespan

anti-: against (e.g., antifungal - against fungal infections)

peri-: around (e.g., perinatal - around the time of birth)

pre-: before (e.g., prenatal - before birth)

-ology: study of (e.g., obstetrics - the study of childbirth and the care of women giving birth)

-itis: inflammation (e.g., arthritis - inflammation of the joints)

-ectomy: surgical removal (e.g., hysterectomy - surgical removal of the uterus)

Chapter 5 Improving Maternal and Child Health Through Integrated Healthcare Services

Mater: Mother (e.g., maternal)

Neo: New (e.g., neonatology)

Ped: Child (e.g., pediatrics)

Gyne: Woman (e.g., gynecology)

Obstet: Midwife or childbirth (e.g., obstetrics)

Natal: Birth (e.g., neonatal)

Ante-: Before (e.g., antepartum - before childbirth)

Post-: After (e.g., postpartum - after childbirth)

Pre-: Before (e.g., prenatal - before birth)

Intra-: Within (e.g., intrapartum - during labor)

-ology: Study of (e.g., obstetrics - study of childbirth)

-ics: Related to (e.g., pediatrics - related to child health)

-al: Pertaining to (e.g., maternal - pertaining to mother)

-ic: Pertaining to (e.g., perinatal - pertaining to the time around birth)

-gram: Record or picture (e.g., sonogram - picture of the fetus)

Chapter 6 Promoting Health for Older Adults

Geri-: Relating to old age (e.g., gerontology, geriatrics).

Sen-: Related to aging or the elderly (e.g., senescence, senile).

Cardi-: Pertaining to the heart (e.g., cardiovascular, cardiology).

Osteo-: Related to bones (e.g., osteoporosis, osteoarthritis).

Neuro-: Relating to nerves or the nervous system (e.g., neurology, neurodegenerative).

Pre-: Before (e.g., prediabetic, preexisting conditions).

mal (e.g., hypoglycemia, hypotension).

Hyper-: Above normal (e.g., hyperlipidemia, hyperglycemia).

-itis: Inflammation (e.g., arthritis, dermatitis).

-osis: Condition or disease (e.g., osteoporosis, sclerosis).

-pathy: Disease or disorder (e.g., neuropathy, cardiomyopathy).

-algia: Pain (e.g., neuralgia, myalgia).

-ectomy: Surgical removal (e.g., appendectomy, mastectomy).

Chapter 7 Nutrition Disorders in Community: Strategies for Prevention and Management

Mal-: Bad or abnormal (e.g., malnutrition, malabsorption)

Hyper-: Excessive or above normal (e.g., hypervitaminosis, hypercalcemia)

Hypo-: Below normal or deficient (e.g., hypoglycemia, hypovitaminosis)

Pre-: Before (e.g., pre-disease, pre-natal nutrition)

Sub-: Under or below (e.g., subclinical, subnutrition)

-osis: Condition or disease (e.g., ketosis, steatosis)

-emia: Blood condition (e.g., anemia, hyperglycemia)

-pathy: Disease or disorder (e.g., neuropathy, cardiomyopathy)

-itis: Inflammation (e.g., gastritis, enteritis)

-al: Pertaining to (e.g., nutritional, dietary)

Chapter 8 Community Health Policies and Programs

Pre-: Means “before,” as in “preventive” (measures taken before disease occurs).

Inter-: Means “between” or “among,” as in “interventions” (actions taken among individuals or groups to improve health).

Re-: Means “again” or “back,” as in “re-evaluation” (assessing something again).

In-: Means “not” or “into,” as in “inadequate” (not sufficient).

-ic: Means “related to,” as in “health-related” (pertaining to health).

-al: Means “pertaining to,” as in “nutritional” (related to nutrition).

-tion: Indicates an action or process, as in “prevention” (the act of stopping something from happening).

-ing: Indicates an ongoing action or process, as in “promoting” (actively supporting health).

Table of Contents

3 Enhancing Community and Public Health through Nutritional Strategies 53

4 Empowering Women's Health: Understanding, Care, and Wellness Across the Lifespan 91

LIST OF FIGURES

LIST OF TABLES

PREFACE

Health is a more difficult concept than disease. When we try to think of it, our thoughts are usually in negative terms—the absence of disease. We think first of ourselves or a child. Regardless of your interactions with your co-livings, you have an impact on your community. It may be good or bad. We all are in a community together; there is no other way and so is health. Community health is the convergence of healthcare services, economics, and social responsibilities. People residing in a particular region more or less share similar kinds of health risks and social and economic conditions. Community health is a medical practice that focuses on people's well-being in a particular geographical area. This essential public health sector covers programs to help neighborhood members protect and improve their health, deter the transmission of infectious diseases, and plan for natural disasters. For example, a community may be exposed to pollutants from a nearby factory or waste dumping site or groundwater contaminants. Public wellness programs expand access to preventive health services, include people in decision-making on treatment, and seek reduced hospitala costs. Community health is usually confused with population health. However, they are interrelated but have sufficient differences. Where community health refers to the collective efforts of individuals or organizations for the better health of a geographically or culturally defined group of people, while population health uses outcome-driven approaches for the health benefits of a specific group of people typically defined by attribution.

To extend these thoughts beyond ourselves and our families to the whole community—diseases of the community and then community health—is a very necessary exercise for all health workers.

This book attempts to cover all these different aspects of community health in one volume. We know that we have to learn about the structure (anatomy) and function (physiology) of the body before we can understand its malfunction, or disease (pathology). We also know that there are many types of diseases that affect the body in different ways and require to be managed in different ways. Similarly, before we can appreciate the problems of a community we must know something about community structure (demography) and function (sociology). We have to learn about the patterns of disease (epidemiology), and the organization and administration of different services that may be provided for the whole community (e.g., environmental control, immunization, child spacing, nutrition and education) or for special groups in the community (e.g., mothers and young children, school children, workers and the handicapped).

As its title suggests, "Concepts in Community Health" was written to introduce students to community and public health. This book is written to provide a comprehensive overview of key concepts, strategies, and best practices in community health, with a focus on improving health outcomes and addressing health disparities at the local and global levels. It aims to serve as a valuable resource for those working in the field of public health, as well as individuals and organizations seeking to promote health and well-being in communities.

Chapter 1

INTRODUCTION TO COMMUNITY HEALTH

Contents

Introduction

Health in communities is influenced by multiple factors, and various segments of the community can contribute to and share the responsibility for safeguarding and enhancing it. Shifts in public policy, the roles of both public and private sectors in health and healthcare, and changing public expectations are creating both opportunities and challenges for communities as they tackle the overall health of the population and specific health concerns. The appropriate geographic unit for addressing a specific health issue may differ depending on the circumstances, such as the county, city, or census tract. Various individuals, organizations, and agencies, including those outside the conventional scope of healthcare or public health, have an impact on and an interest in the health of a community (Patrick & Wickizer, 1995). The entities encompassed in this category may consist of individual healthcare providers, public health agencies, healthcare organizations, purchasers of health services, and community organizations that are specifically focused on health matters. In addition, they can encompass various government entities such as housing, human services, and public safety, as well as educational institutions, businesses, industries, faith communities, and other community organizations that may not typically be associated with explicit health-related responsibilities. Entities such as state health departments, federal agencies, managed care organizations, and national corporations have a wider range of influence than a single community, but they frequently play a significant role at the local level.

As communities address the complex factors associated with different health issues, all parties will need to clarify their roles and responsibilities. The pattern will fluctuate over time and differ among different communities, contingent upon the combination and interplay of factors that contribute to health. To maximize the distinct contributions of these interconnected sectors, it will be crucial to tackle matters of accountability and collective responsibility for different facets of community health. Most communities have limited experience with widespread collaborative or coordinated efforts among diverse groups. Effective collaboration among community stakeholders can be facilitated by a shared language and a comprehensive understanding of the various factors that influence health. This chapter focuses on the fundamental principles of community health.

Orientation and Directional Terms

Term	Definition	Illustration
Community Health	The branch of medicine that focuses on the health of entire populations, aiming to improve health outcomes through disease prevention and health promotion efforts.	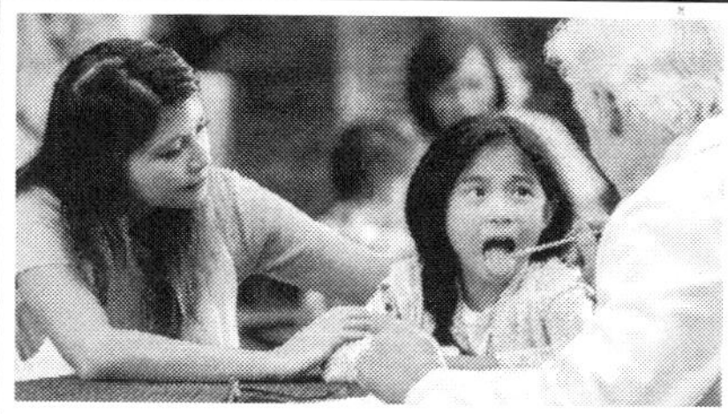
Disease	A pathological condition of a bodily part, an organ, or system resulting from various causes, such as infection, genetic defect, or environmental factors, characterized by an identifiable set of symptoms and signs.	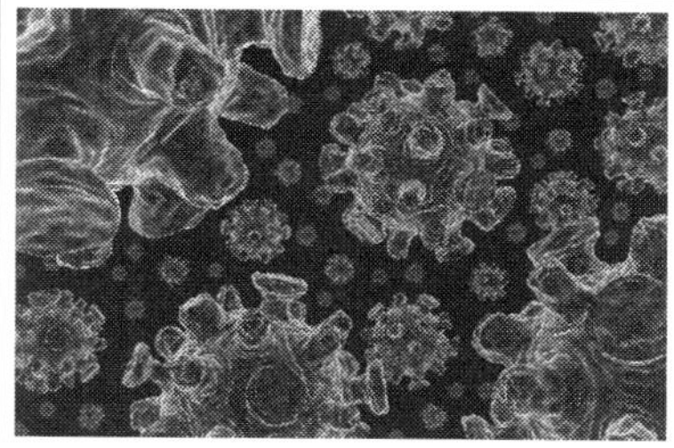
Health Education	The process of providing information and teaching individuals and communities about health topics to promote healthy behaviors and improve health outcomes.	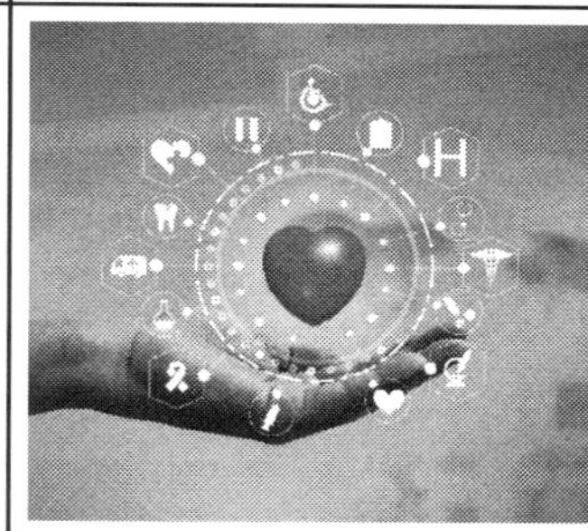
Health Services	The range of services provided to individuals and communities to maintain or improve health, including preventive, diagnostic, therapeutic, and rehabilitative services.	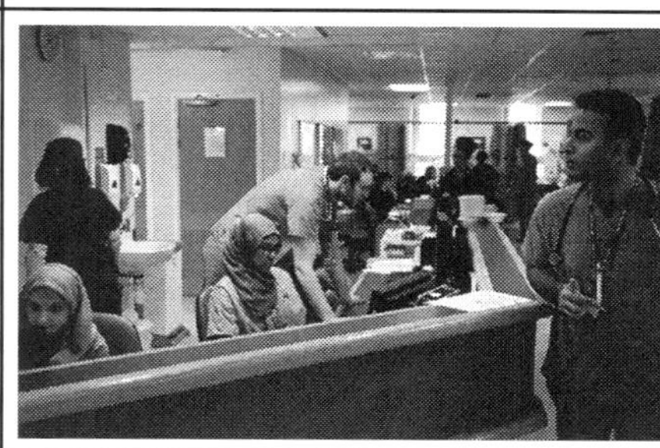
Primary Health Care	Essential health care that is universally accessible to individuals and families in the community at a cost that is affordable, aiming to provide comprehensive, accessible, and community-based care.	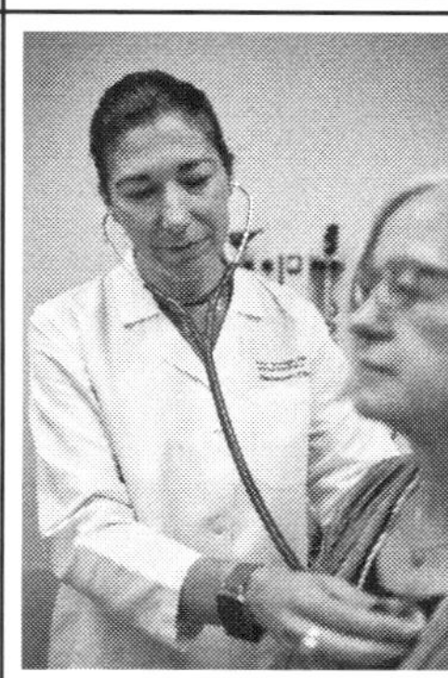

1.1. What Is Community Health?

When it comes to medicine, community health refers to the branch of medicine that focuses on the health of the entire population as well as the prevention of diseases associated with that population. To accomplish this, it first conducts a community diagnosis to determine which diseases are significant and which can be prevented, and then it organizes control programs that are appropriate for the situation. A problem arises when there is only a limited amount of money available to spend on medical services, and that problem is how to accomplish this. Due to the limited amount of money, it is necessary to determine which diseases, among those that are both preventable and significant, are the most important, and then to choose the most effective control programs that are within the financial means of the organization. Medical services have traditionally been structured around curative medicine, such as that which is performed by hospitals, outpatient departments, and dispensaries to treat patients. When sick people come to these services and ask for assistance, they provide it; however, when sick people do not come to these services and do not ask for assistance, they do very little. In the case of those individuals who come, curative medicine has the potential to cure certain diseases, alleviate certain sufferings, and prevent certain deaths; however, it is not capable of significantly affecting the number of new cases of an illness that occur within the community. The treatment of children who have kwashiorkor or gastroenteritis, for example, will not have much of an impact on the number of new cases that occur in the forthcoming years. If we want to reduce the number of new cases, we need to begin taking preventative measures before people become ill. Preventative medicine is what this is. It is necessary to make some basic health services accessible to everyone who has the potential to become ill to accomplish the goal of practicing effective preventive medicine. The stages in the development of diseases, the levels of prevention and the methods that are available, the health needs and demands of a community, the concepts of population coverage and at-risk groups of people, and the organization of basic health services are all discussed in this chapter as part of the presentation of the theory of community health. To determine the order of importance for community health programs, it is necessary to conduct a community diagnosis (Figure 1.1).

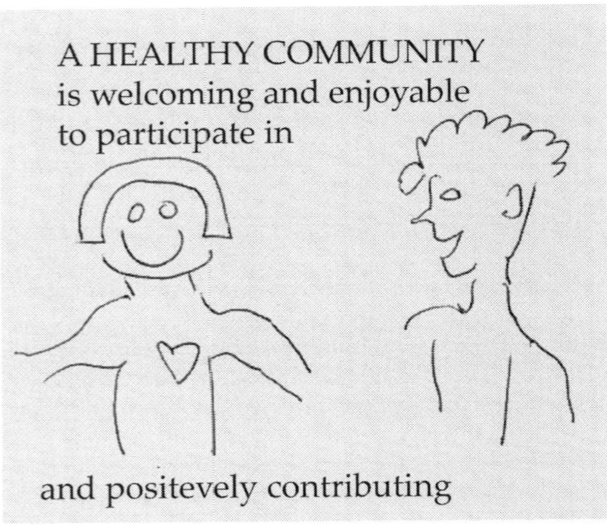

Figure 1.1. *Illustration of community health.*

Source: https://upload.wikimedia.org/wikipedia/commons/4/47/A_healthy_community_is_welcoming_and_enjoyable_to_participate_in_and_positevely_contributing.png.

1.2. Health and the Development of Disease

When people talk about their health, they typically do so in terms of the diseases that they live with. Most people can make a full recovery from diseases; however, some people experience damage to their bodies and may acquire a permanent disability. If the disease is extremely severe, it may become fatal. The individual is initially in good health and well-being. The ideal situation would be for them to continue in this manner throughout their entire lives—on the path to health. However, there are times when something starts to go wrong; for example, a disease process begins within the body for reasons such as an infection with tuberculosis or a lack of food that contains an adequate amount of protein. Initially, the affected individual will be unaware that anything is wrong, even though they have begun the path of disease. This is because the disease is subclinical or pre-symptomatic. As an illustration, if there are bacteria that cause tuberculosis in the lungs, it will take several months before they start to produce symptoms. Similarly, if protein is deficient in the diet, it will take weeks or months before the effects become apparent. Sometimes certain diseases remain subclinical and then heal before they have produced any symptoms at all. This can happen suddenly. This is something that is especially likely to occur with certain infectious diseases, such as cholera, hepatitis, and infections caused by enteroviruses. When a person begins to experience the symptoms of a disease and can identify them, we refer to this as a clinical illness.

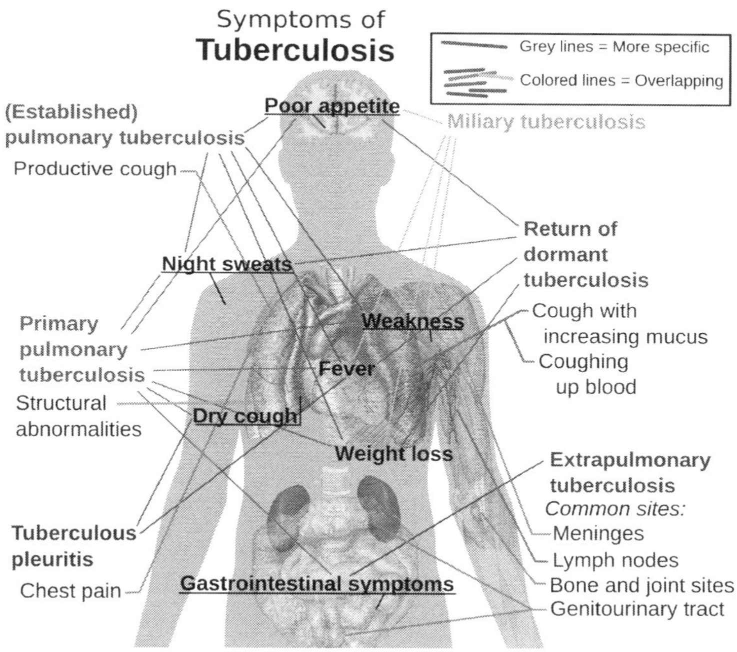

Figure 1.2. *A schematic of disease development.*

Source: https://s3-us-west-2.amazonaws.com/courses-images/wp-content/uploads/sites/1950/2017/05/31184959/76px-tuberculosis-symptoms.png.

Even in the early stages of a disease, when symptoms such as fever, cough, or diarrhea are first appearing, many people choose to disregard them in the hope that they will go away on their own. People may attempt to treat themselves or seek the advice of a local physician if the symptoms continue to be present. It is possible that they do not come from a nearby location, that they are unable to travel due to their illness, that they do not believe that the health services can be of any benefit to them, or that they have a personal dislike for the medical professional. It is possible that people will wait a significant amount of time before seeking assistance for a variety of reasons (Figure 1.2).

Since most outpatients and inpatients are at this stage of illness, the clinical stage is the one that we typically know the most about. Dispensaries, health centers, and hospitals can diagnose and treat patients who are complaining of a wide range of clinical symptoms daily. If the patient's condition is severe and they do not receive the appropriate treatment, they may eventually pass away.

Even if he can recover, he may be left with a disability for the rest of his life. For example, he may have a damaged lung because of pulmonary tuberculosis, a paralyzed arm because of polio, or a leg that has been amputated because of a severe injury. On the other hand, the majority of those who receive care will experience a complete recovery of their health (Centers for Disease Control and Prevention, 2011).

1.3. Methods of Prevention

"Prevention is better than cure" is a proverb that is widely known and widely used. When one considers the three stages that comprise the progression of a disease, it becomes abundantly clear that the most effective method of disease prevention is to treat a person before they become ill, or before they begin the path that leads to the development of a disease. The term for this procedure is primary prevention. Primary prevention can be accomplished through the utilization of a variety of approaches, the primary focus of which is on individuals and the environment in which they reside (Figure 1.2).

Primary prevention methods through people are:

- immunization
- Chemoprophylaxis
- nutrition
- personal hygiene
- good health behavior
- child spacing.

Environmental control methods are:

- safe water supplies
- food hygiene
- excreta and refuse disposal
- disinfection and sterilization
- vector and reservoir control
- good living and working conditions.

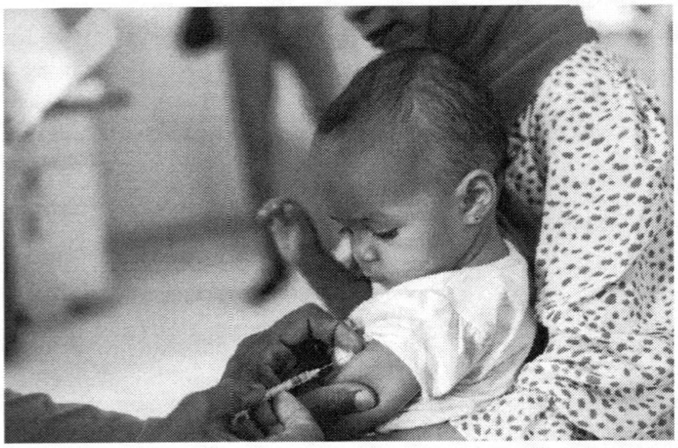

Figure 1.3. *Immunization method of disease prevention.*

Source: https://www.unicef.org/sites/default/files/styles/hero_tablet/public/UN0849186.JPG.webp?itok=cuRAOlD7.

After the disease has begun, but before the symptoms have manifested themselves—that is, before the patient has identified himself as sick—is the next best time to implement disease prevention measures. There are a few different names for this stage of the disease: pre-clinical, subclinical, or pre-symptomatic. The term "secondary prevention" refers to the prevention that occurs at this time. It should come as no surprise that it is frequently impossible to pinpoint the exact moment when a disease began or when the patient first became aware of its symptoms. This holds especially true in the event that there are some of the chronic illnesses that are present, such as tuberculosis, malnutrition, and anemia. Screening is the process that we use to look for these subclinical cases or cases that have not yet reached the clinical stage. The examination of urine and fecal specimens of school children for the presence of parasites, the examination of pregnant women for early signs of complications in their pregnancy, and the calculation of the weight of infants and young children to determine whether or not their weight falls within the nutrition danger area are all examples. If the medical services can aid the affected individual, then screening is only beneficial. It is necessary to have access to a treatment that is effective; if this is not the case, the screening should not have been considered in the first place. Tracing the contacts of a person who has an infectious illness, such as tuberculosis or leprosy, is another method of screening. The purpose of this method is to determine whether or not any other members of the family or friends of the individual in question also have the disease. By maintaining a consistent record of the number of new cases of diseases such as measles or meningitis, it is possible to determine whether or not a control program is effective or to identify an epidemic at an earlier stage. This is an additional form of secondary prevention that is known as surveillance, and it encompasses the whale community. When a person realizes that he or she is sick and that they are experiencing symptoms, diagnosis and treatment, also known as tertiary prevention, become significant. This particular stage of the disease is the focus of the majority of the curative work that is performed by outpatient and inpatient services. Both the diagnosis and the treatment of the disease are the foundations of these methods. The goal is to alleviate any suffering that may be present, to completely cure the disease, and to take measures to prevent disability. On the other hand, if there is a permanent disability such as blindness or paralysis, then it is possible that specialized rehabilitation services will be required. Following is a summary of the various approaches to disease prevention:

1.3.1. Primary Prevention

Preventing disease involves a range of strategies aimed at different stages of disease development. Primary prevention focuses on preventing the occurrence of disease and includes measures such as immunization, which protects individuals from infectious diseases by stimulating the immune system to develop immunity. For example, childhood immunization programs have significantly reduced the incidence of diseases such as measles and polio.

Another aspect of primary prevention is ensuring a safe environment, including access to clean water supplies. This measure prevents waterborne diseases such as cholera and typhoid fever. Similarly, promoting food hygiene practices prevents foodborne illnesses like salmonella infection.

Nutrition plays a crucial role in primary prevention, as a well-balanced diet strengthens the immune system and reduces the risk of chronic diseases such as diabetes and heart disease. Proper excreta and refuse disposal prevent the spread of diseases like cholera and dysentery, which are transmitted through contaminated water and food.

Personal hygiene practices, such as regular handwashing, reduce the transmission of infectious agents. Disinfection and sterilization of medical equipment prevent the spread of infections in healthcare settings. Vector and reservoir control measures, such as insecticide spraying and eliminating standing water, reduce the transmission of diseases like malaria and dengue fever.

Promoting good health behaviors, such as regular physical activity and avoiding tobacco use, reduces the risk of chronic diseases. Child spacing, through family planning methods, reduces maternal and infant mortality rates and improves maternal health.

Finally, ensuring good living and working conditions, such as adequate housing and workplace safety standards, reduces the risk of various diseases and injuries. These primary prevention strategies, when implemented effectively, can significantly reduce the burden of disease and improve overall health outcomes.

1.3.2. Secondary Prevention

Secondary prevention refers to the stage of healthcare that focuses on early detection and intervention in the progression of a disease or condition. It aims to identify individuals who already have an asymptomatic or early-stage disease, often through screening programs, and provide them with prompt and effective treatment to prevent the development of complications or further progression of the disease.

For example, in the case of breast cancer, secondary prevention may involve regular mammograms for women over a certain age to detect any abnormalities in the breast tissue at an early stage. If a suspicious lesion is found, further diagnostic tests and prompt treatment can be initiated to prevent the cancer from spreading or becoming more advanced.

Another example of secondary prevention is contact tracing in the context of infectious diseases. When a person is diagnosed with a contagious disease such as tuberculosis or COVID-19, public health authorities may conduct contact tracing to identify and notify individuals who may have been exposed to the disease. These individuals can then be offered testing and, if necessary, treatment to prevent further transmission of the disease within the community.

Surveillance is also an important component of secondary prevention, as it involves the systematic collection, analysis, and interpretation of health data for early detection of disease outbreaks or trends. By monitoring the incidence and prevalence of certain diseases or conditions, public health authorities can implement targeted interventions to prevent the spread of disease and reduce its impact on the population.

1.3.3. Tertiary Prevention

Tertiary prevention is the stage of healthcare that focuses on reducing the impact of a disease or condition once it has been diagnosed and treated, aiming to improve the quality of life and prevent further complications. This stage typically follows diagnosis, treatment, and initial management.

Diagnosis involves identifying the specific disease or condition affecting an individual. This can be done through various means, including medical history, physical examinations, and diagnostic tests such as blood tests, imaging scans, and biopsies. For example, in the case of osteoarthritis, diagnosis may involve assessing symptoms, performing physical exams to evaluate joint function, and using imaging techniques like X-rays or MRIs to visualize joint damage.

Treatment refers to the interventions used to address the diagnosed disease or condition. This can include medications, surgery, and other medical procedures aimed at controlling symptoms, slowing disease progression, or curing the condition altogether. For instance, diabetes treatment may involve medications such as insulin, lifestyle changes like diet and exercise, and regular monitoring of blood sugar levels.

Management involves the ongoing care and support provided to individuals with a disease or condition to help them maintain health and well-being. This can include monitoring symptoms, adjusting treatment as needed, and providing education and resources to help individuals manage their condition effectively. For example, management of asthma may involve regular check-ups, medication adjustments, and education on avoiding triggers and using inhalers correctly.

Rehabilitation focuses on restoring function and improving the quality of life for individuals who have experienced a loss of function due to a disease, injury, or other health condition. This can include physical therapy, occupational therapy, and other forms of rehabilitation to help individuals regain skills and independence. For example, rehabilitation after a stroke may involve physical therapy to improve movement and strength, speech therapy to regain communication skills, and occupational therapy to relearn daily activities like dressing and eating.

1.4. Health Education and Prevention

If people want to learn how to live a healthy life and learn how to avoid diseases, then health education is absolutely necessary. It encourages individuals to take responsibility for their own health and to participate in the organization of health services and programs to control disease. People may be able to gain a better understanding of the significance of health services for development and the realization that health and health services are fundamental human rights for all individuals through the process of health education. In the context of primary prevention, health education gives individuals the ability to recognize the importance of their own health, as well as to gain knowledge about diseases and the most effective ways to utilize organized health services, such as MCH clinics. It has the potential to inspire them to engage in hygienic personal habits and healthy behaviors for themselves, such as the utilization of safe water, mosquito nets, and physical separation between children. It has the potential to educate people about the importance of taking care of their own environment, including the disposal of waste and water supplies (Figure 1.4).

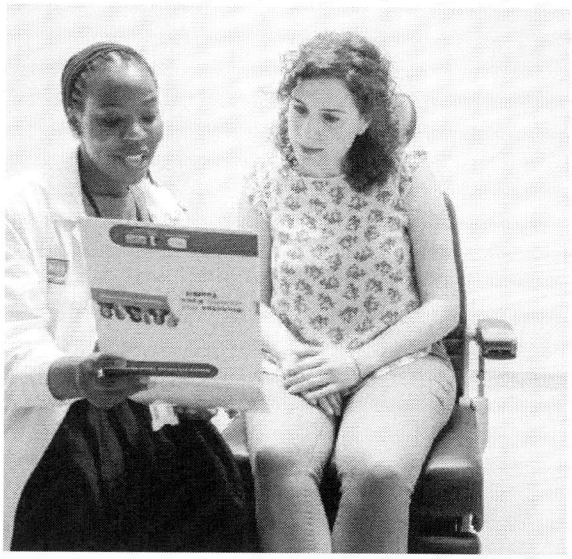

Figure 1.4. *Health education for disease prevention.*

Source: https://www.nei.nih.gov/sites/default/files/styles/400px_square_crop/public/2019–10/NEI-medialibrary-2487101.jpg?itok=rbu1DQ-i.

Education about health can also assist medical professionals in comprehending the desires of the general public, and by cooperating with one another, they can create a healthier way of life.

The purpose of health education in secondary prevention is to assist individuals in comprehending and appreciating various screening procedures, such as those that are involved in mental health services. It can assist individuals in recognizing the symptoms and signs of significant diseases such as leprosy and tuberculosis at an earlier stage, and it can also assist individuals in cooperating with surveillance programs for diseases such as measles, rabies, and malaria. People who receive health education in tertiary prevention may have a better understanding of diseases and may be more willing to cooperate with medical services to ensure that they receive the appropriate treatment.

For instance, they may continue to receive treatment for tuberculosis until they complete their treatment. People can learn new information about how to prevent diseases like malaria and gastroenteritis through health education while they are receiving treatment. This happens while people are receiving treatment. There is no such thing as a one-way process when it comes to health education; it is not simply the medical staff telling people what to do. People can assist us in better comprehending their circumstances, their requirements and requirements, their culture, and their environment. By gaining this further understanding, we can assist them in leading a healthier life (Centers for Disease Control and Prevention, 2011).

1.5. Need and Demand for Health Services

When we refer to the "population" of a health center, what categories of people do we actually mean to refer to? Do you mean the people who visit the outpatient clinics or the staff members who work at the center? Not at all; approximately 50,000 people are living in the vicinity of the health center. The community that is supposed to receive assistance from the health center, dispensaries, and village health workers is in this particular community. Why should the health center bother with all of the 50,000 people when it is already busy enough to take care of those individuals who do attend? (Figure 1.5)

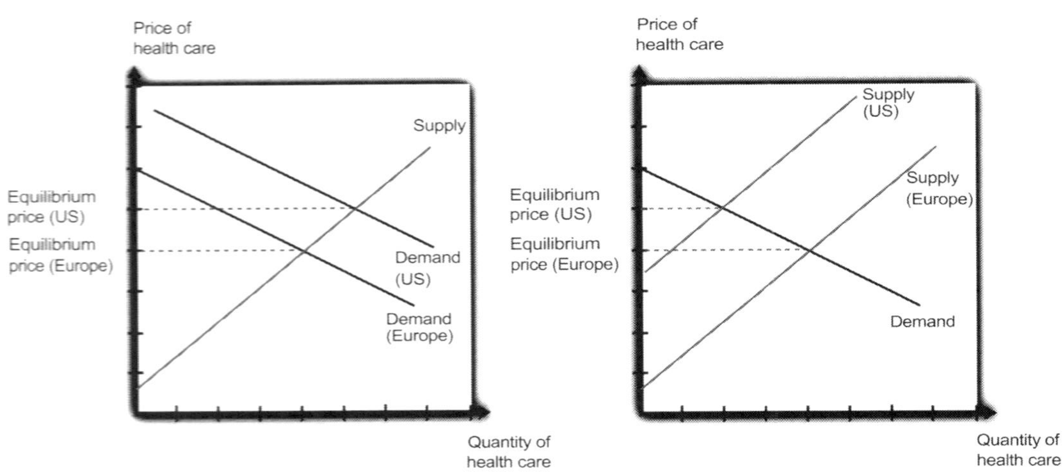

Figure 1.5. *Illustrations for why healthcare in the United States is more expensive than in Europe.*

Source: *https://saylordotorg.github.io/text_microeconomics-theory-through-applications/section_19/ac51917bb735ba93efd7623dbbacdc8d.jpg.*

The following are some of the possible responses to this question:

1. There are many more people who do not take advantage of the health center and dispensary for a variety of reasons than there are people who visit these establishments. It is possible that these individuals, who are not attending, require medical attention as well; however, they may not get it for a variety of reasons, including the fact that they live too far away, there is no one to look after the children or shamba, they are too sick to travel, or they have a negative perception of the medical services. It is equally important for these individuals who do not come to receive medical attention as it is for those who do come.
2. By the time a person experiences symptoms and goes to the health center for treatment, the disease has already begun to manifest throughout the body. A better course of action would have been to take measures to stop the disease from occurring in the first place. It is possible that the number of people who suffer from measles and its complications, such as pneumonia and diarrhea, could be significantly reduced if immunization against measles were administered to all of the elderly children in a village. To achieve the best possible results in disease prevention, it is essential to reach out to the healthy members of the entire community beforehand.
3. Unless the majority of people in a community make changes to the way they live, it is impossible to successfully prevent certain diseases and certain services from functioning effectively in a community. If a village decides to enhance its water supply or to assist in the operation of its own medical community health clinic, it requires the cooperation of the entire community. The only way for this cooperation to actually take place is if everyone is involved, and not just a select few individuals who are sick and actually go to the clinics.

   When looking at a community, it is helpful to take into consideration both the needs and the demands that the community has for health services. The symptoms that they are experiencing are already a sign that their illnesses have progressed. The existence of such a large number of health issues in a community of approximately 50,000 people is the source of the demand for health services.

It is necessary to take action in response to all of these issues, whether it be by the people themselves, by the health services, or by both sets of individuals working together. This course of action is not necessarily being demanded, but it may include things like addressing infections that have not been diagnosed or treated, addressing difficulties with deliveries, addressing infant feeding and malnutrition, addressing immunization, addressing the disposal of refuse, or controlling mosquitoes. The community's health needs are comparable to a hippopotamus with its head submerged in water.

1.6. Population Coverage

The objective of community health is to diminish and subsequently maintain a low incidence of new disease cases within the entire population. Curative services exclusively focus on unwell individuals. As we regress toward the initial phases of the disease progression, it becomes increasingly crucial to engage the entire community, especially individuals who have a higher susceptibility to contracting the disease. To prevent disease and maintain the overall health of the community, it is essential to consider the healthcare requirements of the entire population, rather than solely focusing on individuals seeking services at clinics. Population coverage is the concept that is relevant here. We need to determine the proportion of the population with a health requirement who are effectively receiving assistance from various health services. For example, what proportion of pregnant women attend the antenatal clinic? What is the vaccination rate for two-year-old for measles? What is the proportion of the global population that has access to a sufficient water supply? What is the proportion of the community that resides within a 5 km radius of a dispensary or health center? The incidence of common diseases can be reduced by effectively implementing preventive medicine, particularly primary prevention, and ensuring that all individuals at risk in the community receive adequate population coverage. This statement holds especially true when it comes to infectious diseases and malnutrition. The significance of understanding the entire population and subsequently approximating the population coverage becomes evident when considering the reduction of new cases. It is crucial to ensure that health center services are founded on a comprehensive understanding of the local population (Centers for Disease Control and Prevention, 2011).

1.7. High-Risk Groups in the Population

Every individual, regardless of gender or age, is susceptible to illness and mortality, although certain demographics face a higher level of risk than others. These groups have been carefully selected as being at high risk. Certain individuals not only have a higher susceptibility to certain diseases, but they also exhibit lower utilization of healthcare services, putting them at a heightened risk of not receiving proper treatment. These high-risk groups can be characterized by specific attributes that are shared among the members of the group. These features can pertain to individuals, their habitats, or specific periods within a day, month, or year. Certain individuals, such as young children, leprosy patients, and those residing in remote areas, may underutilize healthcare services. By identifying these specific groups, health services can allocate additional resources, such as time, personnel, infrastructure, mobile clinics, dedication, and funding, to aid them. This approach ensures that the limited resources are not solely focused on providing care to nearby outpatients. Consequently, we can allocate a greater portion of our medical efforts towards individuals who genuinely require them.

Which groups are considered high-risk? (Examples 1 to 8 pertain to individuals, while examples 9 and 10 relate to locations, and example 11 pertains to time.)

1. Approximately 20% of the population, specifically mothers, have a higher likelihood of experiencing complications during pregnancy and facing mortality during childbirth.
2. Infants and young children, who make up one-fifth of the total population, experience a disproportionately high mortality rate due to malnutrition and a range of infections such as measles, gastroenteritis, and malaria.
3. Approximately 20% of the total population, specifically school children, have a high probability of contracting childhood illnesses.
4. Certain workers may be exposed to additional risks or hazards, such as

accidents in industrial settings or incidents involving agricultural machinery, as well as the potential for insecticide poisoning among crop sprayers.

5. Elderly individuals experience chronic and degenerative conditions, such as bronchitis and heart failure.
6. Individuals who have been exposed to a contagious illness such as tuberculosis or leprosy.
7. Diverse cultural and economic groups, such as those engaged in subsistence farming, are at a higher risk of experiencing famine in the event of crop failure. Life in rural areas clearly contrasts with life in urban areas.
8. Local beliefs and customs have a significant impact on how individuals prioritize their health, manage illness, and utilize healthcare services.
9. Specific diseases are more prevalent in different geographical regions, such as trypanosomiasis in Tabora.
10. People residing in remote areas face a significant risk due to limited access to medical services, resulting in lower utilization rates. The presence of roads and transportation infrastructure will significantly impact the situation. Inclement weather during the rainy seasons can pose challenges for accessing clinics.
11. Certain diseases, such as malaria, are more likely to occur after periods of rainfall, while road accidents are more common on weekends when people have been drinking.

1.8. The Organization of Health Services

Every nation lacks sufficiently trained medical personnel and financial resources to fully operate all desired healthcare services. The allocation of resources for the advancement of health services is constrained, necessitating competition with other key sectors such as education, agriculture, and water. The challenge lies in effectively allocating these finite resources to ensure equitable distribution of benefits among the entire population, with a particular focus on individuals at elevated risk of contracting diseases. Constructing and upkeeping hospitals incur significant costs, and their focus on tertiary prevention limits their impact on the occurrence of common diseases. Nevertheless, hospitals are indispensable for the minority of individuals in the community who are severely ill. The organization of health services plays a significant role in determining the level of importance placed on preventive medicine and the effectiveness of community health programs.

1.9. The Basic Health Services

Basic health services encompass the essential medical care that dispensaries and health centers are responsible for delivering. They embody the essential threshold of healthcare services that ought to be accessible to most of the population. These services have also been referred to as 'essential health services' and are included in the widely used term 'primary health care.' They provide specialized care for women and children, who are the most significant high-risk populations. There is a consensus that fundamental health services should encompass the identification and treatment of common and less severe ailments, while severe or complicated cases should be referred to a hospital. These services are fundamental components of primary healthcare, aimed at meeting the basic health needs of the population.

Firstly, comprehensive health education is a cornerstone of basic health services. It involves raising awareness among community members about prevalent diseases, their prevention strategies, and the importance of utilizing available health services. This empowers individuals to take proactive steps in managing their health and preventing illnesses.

Environmental regulation is another critical aspect covered by basic health services. This includes monitoring and ensuring the safety of food, water, waste disposal, shelter conditions, disease carriers, and infected animals. By controlling these environmental factors, health centers contribute to preventing the spread of diseases and promoting a healthier living environment.

The management of contagious diseases is also a key responsibility. Basic health services address common infectious diseases such as measles, tuberculosis, malaria, and schistosomiasis through prevention, diagnosis, and treatment. Early detection and intervention are essential in controlling outbreaks and reducing the burden of these diseases on the community.

Gathering fundamental statistical data is vital for assessing community health needs and evaluating the effectiveness of healthcare interventions. Basic health services collect data on prevalent health issues, healthcare utilization, and health outcomes. This information guides healthcare planning and resource allocation to address priority health concerns effectively.

In practice, dispensaries and health centers integrate these services into a cohesive healthcare delivery system. While each service is interconnected, coordination at the national level is crucial. Ministries of Health oversee and coordinate nationwide initiatives across various departments, including medical treatment, health promotion, maternal and child health, nutrition, family planning, environmental health, infectious disease control, and statistical analysis. This centralized coordination ensures that basic health services are delivered efficiently and equitably across different regions.

1.10. Primary Health Care

The most widely accepted definition of primary care is the one recently formulated by the World Health Organization (WHO):

Primary healthcare is a pragmatic method of ensuring that necessary healthcare is accessible to all individuals and families in the community, in a manner that is both acceptable and affordable, and with their active involvement.

The individuals responsible for providing crucial primary healthcare services are known as village health workers (VHW), formerly referred to as village medical helpers (VMH), who operate in each village. Additionally, there are rural medical aids (RMA) and maternal and child health aids (MCH Aid) stationed at the dispensary, as well as medical assistants (MA) and other personnel at the health center. The Village Headman (VHW) is elected by the villagers and is accountable to them. The active involvement of individuals in their local community health initiatives is a crucial component of primary healthcare. The VHW primarily belongs to the village rather than the government health services, although the district medical officer professionally supervises the entire health program in the district. He should also engage in the health components of rural development. Male VHWs may lack the ability to coordinate village MCH activities, but they can exert significant influence on local environmental health. Individuals should have convenient access to primary healthcare services, such as a Village Health Worker (VHW), dispensary, or primary health center, located within a short distance from their residences. Furthermore, it is generally expected that these services will be provided free of charge.

1.11. Individual Sickness and Community Health

When contemplating health and disease, our thoughts typically revolve around ourselves or individuals we are acquainted with, including children. Is that individual in good health or afflicted with a medical condition? Is the condition considered severe or mild? Is the disease recent or long-standing, and is the prognosis for recovery expected to be protracted? Has anyone else in the family or community contracted a similar illness? Certain individuals, families, or communities exhibit a higher prevalence of illness and mortality compared to others, including a greater number of children suffering from malnutrition, or a higher incidence of tuberculosis or anemia among young people. These observations regarding the patterns of health and disease within a community and the corresponding actions that can be taken have given rise to the field of community health, also known as public health. To assist an individual, it is imperative to gather fundamental data regarding their health condition, including the current stage of any diseases they may be afflicted with. This is accomplished through the process of obtaining a patient's medical history, conducting a thorough physical examination, and performing necessary diagnostic tests. Next, the process involves establishing a diagnosis to determine the underlying issue. Once the available assistance is identified, a comprehensive strategy is devised to effectively support and rehabilitate the patient, which is referred to as management and rehabilitation. Subsequently, it is necessary to monitor his progress to ensure the efficacy of the treatment. The identical procedure is suitable for the community. Initially, it is imperative to gather fundamental data of the entire community. First, conduct a community diagnosis to identify the primary issues affecting the community. Next, determine the most suitable community health programs for addressing these issues. Finally, monitor and assess the effectiveness of these programs in improving the overall health of the community (Centers for Disease Control and Prevention, 2011).

1.12. Basic Information for Community Health

Where can I locate the information? What is the method of collection? An abundance of information is readily accessible to those who are aware of where to find it. In cases where the desired information is not readily available, conducting straightforward surveys can often yield the desired results. Data can be acquired from individuals and documents within the immediate vicinity, the healthcare facility, the region, and other establishments such as the Ministry of Health. Data should be gathered regarding:

- The local people and their environment – the individual, family and community.
- The number of people and their distribution.
- The diseases they suffer from-the local patterns of diseases and deaths.
- The organization of the local health services that handle these diseases in that community.

1.13. The Community Diagnosis

This is a method of determining, through collaboration with the community, which local diseases or health issues are significant and should be prioritized in the efforts of healthcare professionals. By understanding the specific factors that contribute to illness (morbidity) and death (mortality) in a particular area, we can provide answers to the following inquiries.

- What are the ten most prevalent diseases observed in outpatients?
- What is the prevalence of common diseases in the area?
- What is the geographical prevalence of rare yet significant diseases?
- Which diseases have previously experienced an epidemic in this region?
- Which disease is the primary focus of concern within the community?
- What are the primary local issues affecting the community?

The next step entails identifying the diseases that can be controlled and the health problems that can be resolved. Give priority to diseases and health issues that can be efficiently and feasibly tackled by the local community, dispensary, health center, or district health staff. Conducting a community diagnosis is a technique used to determine the most effective distribution of efforts and resources by health center services.

1.14. Community Health Programs

Once the community diagnosis has facilitated the identification of local priorities, the subsequent step involves determining the optimal utilization of the health team's efforts and resources to achieve the most significant impact. Community health programs typically have one of the following objectives:

- Specific disease control such as leprosy, measles, malaria, schistosomiasis, or tuberculosis
- General disease control such as that achieved by environmental health and nutrition programs
- High-risk groups of people such as mothers and children and other special groups.

In practice, the services are integrated in such a way that all three approaches are often combined, as is seen in the work of the MCH services.

1.15. Assessment of Community Health Programs

It is crucial to ascertain the effectiveness of community health programs in achieving their intended goals. The primary objective of any community health program is to enhance the well-being of the community by diminishing the occurrence of new cases to a level where a disease ceases to be a significant concern. Quantifying this is challenging. Frequently, the efforts of dispensaries and health centers are not quantified; it is presumed that they decrease the incidence of illness and death. It is crucial to avoid making risky assumptions and instead make a diligent effort to assess, as accurately as possible, whether the program is achieving its specific objectives. Measurement can be conducted by approximating:

1.15.1. Population Coverage

What percentage of the total population is under the care of the services efficiently? The services were not involved with what percentage of the births and deaths that occurred in the community? What percentage of the population lives within ten kilometers of a health center or dispensary?

1.15.2. Work Load of the Dispensary and Health Center Services

When it comes to those individuals who do attend the services, what are they doing? During each month, how many new cases of diseases that are either common or significant, such as gastroenteritis and hookworm, were there? What transpires over the course of a certain amount of time about the total number of outpatient attendances? What number of injections are being administered? What is the total number of laboratory investigations that have been carried out? As a result, how much does health education cost?

- **Effects of the Treatments Given:** Is the prevalence of common diseases decreasing? What was the distribution of patients among those who were cured, disabled, or died? For example, what is the status of the statistics regarding gastroenteritis and measles fatalities, as well as maternal and neonatal mortalities? What is the total number of referrals from the dispensaries to the health center, and how many individuals were subsequently referred to the district hospital?

Assessing our actions is necessary to determine if we are making any positive impact.

1.16. Community Health Techniques and Administration

Proficiency in community health work necessitates the acquisition of specific skills, analogous to the process of learning how to conduct a patient examination. There are specific indispensable methodologies for engaging with the local community that are necessary for gathering fundamental data, conducting a community assessment, implementing community health initiatives, and assessing their effectiveness. In addition to possessing knowledge of the techniques, it is equally crucial to have the ability to strategize and manage health services. The clinical and community health skills possessed by medical workers will be rendered ineffective if they are unable to efficiently manage the delivery of services.

1.17. Value of Community Health

Attempting to divide between preventive and curative medicine, as well as individual and community health, is both impractical and unproductive. When a mother brings a sick child with diarrhea, you guide both the treatment of the child's illness and the prevention of future occurrences. Providing treatment to individuals with pulmonary tuberculosis is effective in preventing the transmission of the disease to others in the community. Similarly, when we administer immunization to one child, we do not neglect the health of their sick sister or brother. Frequently, the allocation of resources towards disease prevention in the community through means such as education, immunization, environmental health, and child spacing yields significantly superior outcomes compared to the alternative approach of waiting for individuals to fall ill and subsequently investing time and money in their treatment.

While there is a consensus that preventive measures have a greater impact on the community compared to individual treatment, the implementation of prevention strategies can be challenging. Firstly, it is essential to possess the foundational knowledge and skills that form the basis of community health. Secondly, it is crucial to hold a strong belief in the significance of community health. Lastly, it is necessary to effectively allocate the available time, money, and other resources between treatment and prevention.

1.18. Health and Development

It is widely recognized that individuals with lower socioeconomic status experience higher rates of illness and disease compared to those with higher socioeconomic status. Additionally, they tend to utilize healthcare services less frequently. There is a correlation between the wealthier regions of a country and the presence of healthier individuals and superior medical facilities. Here are two examples illustrating the correlation between economic development and good health. However, if national economic development is not accompanied by an equitable distribution of wealth and resources, a small group of wealthy individuals will profit while many people remain impoverished. The objective of villagization and other development policies is to facilitate the consolidation of rural populations to actively engage them in their own development. Enhancing health should be an integral component of this progress. Health services, education, water supplies, sufficient food, and adequate housing are key focal points for rural development. There is a growing belief that medical services, particularly those focused on treatment, have a limited impact on enhancing the health of a community. Significant progress can be made by ensuring that everyone has an adequate supply of nutritious food and by implementing basic measures to manage the environment. The significance of village health services lies in the crucial role played by improved nutrition and favorable environmental conditions. Furthermore, the establishment of a monetary system, enhanced farming techniques, equitable land distribution, elevated educational attainment, high rates of adult literacy, and upgraded transportation infrastructure collectively contribute to enhanced health outcomes. Enhancing living conditions by involving individuals in development initiatives will result in the establishment of healthier communities. It is imperative for all healthcare professionals to actively participate in local political and development matters, collaborating with the community and other workers to facilitate positive progress. It is crucial for all healthcare professionals to recognize that health is a significant aspect of rural development and that medical services play a vital role in this process. It is essential to incorporate development plans and services with those from other sectors such as agriculture, water, and education (Zingg et al., 2015; Vasile et al., 2018).

A Closer Look

Child Spacing

Child spacing, also known as birth spacing, refers to the practice of timing the intervals between the births of children. This practice has significant implications for the health and well-being of both mothers and children, as well as for broader socio-economic factors.

Health professionals advocate for a minimum of 18 to 24 months between pregnancies. This interval allows a mother's body adequate time to recover and replenish nutrients lost during pregnancy and breastfeeding. Shorter intervals between pregnancies can increase the risk of adverse outcomes such as preterm births, low birth weight, and maternal complications including anemia and uterine rupture. On the other hand, excessively long intervals, particularly beyond five years, may also pose risks, though the evidence here is less clear-cut.

For children, appropriate spacing is associated with better health and development outcomes. Sufficient intervals between births reduce the likelihood of sibling rivalry and ensure that parents can provide adequate attention and resources to each child during their critical early years of development. From a nutritional standpoint, proper spacing allows each child to benefit fully from breastfeeding, which is crucial for their immunity and growth.

Beyond health, child spacing has economic and social dimensions. Families can better manage resources and provide for their children's education and other needs when births are adequately spaced. For women, planned spacing can improve their ability to participate in the workforce and pursue educational opportunities, contributing to their personal empowerment and overall family welfare.

Effective child spacing often requires access to reliable contraception and comprehensive family planning services. Education and counseling play critical roles in helping couples understand the benefits of birth spacing and make informed choices. Additionally, cultural and societal norms can influence decisions about child spacing, highlighting the need for culturally sensitive health education and policies.

Therefore, child spacing is a critical aspect of reproductive health with far-reaching benefits. It supports the health and well-being of mothers and children, promotes economic stability, and empowers women, underscoring the importance of accessible family planning services and education.

Summary

Community health refers to the well-being of a group of individuals within a specific geographic area or shared identity. It encompasses various aspects of health, including physical, mental, and social well-being, and is influenced by factors such as genetics, environment, lifestyle, and healthcare services.

One of the key principles of community health is prevention, which aims to reduce the risk of disease and promote overall health. This includes efforts such as vaccinations, health education, and promoting healthy behaviors like exercise and proper nutrition. By focusing on prevention, community health initiatives can reduce the burden of disease and improve quality of life.

Community health also emphasizes the importance of addressing health disparities, which are differences in health outcomes between different populations. This includes addressing social determinants of health, such as income, education, and access to healthcare, which can impact an individual's health.

Health promotion is another important aspect of community health, which involves empowering individuals and communities to take control of their health. This can include providing resources and education on topics such as smoking cessation, mental health awareness, and healthy eating.

In summary, community health focuses on improving the health and well-being of a group of individuals within a community through prevention, addressing health disparities, and promoting health. By taking a holistic approach to health and involving the community in the process, community health initiatives can have a positive impact on the overall health of a population.

References

1. Allegranzi, B., Nejad, S. B., Combescure, C., Graafmans, W., Attar, H., Donaldson, L., & Pittet, D. (2011). Burden of endemic health-care-associated infection in developing countries: Systematic review and meta-analysis. *Lancet, 377*(9761), 228–241.
2. Baid, H. (2016). Patient safety: Identifying and managing complications of mechanical ventilation. *Critical Care Nursing Clinics, 28*(4), 451–462.
3. Benet, T., Ecochard, R., Voirin, N., Machut, A., Lepape, A., Savey, A., & Vanhems, P. (2014). Effect of standardized surveillance of intensive care unit-acquired infections on ventilator-associated pneumonia incidence. *Infection Control & Hospital Epidemiology, 35*(10), 1290–1293.
4. Bernard, M. S., Hunter, K. F., & Moore, K. N. (2012). A review of strategies to decrease the duration of indwelling urethral catheters and potentially reduce the incidence of catheter-associated urinary tract infections. *Urologic Nursing, 32*(1), 29–37.
5. Bouza, E., San Juan, R., Munoz, P., Voss, A., Kluytmans, J., & on behalf of the Co-operative Group of the European Study Group on Nosocomial Infections (ESGNI). (2001). European perspective on nosocomial urinary tract infections II. Report on incidence, clinical characteristics and outcome (ESGINI–04 study). *Clinical Microbiology and Infection, 7*(10), 532–542.
6. Cassini, A., Plachouras, D., Eckmanns, T., Abu Sin, M., Blank, H. P., Ducomble, T., & Monnet, D. L. (2016). Burden of six healthcare-associated infections on European population health: Estimating incidence-based disability-adjusted life years through a population prevalence-

based modelling study. *PLoS Medicine, 13*(10), e1002150. https://doi.org/10.1371/journal.pmed.1002150.

7. Centers for Disease Control and Prevention. (2011). Vital signs: Central line-associated bloodstream infections—United States, 2001, 2008, and 2009. *Annals of Emergency Medicine, 60*(2), 243.
8. Choi, J. Y., Kwak, Y. G., Yoo, H., Lee, S. O., Kim, H. B., Han, S. H., & Kim, Y. K. (2015). Trends in the incidence rate of device-associated infections in intensive care units after the establishment of the Korean nosocomial infections surveillance system. *Journal of Hospital Infection, 91*(1), 28–34.
9. Chopra, V., Krein, S. L., Olmsted, R. N., Safdar, N., & Saint, S. (2013). Prevention of central line associated bloodstream infections: Brief update review. Retrieved from: http://www.ncbi.nlm.nih.gov/books/NBK133363/pdf/Bookshelf_NBK133363.pdf (accessed on 11 July 2024).
10. Eom, J. S., Lee, M. S., Chun, H. K., Choi, H. J., Jung, S. Y., Kim, Y.-S., & Oh, G.-B. (2014). The impact of a ventilator bundle on preventing ventilator-associated pneumonia: A multicenter study. *American Journal of Infection Control, 42*(1), 34–37.
11. Fagan, R. P., Edwards, J. R., Park, B. J., Findkin, S. K., & Magill, S. S. (2013). Incidence trends in pathogen-specific central line—Associated bloodstream infections in US intensive care units, 1990–2010. *Infection Control & Hospital Epidemiology, 34*(9), 893–899.
12. Fattorini, M., Rosadini, D., Messina, G., Basagni, C., Tinturini, A., & De Marco, M. (2018). A multidisciplinary educational programme for the management of a carbapenem-resistant Klebsiella pneumoniae outbreak: An Italian experience. *Journal of Hospital Infection, 99*(4), 427–428.
13. Furmenti, M. F., Rossello, P., Bianco, S., Olivero, E., Thomas, R., Emelurumonye, I. N., & Zotti, C. M. (2019). Healthcare-associated infections and antimicrobial use in long-term care facilities (HALT3): An overview of the Italian situation. *Journal of Hospital Infection, 102*(4), 425–430.
14. Gastmeier, P., Geffers, C., Brandt, C., Zuschneid, I., Sohr, D., Schwab, F., & Rüden, H. (2006). Effectiveness of a nationwide nosocomial infection surveillance system for reducing nosocomial infections. *Journal of Hospital Infection, 64*(1), 16–22.
15. Kariya, X. N., Sakon, N., Komano, J., Tomono, K., & Iso, H. (2018). Current prevention and control of health care-associated infections in long term care facilities for the elderly in Japan. *Journal of Infection and Chemotherapy, 24*(5), 347–352.
16. Magill, S. S., Edwards, J. R., Bamberg, W., Beldavs, Z. G., Dumyati, G., Kainer, M. A., & Bell, J. M. (2014). Multistate point-prevalence survey of health care—Associated infections. *New England Journal of Medicine, 370*(13), 1198–1208.
17. Moro, M. L., Ricchizzi, E., Morsillo, F., Marchi, M., Puro, V., Zotti, C. M., & Privitera, G. (2013). Infections and antimicrobial resistance in long term care facilities: A national prevalence study. *Annali di Igiene, 25*(2), 109–118.
18. National Institute for Health and Clinical Excellence (NICE). (2008). Surgical site infection: Prevention and treatment of surgical site infection. Retrieved from: https://www.nice.org.uk/guidance/cg74 (accessed on 11 July 2024).

19. Rosenthal, V. D., Bijie, H., Maki, D. G., Mehta, Y., Apisarnthanarak, A., Medeiros, E. A., & Khader, A. I. (2012). International Nosocomial Infection Control Consortium (INICC) report, data summary of 36 countries, for 2004–2009. *American Journal of Infection Control, 40*(5), 396–407.

20. Russo, P. L., Cheng, A. C., Richards, M., Graves, N., & Hall, L. (2015). Healthcare-associated infections in Australia: Time for national surveillance. *Australian Health Review, 39*(1), 37–43.

21. Saleem, Z., Hassali, M. A., Godman, B., Hashmi, F. K., & Saleem, F. (2019). A multicenter point prevalence survey of healthcare-associated infections in Pakistan: Findings and implications. *American Journal of Infection Control, 47*(4), 421–424.

22. Salmanov, A., Vozianov, S., Kryzhevsky, V., Litus, O., Drozdova, A., & Vlasenko, I. (2019). Prevalence of healthcare-associated infections and antimicrobial resistance in acute care hospitals in Kyiv, Ukraine. *Journal of Hospital Infection, 102*(4), 431–437.

23. Schumacher, M., Allignol, A., Beyersmann, J., Binder, N., & Wolkewitz, M. (2013). Hospital-acquired infections—Appropriate statistical treatment is urgently needed! *International Journal of Epidemiology, 42*(5), 1502–1508.

24. Scott, R. D. (2009). The direct medical costs of healthcare-associated infections in US hospitals and the benefits of prevention. Retrieved from: https://stacks.cdc.gov/view/cdc/11550.

25. Suetens, C., Latour, K., Karki, T., Ricchizzi, E., Kinross, P., Moro, M. L., & Lyytikäinen, O. (2018). Healthcare-associated infections prevalence study group, prevalence of healthcare-associated infections, estimated incidence and composite antimicrobial resistance index in acute care hospitals and long-term care facilities: Results from two European point prevalence surveys, 2016 to 2017. *Eurosurveillance, 23*(46).

26. Van der Kooi, T., Sax, H., Pittet, D., van Dissel, J., van Benthem, B., Walder, B., & Wolkewitz, M. (2018). Prevention of hospital infections by intervention and training (PROHIBIT): Results of a pan-European cluster-randomized multicenter study to reduce central venous catheter-related bloodstream infections. *Intensive Care Medicine, 44*(1), 48–60.

27. Vasile, C., Azoicăi, D., Iancu, L. S., Trifan, M., Duca, E., Fochi, M., & Iacob, O. (2017). *Guide for the Management of Infections Associated with Healthcare, 2nd Edition*. Global Arts Management Publishing House, Bucharest. Retrieved from: https://sanatateromania.ro/ghid-de-management-al-infectiilor-asociate-asistentei-medicale/ (accessed on 11 July 2024).

28. Yazdani, M., Sabetian, G., Ra'Ofi, S., Roudgari, A., & Feizi, M. (2015). A comparative study of teaching clinical guideline for prevention of ventilator-associated pneumonia in two ways: Face-to-face and workshop training on the knowledge and practice of nurses in the intensive care unit. *Journal of Advanced Medical Education & Professionalism, 3*(2), 68–71.

29. Zarb, P., Coignard, B., Griskeviciene, J., Muller, A., Vankerckhoven, V., Weist, K., & Catry, B. (2012). The European center for disease prevention and control (ECDC) pilot point prevalence survey of healthcare-associated infections and antimicrobial use. *Eurosurveillance, 17*(46), 20316.

30. Zimlichman, E., Henderson, D., Tamir, O., Franz, C., Song, P., Yamin, C. K., & Bates, D. W. (2013). Health care-associated infections: A meta-analysis of costs and financial impact on the US healthcare system. *JAMA Internal Medicine, 173*(22), 2039–2046.

31. Zingg, W., Holmes, A., Dettenkofer, M., Goetting, T., Secci, F., Clack, L., & Pittet, D. (2015). For the systematic review and evidence-based guidance on organization of hospital infection control programs (SIGHT) study group. Hospital organization, management, and structure

for prevention of health-care-associated infection: A systematic review and expert consensus. *The Lancet Infectious Diseases, 15*(2), 212–224.

32. Zingg, W., Hopkins, S., Gayet-Ageron, A., Holmes, A., Sharland, M., & Suetens, C. (2017). Health-care-associated infections in neonates, children, and adolescents: An analysis of pediatric data from the European Centre for Disease Prevention and Control point-prevalence survey. *The Lancet Infectious Diseases, 17*(4), 338–381.

Chapter 2

INFECTIOUS DISEASE EPIDEMIOLOGY

Contents

Introduction

Infectious diseases have played a significant role in shaping human history, influencing population dynamics, societal structures, and even the course of wars. These diseases, caused by pathogenic microorganisms such as bacteria, viruses, parasites, and fungi, have posed persistent challenges to human health and well-being. Understanding their mechanisms of transmission, pathogenesis, and epidemiology is crucial for developing effective prevention and control strategies. As stated by Jones et al. (2019), infectious diseases are responsible for a substantial burden of morbidity and mortality globally, particularly in low- and middle-income countries where access to healthcare resources may be limited. The emergence and reemergence of infectious diseases, driven by factors such as urbanization, globalization, antimicrobial resistance, and environmental changes, further complicate efforts to control them (Morens et al., 2004). The study of infectious diseases encompasses a wide range of disciplines, including microbiology, immunology, epidemiology, and public health. Researchers in these fields collaborate to investigate the complex interactions between pathogens, hosts, and the environment, intending to develop effective strategies for disease prevention, diagnosis, and treatment.

Infectious diseases continue to pose significant challenges to global health security, as highlighted by recent outbreaks of diseases such as Ebola, Zika, and COVID-19. These events underscore the importance of ongoing research and preparedness efforts to address both known and emerging infectious threats.

Infectious Disease Epidemiology is a field of study that examines the patterns, causes, and effects of infectious diseases within populations. It encompasses a broad range of topics, including the transmission dynamics of infectious agents, the impact of social, environmental, and behavioral factors on disease spread, and the design and evaluation of interventions to control and prevent infectious diseases.

As described by Murray et al. (1991), infectious disease epidemiology is "the study of the occurrence and distribution of health-related states or events in specified populations, including the study of the determinants influencing such states, and the application of this knowledge to control the health problems."

Infectious diseases have shaped human history in profound ways, as highlighted by McNeill (1976), who noted that epidemics have been major factors in societal change, affecting population size, migration patterns, and even the outcomes of wars.

In recent years, the field of infectious disease epidemiology has become increasingly important due to emerging infectious diseases such as SARS-CoV-2, the virus responsible for the COVID-19 pandemic. As noted by Morse (1995), emerging infectious diseases pose unique challenges due to factors such as global travel, urbanization, and microbial evolution.

This chapter presents the principles and concepts of modern infectious disease epidemiology. We define the function of epidemiology in relation to public health and examine the specific attributes of infectious disease epidemiology. This chapter also contains precise explanations of significant terminology utilized in the field of infectious disease epidemiology.

Orientation and Directional Terms

Term	Definition	Illustration
Epidemiology	The branch of medicine that studies the distribution, patterns, and determinants of health and disease conditions in populations. It aims to understand the causes and effects of diseases to inform public health interventions and policies.	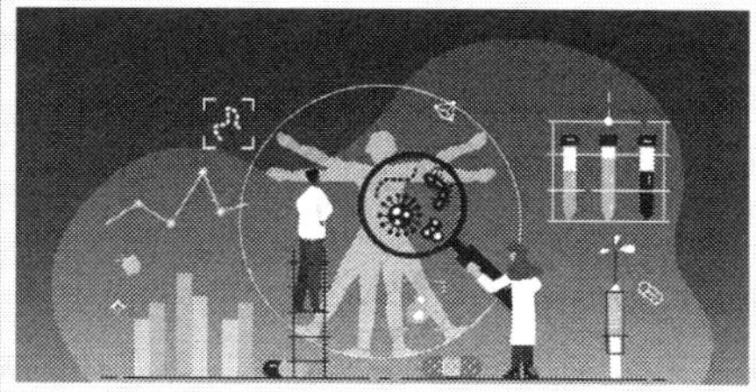
Aetiology	The study of the cause or origin of a disease. In medical terms, it refers to the factors that contribute to the development of a disease, including biological, environmental, and lifestyle factors.	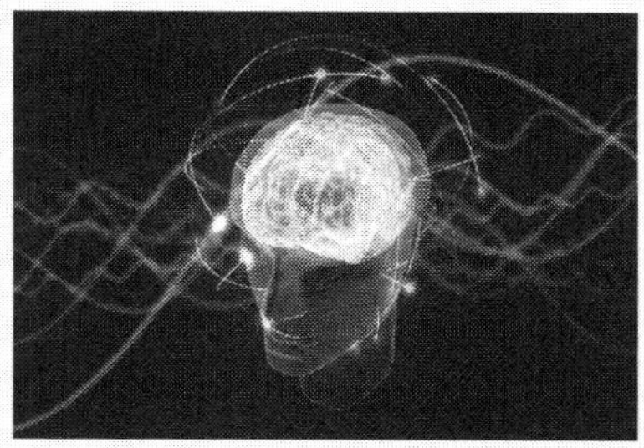
HIV/AIDS Epidemic	A global health crisis characterized by the widespread prevalence of HIV (Human Immunodeficiency Virus) and AIDS (Acquired Immunodeficiency Syndrome), which has caused a significant impact on public health, economies, and societies worldwide.	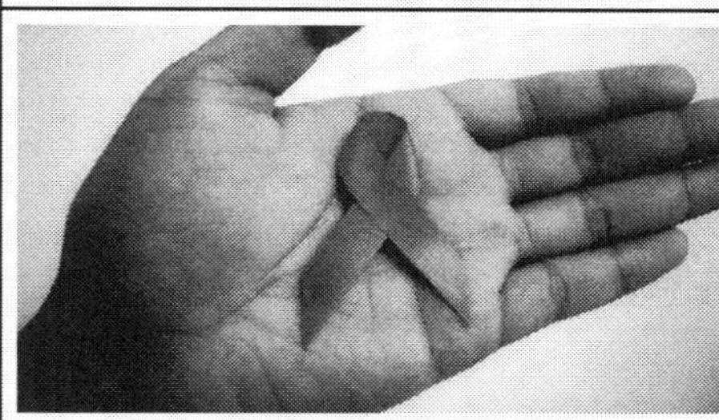
Pathogenicity	The ability of an organism to cause disease. It involves factors such as the organism's ability to invade host tissues, evade immune responses, and produce toxins that contribute to disease.	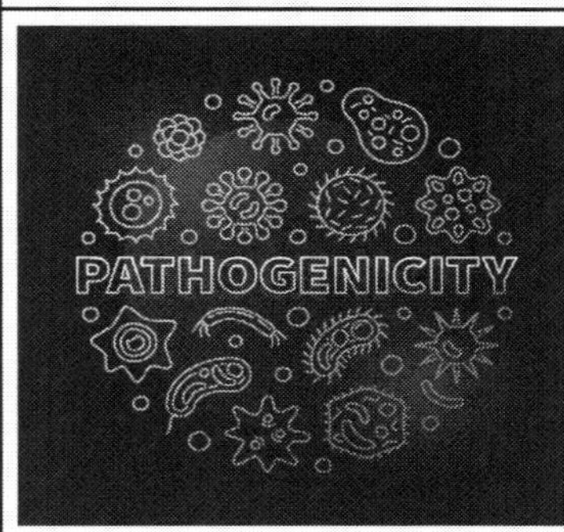
Immunogenicity	The ability of a substance, such as an antigen or vaccine, to induce an immune response in the body. This includes stimulating the production of antibodies and activating immune cells to recognize and combat pathogens.	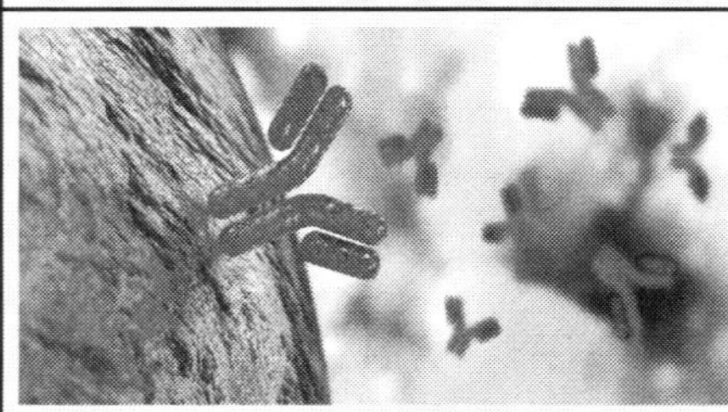

2.1. Definition and Aims of Epidemiology

Providing a universally applicable definition of epidemiology is challenging. Epidemiology lacks a clearly delineated scope of application, unlike anatomy or gastroenterology, which focus on specific regions or aspects of the human body. Instead, it is a systematic approach that can be utilized to address a wide array of health and medical issues, spanning from infectious diseases to healthcare. Epidemiology is a dynamic scientific field that undergoes continuous evolution due to emerging inquiries in population health and the development and integration of novel statistical methodologies from other disciplines. In the era of modern information technologies and high-speed computers, there are new possibilities for collecting and storing large amounts of data, as well as for using advanced bio-informatic and modeling techniques. Amidst the era of globalization, numerous health issues hold significance on a worldwide level, necessitating the formulation of intervention strategies at an international scale. Specifically, in the field of infectious disease epidemiology, the significance of global spread is becoming more prominent, as evidenced by the dissemination of the human immunodeficiency virus (HIV) and the widespread occurrence of influenza A pandemics.

2.1.1. Definition: Epidemiology

The word "Epidemiology" is derived from Greek words meaning *study upon populations* (epi-upon, demos-people, logos-study).

A broader definition of epidemiology from *A Dictionary of Epidemiology* has been widely accepted. According to this definition, epidemiology is *the study of the distribution and determinants of health-related states or events in specified populations, and the application of this study to control of health problems* (Last, 2001).

Epidemiology focuses on populations or groups of the population, while clinical medicine is concerned with individual patients. Epidemiology is the study of the occurrence and distribution of health and disease factors within a population or a particular subgroup of a population. Epidemiology encompasses the examination of connections between particular diseases and the factors that populations are exposed to. By employing this method, one can identify the risk factors or protective factors that are linked to an individual's health status or certain conditions. These associations can be identified because risk factors and diseases are not randomly distributed in populations. Instead, certain population groups have a higher occurrence of certain diseases and associated factors compared to other population groups. Typically, risk factors are categorized based on age and frequently exhibit variations between genders.

The concept of a "vulnerable" population can be derived by analyzing the distribution of risk factors among different population groups. This particular group is more susceptible to certain conditions due to the presence of a combination of risk factors that strongly predispose them to these conditions.

Epidemiological methods can demonstrate statistical correlations, but establishing causal relationships requires clinical and biological research. Epidemiological studies frequently seek to produce statistical evidence that identifies the factors that significantly contribute to the acquisition of an infection and the development of a disease. The relationship between these factors and the outcome may vary in terms of plausibility and strength. Researchers have developed certain criteria, such as the causal criteria by Hill and the criteria proposed by Rothman and Greenland in 2008, to establish a potential cause-and-effect relationship between identified factors and disease. Epidemiological studies allow us to generate specific hypotheses that identify potential factors that may have a causal role in the development of certain diseases. Verifying the causal relationship of these associations is a responsibility of other disciplines such as clinical medicine or microbiology.

2.2. Epidemiology and Public Health

Epidemiology is a crucial discipline in the field of public health, serving as the cornerstone for evidence-based decision-making and strategy development among public health practitioners (Detels et al., 2002). Epidemiology equips us with the necessary tools to manage and prevent diseases, as well as promote good health. Specifically, epidemiology plays a crucial role in public health by performing important tasks.

- To elucidate the etiology of a disease
- To describe the spectrum of a disease (what kind of symptoms occur and how frequently do they occur)
- To describe the natural history of a disease (what disease stages does a patient typically go through)
- To identify risk factors and protective factors (which factors enhance or prevent the occurrence of a disease)
- To estimate disease burdens and health-care needs of a population
- To predict disease trends (to extrapolate from observations about time trends in risk factors and the future occurrence of the disease)
- To evaluate the effectiveness of interventions and public health programs

Surveillance methods and epidemiological studies can establish the spatial and temporal connections between the distribution of risk factors and the occurrence of disease. By utilizing this method, we can gather data that allows us to identify both risk and protective factors, as well as analyze the patterns of disease occurrence over time and in specific geographic areas. Understanding the geographical and temporal patterns of diseases is crucial for effectively implementing preventive and intervention strategies to reduce the associated disease burdens. We aim to demonstrate the impact of epidemiology on public health by using the case of HIV/AIDS as an illustration.

2.2.1. Epidemiology and the HIV/AIDS Epidemic

An exemplary demonstration of the crucial role of epidemiology in conjunction with other pertinent public health and medical fields is the investigation of the AIDS epidemic. The syndrome of acquired immunodeficiency (AIDS) was initially documented in the United States at the start of the 1980s. The study focused on a cohort of homosexual men residing in California and New York who presented with opportunistic infections and specific tumors.

2.2.2. Elucidating the Aetiology

During that period, multiple theories were proposed to explain the cause of this syndrome. By conducting focused epidemiological studies, researchers discovered that a specific infectious agent was the cause of this syndrome. Sexual contact was determined to be a significant mode of transmission, as homosexual men with a high number of sexual partners were more prone to contracting the disease compared to those with a low number of partners. Subsequently, the human immunodeficiency virus (HIV) was identified in the laboratory as the underlying cause of the disease, and a diagnostic test based on antibodies was created. Epidemiological studies partially served as a filter to understand this novel infectious disease by examining various potential causes and clarifying its infectious nature. Subsequently, this hypothesis was verified in the laboratory and substantiated by the identification of the pathogenic microorganism. Subsequently, epidemiology has maintained its crucial role in studying the HIV epidemic. However, epidemiological studies still have a crucial role in monitoring and preventing this highly destructive infectious disease on a global scale.

2.2.3. Describing the Spectrum of Disease for HIV/AIDS

HIV can cause AIDS, a condition characterized by a variety of symptoms and diseases, including opportunistic infections, tumors, and neurological illnesses. A shared pathogenic characteristic of these clinical conditions is the immunodeficiency caused by HIV, which primarily infects and destroys specific immune system cells known as $CD4^+$ T lymphocytes. The objective of epidemiology is to examine the prevalence and patterns of these clinical manifestations in relation to the population and its associated risk factors.

2.2.4. Describing the Natural History of HIV Infection

Epidemiological studies provide valuable insights into the progression and development of a disease. The natural history of a disease pertains to the progression of the disease in the absence of treatment, a phenomenon that is typically not observed in clinical medicine. The antibody test enabled the examination of specific high-risk populations for HIV infection through screening. It also allowed for the tracking of individuals with and without HIV infection over time in cohort studies. This helped in understanding the risk factors and progression of the infection, as well as identifying factors that predict the development of AIDS. The early stages of HIV infection are marked by acute retroviral syndrome, which includes symptoms such as fever, significant viral damage, and the presence of the virus in the bloodstream. This is followed by a prolonged period of latency, during which there is a balance between HIV and the immune system of the infected person, despite ongoing viral replication. After an initial clinical stage, a severe form of AIDS may occur, characterized by a complete breakdown of the immune system. Within the field of clinical epidemiology, the issue arises regarding the specific phase and timing for administering treatment to patients infected with HIV.

2.2.5. Risk Factors and Protective Factors for HIV Infection

Epidemiology aims to identify the risk and protective factors that are linked to a disease, as well as determine the frequencies and distributions of these factors in the population. Specific public health interventions can be used to decrease the occurrence of relevant risk factors. In the case of HIV, the process of identifying risk factors involves examining sexual behavior and behavior associated with intravenous drug use. On the other hand, the investigation of protective factors includes analyzing the impact of circumcision on the occurrence of HIV.

2.2.6. Predicting Disease Trends

Back calculation methods and time series analysis are applicable for forecasting epidemiological patterns. Back calculation approaches were commonly employed during the HIV epidemic prior to the widespread implementation of antiretroviral therapy (Rosenberg et al. 1991; Seydel et al. 1994; Verdecchia and Mariotto 1995). In recent times, there has been a growing significance placed on incidence-based measures due to the rise in testing rates and the development of methods to identify early HIV infection.

2.2.7. Estimate Disease Burdens and Health-Care Needs of a Population

Forecasting the prevalence of infectious diseases is challenging due to their ever-changing nature. However, it is projected that by 2030, HIV/AIDS will rank as the third most common cause of death and the primary cause of disability-adjusted life years globally (Mathers and Loncar 2006). According to the authors' estimation, HIV/AIDS will account for 12.1% of all disability-adjusted life years in 2030. These findings have significant ramifications for the demand for healthcare, specifically the demand for antiretroviral treatment (ART) on a global scale. Moreover, they may undermine the goals of the World Health Organization (WHO) to provide ART to individuals living with HIV, particularly in low-income nations.

2.2.8. To Test the Effectiveness of Interventions

A comprehensive analysis has been conducted to assess the efficacy of different prevention strategies in mitigating the transmission of HIV. Some prevention strategies that have been examined in extensive epidemiological studies include mass treatment for sexually transmitted infections (Korenromp et al. 2005) and the impact of circumcision on HIV transmission (Auvert et al. 2005; Gray et al. 2007). Although mass treatment for sexually transmitted infections did not demonstrate long-term effectiveness, the outcomes of the circumcision trials have shown great promise.

2.3. Infectious Disease Epidemiology

Infectious diseases result from the transmission of pathogens, which can occur either through direct contact between individuals or indirectly through a vector or the environment. These diseases are commonly referred to as "communicable diseases" because they are transmitted through contact between individuals in a population. The presence of transmission distinguishes the epidemiology of infectious diseases from that of non-communicable diseases, as the likelihood of contracting the disease is influenced by its prevalence in the population.

The transmission of an infectious disease across populations is influenced by the attributes of the infectious agent, the host, and the surrounding environment. Infectious agents possess distinct biological properties, exhibit a range of hosts, and occur naturally. Host characteristics, such as susceptibility to particular diseases, immune status, sociodemographic factors, and contact behavior, also play a role. The interaction between a host and a pathogen is influenced, among other factors, by the immune response, the virulence of the pathogen, the behavioral responses to disease symptoms, and the pathogen's ability to adapt to treatment. Environmental factors dictate the circumstances in which the interaction between the host and the pathogen occurs, and they have an impact on the survival of the pathogen and the behavior of the host. Environmental factors encompass various elements, including physical factors like climate, biological factors such as insects that transmit the infectious agent, and social factors like sanitary conditions and quality of health-care services.

- **Definition: Infectious Disease:** An infectious disease is defined as a disease caused by an infectious agent or its toxic products. This agent can be transmitted by an infected person, an animal or a reservoir directly or indirectly through a vector (e.g., alternate host).

Infectious disease epidemiology, like other branches of epidemiology, focuses on populations rather than individual patients. The core of infectious disease epidemiology revolves around the interplay between an infectious agent and its host, the various pathways through which the agent is transmitted, and the specific environmental conditions that facilitate transmission. Unlike non-communicable diseases, an infected individual (case) can serve as an initial source for additional infections, resulting in the spread of the disease through a population. If these occurrences are closely grouped together in time, they will be identified as an outbreak and will necessitate targeted intervention to disrupt the spread of the disease. Unrecognized and asymptomatic infections and individuals who carry the infection may serve as sources for additional infections without being recognized as contagious cases. Certain individuals or demographic groups may possess immunity to an infection as a result of receiving vaccinations or having been previously exposed to the infection.

Infectious disease epidemiology focuses on studying crucial aspects such as the ability of pathogens to spread and cause harm, the progression of infections with or without noticeable symptoms, and the length of time that immunity provides protection. In infectious disease epidemiology, the study of human contact patterns is significant, unlike the epidemiology of non-communicable diseases. These interactions can occur among humans, between humans and animals, between humans and vectors (such as disease-carrying organisms), or between humans and their surrounding environment. Epidemiological studies aim to ascertain the underlying reasons for the endemic or epidemic occurrence of infectious diseases, as well as the factors that contribute to variations in infection rates between and within populations.

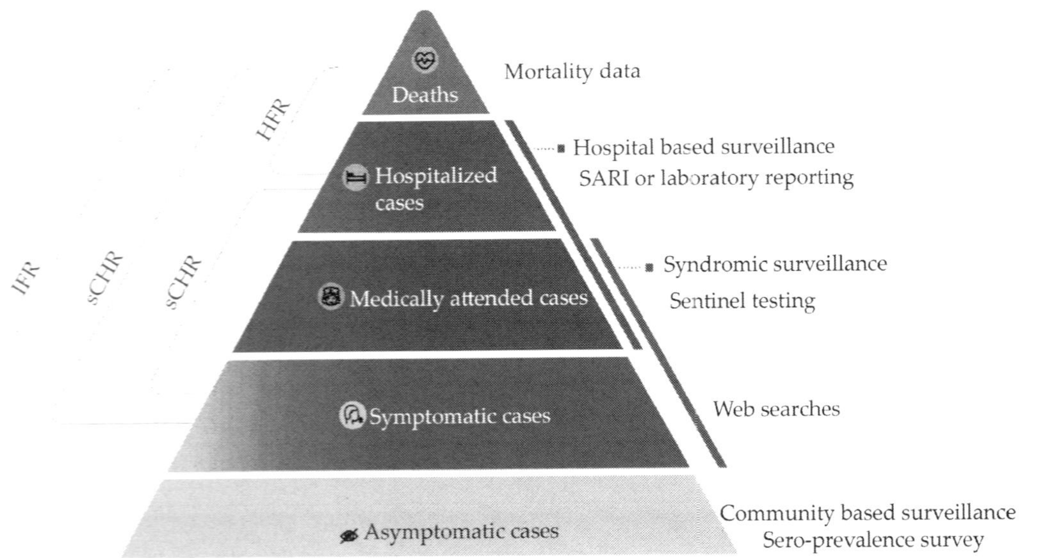

Figure 2.1. *The chain of infection.*

Source: *Ryu S, Chun JY, Lee S, Yoo D, Kim Y, Ali ST, & Chun BC. (2022). Epidemiology and transmission dynamics of infectious diseases and control measures. Viruses, 14(11), 2510. https://doi.org/10.3390/v14112510.*

Page et al. (1995) outline a conceptual framework consisting of six essential components that must be present for the transmission of infectious diseases and the subsequent development of illness in an individual. The process of transmission is commonly known as the "chain of infection" (Figure 2.1). For an infection to occur, it is necessary for each element to be present and arranged in a sequential order. Intervention can address any of the six components of the cycle.

The portal of entry refers to the specific route through which an infectious agent gains access to a vulnerable host. The point of entry typically corresponds to the point of departure from the host (Timmreck 1994). As an illustration, the measles virus leaves the respiratory tract of the infected individual and enters the respiratory tract of a different individual. In gastrointestinal infections, the infectious agent is present in feces and can be transmitted to the mouth of a new host through inadequately washed hands. Additional routes of entry include the integumentary system (such as schistosomes), the mucous membrane (for sexually transmitted diseases), the circulatory system (for HIV), and the transplacental mode of entry (for toxoplasmosis).

The portal of exit refers to the pathway through which the infectious agent departs from the host. The exit point typically relies on the location of the infectious agent within the host. The primary routes of exit include the respiratory tract (such as influenza, measles, mumps, and rubella), genitourinary tract (HIV, syphilis), gastrointestinal tract (hepatitis A, Salmonella), transmission through the skin (hepatitis B through needles), and the placenta (toxoplasmosis).

Below, we present several key concepts in the field of infectious disease epidemiology.

2.3.1. Exposure

An essential principle in epidemiology is the individual's contact with a potential pathogen or harmful substance that can cause disease. If an individual is exposed to infectious agents, also known as pathogens, during an infectious disease, it can result in an infection, but it does not always result in the development of a disease. Prions, viruses, bacteria, fungi, and parasites are all examples of infectious agents. The disease can be caused by either the pathogens themselves, once they have replicated in the infected host, or by the toxic substances they produce.

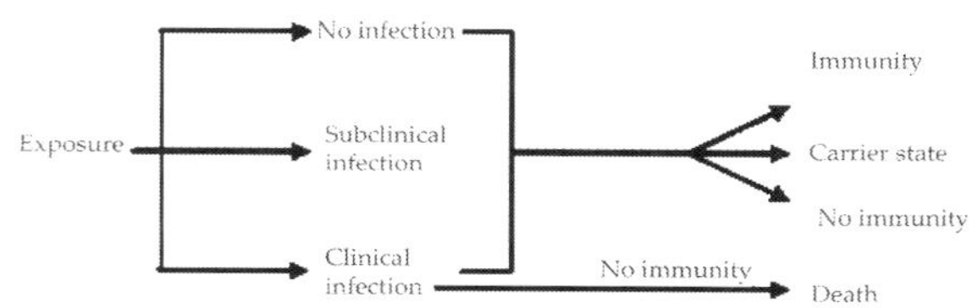

Figure 2.2. *The different outcomes of an exposure to an infectious agent.*

Source: Giesecke 1994.

The level of contact with an infectious agent is determined by the method through which it is transmitted. Various outcomes resulting from exposure to an infectious agent can be observed (Figure 2.2). The result may or may not be influenced by the amount of infectious material or the size of the initial inoculation. Highly contagious pathogens can infect the host with a small amount, whereas less contagious pathogens require a larger amount of the pathogen for infection to occur. For instance, the likelihood of contracting an infection is significantly greater when exposed to the hepatitis B virus through sexual contact compared to exposure to HIV. The relationship between the amount of infectious material and the likelihood of infection can be measured using dose-response relationships (Teunis et al. 1999).

2.3.2. Infection

What is the precise definition of infection? In the case of most pathogens, infection refers to the occurrence when the pathogen is able to successfully settle in the host organism and reproduce itself or certain stages of its life cycle. In the case of certain pathogens, it is necessary to differentiate between colonization, which refers to the pathogen settling on the skin or other body tissues without causing any clinical signs or symptoms of disease, and invasive infection, which occurs when the pathogen penetrates through specific barriers of the host (such as the skin or mucous membrane) and causes symptomatic infection. In the field of pathology, an inflammation caused by an infectious pathogen or other harmful agents is distinguished by four specific phenomena: the affected skin areas exhibit redness and increased temperature, followed by swelling, pain, and a decrease or impairment in function.

Infections caused by various pathogens, as well as infections caused by the same pathogen in different individuals, can exhibit significant variations in their natural progression. Certain infections have an acute nature and last for a brief period of time, ranging from a few hours to days or weeks. Examples of such infections include measles, mumps, influenza, and diarrhea. On the other hand, some infections initially have a short acute phase but can later become chronic, persisting and being detectable for many years. Examples of these chronic infections include hepatitis B and C, as well as HIV. The variations observed are a result of the ability of the human immune system to respond to various pathogens. This ability is influenced by the genetic diversity of the pathogens and their specific location within the host.

The symptoms of an infection can vary significantly among individuals. An infection can result in a carrier phase, during which an infected person exhibits no symptoms. However, the presence of pathogens can be identified in carriers through microbiological tests, such as serological tests or direct methods for detecting the presence of pathogens. Carriers play a significant role in the transmission of infections and in implementing interventions, as they are not readily identifiable or detectable. An individual who is carrying an infection is typically unaware of their infection and the potential danger they present to those they come into direct contact with. Consequently, individuals who are vulnerable to infection do not take preventive measures. Targeting public health measures to prevent risky contacts and identify sources of infection, such as hepatitis B and HIV, poses a challenging task. Only by systematically screening entire population groups can we ensure the implementation of effective interventions under these circumstances.

Infections that present with noticeable or observable symptoms can exhibit a wide range of variations in the symptoms displayed. These symptoms can be highly distinctive for certain infectious diseases (e.g., characteristic rash and pustules in smallpox) or they can be more nonspecific, such as respiratory tract infections (fever and cough) or gastrointestinal infections (diarrhea), which can have multiple possible causes. In the latter scenario, a conclusive diagnosis can only be made through laboratory testing of a specimen.

The protective effect of immunity acquired after infection can vary and its duration can be unpredictable. Certain infectious diseases provide lifelong immunity, such as measles. Others provide some level of immunity against severe symptomatic infection, but offer much less protection against sub-clinical infection, like pertussis. There are also some diseases, such as Chlamydia infection, that provide little to no immunity. Some pathogens can invade the immune system, which not only weakens the host's immune response against them but also allows other pathogens to invade the infected host. Examples of such pathogens include HIV and opportunistic infections. Immunity can be obtained either through natural infection or indirectly. Maternal antibodies provide immunity to the newborn against numerous infections during the initial months of its existence. Subsequently, vaccination can be utilized to achieve immunization against certain infectious diseases. Vaccine-induced immunity can either be long-lasting or temporary. In the latter scenario, it is imperative to administer multiple booster vaccinations to guarantee immunity against the infection.

2.3.3. Stages of Infection and Disease

During the course of an infection, different stages or time periods can be distinguished regarding the infectivity and manifestations of symptoms in the infected individual. The *latent period* is the time interval from infection to the start of the infectious period; the *incubation period* is the time interval from infection to the onset of clinical symptoms (Figure 2.3). The *infectious period* is the time interval during which an infected person can transmit an infection to other susceptible persons.

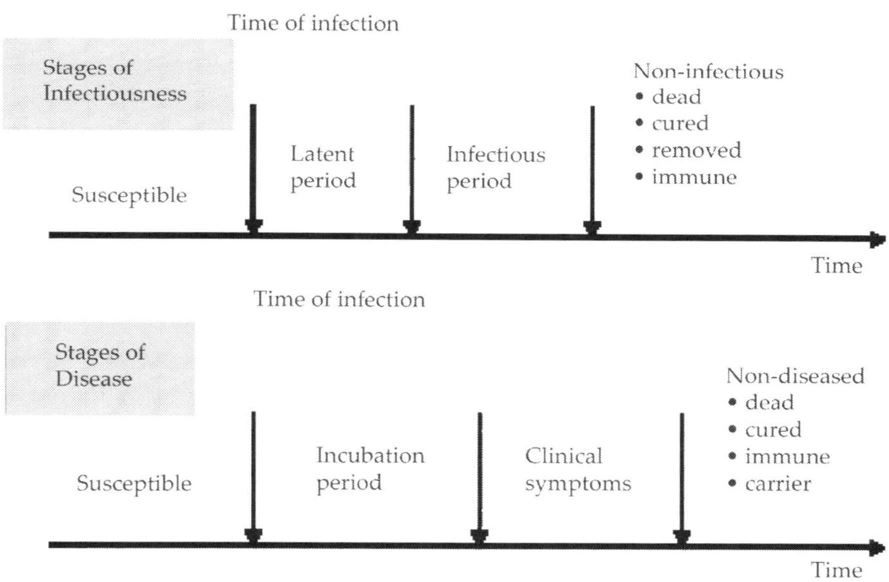

Figure 2.3. *Stages of infection and disease.*

Source: Halloran 1998.

The incubation period of a particular infectious disease can vary significantly among individuals. Thus, incubation periods can be more accurately characterized as incubation time distributions that include a minimum, a mean or median, and a maximum incubation time (Figure 2.4). During outbreaks, it is common to see multiple generations of an infection, which refers to groups of cases that have a consistent time interval between the days when symptoms first appear (Figure 2.5). The initial case, also known as the index case, holds significant significance in an outbreak as they introduce the infectious disease into the community. Secondary cases refer to individuals who have been infected by the primary case, while tertiary cases are individuals who have been infected by a secondary case, and so on. The generation interval or serial interval refers to the typical time interval between the onset of symptoms in a case and the onset of symptoms in the cases infected by that individual. The distribution of this interval is influenced by the durations of the latent period and infectious period, as well as the contact rates of infectious individuals (Fine, 2003).

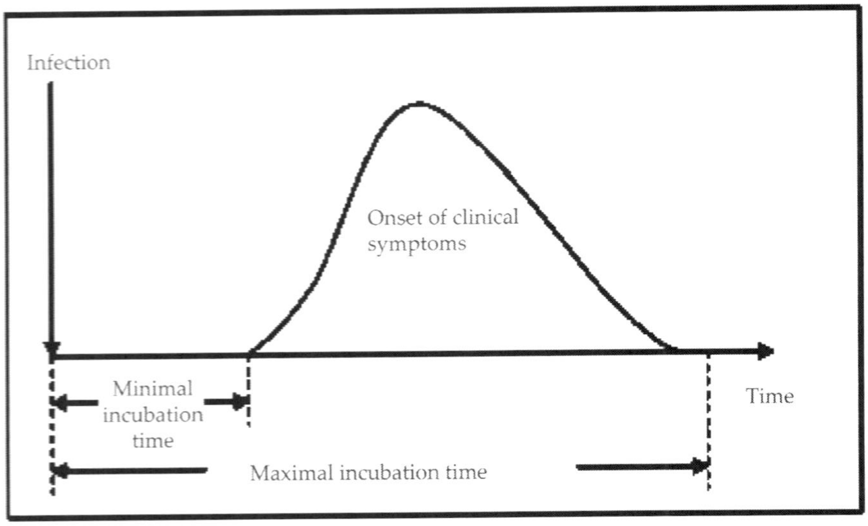

Figure 2.4. *Incubation time distribution.*

Source: NCBI.

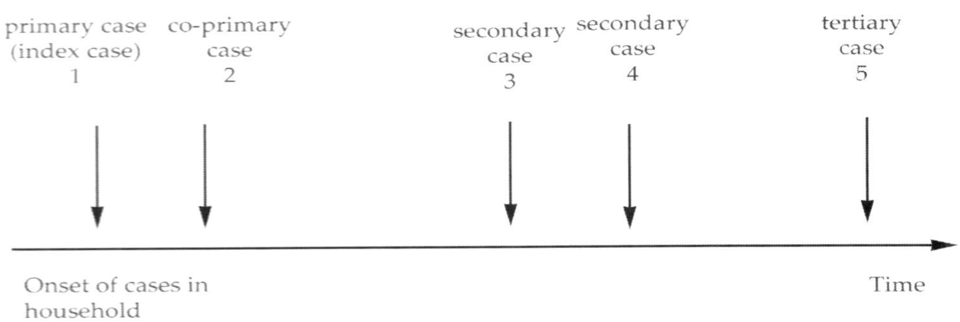

Figure 2.5. *Generations of an infection.*

Source: *Halloran, 1998.*

The reproduction number, also known as the reproductive rate, refers to the capacity of an infection to propagate within a population following its introduction. The outcome is contingent upon the ratio of immune individuals in the population, the length of time during which the infection can be transmitted, the frequency of interactions, and the likelihood of transmission when an infected person comes into contact with a susceptible individual.

2.3.4. Virulence, Pathogenicity and Immunogenicity

Various definitions of virulence can be found in the literature, primarily focusing on the pathogen's capacity to induce host mortality. Nevertheless, in numerous cases of infectious diseases, a virulence definition predicated on host mortality proves impractical, as our primary concern lies in the intensity of symptoms rather than fatality. Pathogenicity refers to the inherent ability of a pathogen to induce symptoms in a host. Virulence typically refers to the relative pathogenicity of one strain of a pathogen compared to another. According to Casadevall and Pirofski (1999), we define virulence as the comparative ability of a pathogen to inflict harm on the host.

The pathogenicity and virulence of a pathogen are determined by the interaction it has with the host. The virulence of infectious agents is influenced by their capacity to replicate, infiltrate organisms, and harm the host. The occurrence of these effects may rely on the infective dose, which refers to the minimum number of organisms required to initiate an infection. A highly infectious pathogen can infiltrate the host organism with a minimal amount of infectious particles. The pathogenicity and virulence of a pathogen are influenced by various factors, including the characteristics of the host such as resistance, immune system function, genetic factors, age, gender, and physiological conditions like pregnancy.

Immunogenicity refers to the capacity of a pathogen or vaccine to stimulate an immune response following infection or vaccination, potentially resulting in protection against subsequent infections caused by the same or similar pathogen. Certain infections, such as measles or polio virus, provide lifelong immunity after natural infection, whereas others, like pertussis, offer only temporary immunity or immunity specific to certain strains, as is the case with influenza. In certain infections, immunity is obtained only through multiple re-infections and diminishes if additional infections that boost immunity do not occur (such as in the case of malaria). In certain cases, the body develops immunity against noticeable infection, but there is still a possibility of experiencing unnoticed infection.

2.3.5. Routes of Transmission

An infectious pathogen can be transmitted to a vulnerable recipient through various means. The routes of transmission are categorized as direct and indirect transmission (Giesecke, 1994). Direct transmission involves direct contact between skin surfaces and close proximity that allows transmission through droplets and aerosols. Droplet transmission occurs through the expulsion of respiratory droplets during sneezing, coughing, or speaking in close proximity. Droplet spread is classified as direct transmission due to its transmission through a direct spray that covers a short distance of a few meters before the droplets descend to the ground. Indirect transmission occurs through vectors or the environment. A vector is a parasitic organism that acquires an infection from infected animals or individuals and then transmits the infection to other individuals. An example of this is the Anopheles mosquitoes, which transmit malaria parasites from one person to another. Vectors are commonly insects or arthropods. Furthermore, medical devices such as injection syringes have the potential to serve as carriers for the transmission of diseases. Moreover, pathogens can be transmitted through various environmental mediums such as water, food, soil, air, and solid surfaces, depending on the conditions that allow them to thrive outside of their host.

The source of infection is the primary location from which the infection is transmitted to an individual. In cases of directly transmitted infections, the origin can be traced back to an individual who is already infected. Indirectly transmitted infections can arise from various sources in the environment, such as objects, soil, water, as well as contaminated or infected foods and animal vectors. A reservoir of infection refers to a living organism or material that serves as a habitat for an infectious agent, allowing it to live and reproduce.

Examples of directly transmitted infections include sexually transmitted infections (transmitted through contact with mucous membranes), toxoplasmosis (transmitted through the placenta), HIV and hepatitis B (transmitted through sexual contact and blood), herpes virus type 1 infection (transmitted through skin-to-skin contact), and influenza (transmitted through coughing and sneezing, known as droplet spread). Indirectly transmitted infections include hepatitis A (transmitted through contact with feces), Salmonella (transmitted through contaminated food), malaria (transmitted through mosquito bites), and schistosomiasis (transmitted through contaminated water) (Table 2.1).

Table 2.1. Frequent Media of Transmission and Transmission Routes for Some Infectious Agents

Transmission Medium	**Pathogen**	**Transmission Route**
Foods	*Salmonella* *Campylobacter* Hepatitis A	Foodborne Fecal–oral
Water Sputum droplets Air/aerosols	Cholera Influenza Tuberculosis Chickenpox, *Legionella* infection	Water-borne Close contact Airborne
Organ transplants Blood Sperm, body fluids	Cytomegalovirus HIV, hepatitis C Hepatitis B	Transplant-borne Blood-borne Sexual contact

Source: *Adapted from "Control of Communicable Diseases Manual" by David L. Heymann, American Public Health Association, 2015.*

Some pathogens have one or several intermediate hosts, such as arthropods, in which they undergo multiplication and development, in addition to their primary host, which is usually a human or vertebrate animal. During a malaria infection, humans serve as intermediate hosts, while the Anopheles mosquito is responsible for the sexual reproduction of the pathogen.

Humans can also inadvertently become hosts through atypical contact with an infectious agent primarily hosted by animals, such as hantavirus pulmonary syndrome. Zoonosis refers to any infection that is transmitted from an animal to a human. Many newly emerging infections in humans are thought to originate from zoonoses.

2.3.6. Endemic Infectious Diseases and Epidemic Outbreaks

An outbreak is characterized by the occurrence of an infection in a population that surpasses the anticipated level of cases in terms of both space and time. An outbreak can range in size, with even just two connected cases being considered an outbreak, or it can have a significant impact on a large portion of the population. An epidemic refers to a more extensive outbreak that impacts a significant portion of a population. A pandemic refers to a worldwide outbreak that impacts numerous or all countries.

An infectious disease that can establish a permanent presence in a population is referred to as endemic. The prevalence of many endemic infections remains relatively stable over time if there are no alterations in intervention or prevention strategies. Through the implementation of preventive measures or timely intervention, it is possible to strive for the complete eradication of an endemic infection from a population. Eradication refers to the complete elimination of something on a worldwide level. Elimination refers to the absence of natural transmission of a pathogen within a population, while eradication refers to the complete absence of circulation of a pathogen in the human population. Currently, smallpox is the sole infectious disease that has been successfully eradicated.

Several infectious diseases that are unique to a particular region have incidence rates that vary throughout the year (Fisman, 2007). The seasonality is a result of climate conditions, which impact the ability of pathogens to survive in the environment, and human contact patterns, which vary due to activity patterns such as school holidays.

2.4. Challenges in the Field of Infectious Disease Epidemiology

The challenges of modern infectious disease epidemiology include transnational migration, shifts in human behavior, rapid urbanization, and the emergence of new infectious diseases like SARS and BSE (mad cow disease). During the era of globalization, the movement of people across national borders plays a significant role in the transmission of infectious diseases. The border is no longer perceived as an effective barrier due to the presence of infectious diseases with extended incubation periods, which poses challenges in containing their spread. Conversely, migrant populations frequently experience social marginalization, rendering them susceptible to specific diseases (Tselmin et al., 2007). Socioeconomic disparities significantly contribute to the transmission of infectious diseases. The impoverished population frequently resides in densely populated dwellings with insufficient sanitation facilities. These individuals typically have a poorer nutritional status, rendering them more susceptible to infectious diseases. Individuals belonging to lower socio-economic classes may face restricted availability of primary healthcare services.

Educational interventions aimed at improving knowledge, beliefs, and attitudes regarding prevention can be advantageous for population groups vulnerable to infectious diseases. These endeavors are vital in halting the dissemination of infections. To foster greater engagement between academic research and vulnerable populations, the community-based participatory research (CBPR) approach can be employed. This approach actively involves the community being studied in the research process (Israel et al., 1998). The advantages of this form of research are as follows: (a) Community members are regarded as study collaborators rather than mere subjects of research; (b) The community's knowledge is utilized to gain a deeper understanding of health issues within the community; (c) Interventions can be implemented directly within the community. Effective public health strategies that address community concerns require close collaboration between communities and researchers (Kone et al., 2000). This method is particularly suitable when researching sensitive topics like HIV/AIDS or sexually transmitted diseases and has been effectively utilized in the field of infectious disease epidemiology.

Additional complexities in the field of infectious disease epidemiology arise from the swift advancements in genetic typing techniques. These methods enable a more comprehensive understanding of the genetic relationships between different strains of pathogens and the potential pathways through which they may have disseminated within a population. Currently, there is a substantial amount of genotyping data accessible. However, there is a lack of epidemiological studies that investigate the connection between transmission risks and the distribution of genotypes.

Another urgent research area in infectious disease epidemiology arises from the pathogens' capacity to evade intervention pressure through evolutionary adaptation. An instance of this is the emergence of pathogen resistance to treatments, such as antibiotic resistance and resistance to antiviral medication. This phenomenon is leading to growing challenges, not only within hospitals where there is a prevalence of multi-resistant strains of pathogens but also in the management of tuberculosis and chronic hepatitis B.

A Closer Look

Polio Virus

Poliovirus, a member of the Enterovirus genus within the Picornaviridae family, is the causative agent of poliomyelitis, a disease that has profoundly affected human populations throughout history. The virus is an RNA virus with a single-stranded positive-sense genome encapsulated in a protein shell called a capsid. This virus primarily targets the nervous system, leading to severe complications, including paralysis and even death in some cases.

Poliovirus is transmitted primarily through the fecal-oral route, where contaminated food and water become the vectors for its spread. Once ingested, the virus multiplies in the intestines and can enter the bloodstream, subsequently targeting motor neurons in the spinal cord and brainstem. The destruction of these neurons leads to the characteristic symptoms of poliomyelitis, including acute flaccid paralysis.

The clinical manifestations of polio can vary significantly. While the majority of infections are asymptomatic, a fraction of individuals may develop non-paralytic polio, characterized by flu-like symptoms, or the more severe paralytic polio, which can lead to permanent disability. Bulbar polio, a subtype of paralytic polio, affects the brainstem, causing difficulties in breathing, swallowing, and speaking, and can be fatal if respiratory muscles become paralyzed.

The development of effective vaccines has been a pivotal moment in the fight against polio. The two main types of vaccines are the inactivated poliovirus vaccine (IPV) and the oral poliovirus vaccine (OPV). IPV, developed by Jonas Salk, uses inactivated virus particles and is administered via injection, providing immunity without the risk of vaccine-derived virus. OPV, developed by Albert Sabin, contains live attenuated virus and is administered orally. OPV has the advantage of inducing gut immunity and being easier to administer, making it a crucial tool in mass immunization campaigns.

Global vaccination efforts have drastically reduced the incidence of polio. The World Health Organization (WHO) launched the Global Polio Eradication Initiative (GPEI) in 1988, which has led to the eradication of wild poliovirus type 2 and type 3. However, wild poliovirus type 1 (WPV1) remains endemic in a few countries, including Afghanistan and Pakistan, posing a significant challenge to global eradication efforts. Additionally, vaccine-derived polioviruses (VDPVs) can emerge in under-immunized populations, highlighting the need for continued vigilance and comprehensive immunization coverage.

Despite the significant strides made in controlling polio, complete eradication remains elusive. Political instability, logistical challenges, and vaccine hesitancy are significant barriers that need to be addressed. Continued global cooperation, sustained funding, and innovative strategies are essential to achieve the ultimate goal of a polio-free world.

Summary

- Infectious disease epidemiology is the study of the patterns, causes, and effects of infectious diseases in populations.
- It involves investigating how diseases are transmitted, who is at risk, and why some individuals or communities are more susceptible than others.
- Epidemiologists use various methods, such as surveillance, outbreak investigation, and statistical modeling, to track and understand the spread of infectious diseases.
- The field also focuses on developing strategies to prevent and control infectious diseases, including vaccination programs, vector control, and health education.
- Infectious disease epidemiology plays a crucial role in public health, helping to inform policies and interventions aimed at reducing the burden of infectious diseases on society.
- Recent advances in technology and data analysis have improved our ability to study and respond to infectious disease outbreaks, but challenges such as antimicrobial resistance and emerging pathogens continue to pose significant threats to global health.

References

1. Abbotts, R., Harrison, S. E., & Cooper, G. L. (2007). Primary blast injuries to the eye: A review of the evidence. *Journal of the Royal Army Medical Corps, 153*(2), 119–123.
2. Abdellatif, M. Z., Elmazar, H. M., & Essa, A. B. (2011). *Oestrus ovis* as a cause of red eye in Aljabal Algharbi, Libya. *Middle East African Journal of Ophthalmology, 18*(4), 305–308. Erratum in *Middle East African Journal of Ophthalmology, 23*(3), 332.
3. Abihaidar, N., & Garcin, T. (2022). External ophthalmomyiasis due to *Oestrus ovis*. *New England Journal of Medicine, 386*, e35.
4. Abuelhassan, A. A. (2010). External ophthalmomyiasis due to *Oestrus ovis*: A case report from Oman. *Oman Medical Journal, 25*, e014.
5. Ahaduzzaman, M. (2019). The global and regional prevalence of oestrosis in sheep and goats: A systematic review of articles and meta-analysis. *Parasites & Vectors, 12*, 346.
6. Akbarzadeh, K., Rafinejad, J., Alipour, H., & Biglarian, A. (2012). Human myiasis in Fars Province, Iran. *Southeast Asian Journal of Tropical Medicine and Public Health, 43*(5), 1205–1211.
7. Akçakaya, A. A., Sargın, F., Aslan, Z. I., Sevimli, N., & Sadikov, F. (2014). External ophthalmomyiasis seen in a patient from Istanbul, Turkey. *Acta Parasitologica Turcica, 38*, 205–207.
8. Akdemir, M. O., & Ozen, S. (2013). External ophthalmomyiasis caused by *Oestrus ovis* misdiagnosed as bacterial conjunctivitis. *Tropical Doctor, 43*(3), 120–123.
9. Alameri, O. H. (2014). External ophthalmomyiasis report in Jordan valley. *Veterinary Science Development, 4*, 5628.
10. Al-Amry, M., Al-Saikhan, F. I., & Al-Dahmash, S. (2014). External ophthalmomyiasis: A case report. *Saudi Journal of Ophthalmology, 28*, 322–324.
11. Albaroudi, N., Tijani, M., & Daoudi, R. (2016). Ophtalmomyiase externe au Maroc: À props d'un cas en milieu urbain [External ophthalmomyiasis in Morocco: About a case in an urban area]. *Journal Français d'Ophtalmologie, 39*(3), 320–321. (In French)

12. Alcaide, M., Reina, D., Sánchez-López, J., Frontera, E., & Navarrete, I. (2005). Seroprevalence of *Oestrus ovis* (Diptera, Oestridae) infestation and associated risk factors in ovine livestock from southwestern Spain. *Journal of Medical Entomology, 42*(3), 327–331.
13. Alhady, M., Zabri, K., & Chua, C. N. (2008). Ophthalmomyiasis from Chrysomyia bezziana (screwworm fly). *Medical Journal of Malaysia, 63*(3), 269–270.
14. Ali, A., Feroze, A. H., Ferrar, P., Abbas, A., & Beg, M. A. (2006). First report of ophthalmomyiasis externa in Pakistan. *Journal of the Pakistan Medical Association, 56*(2), 86–87.
15. Alsaif, N., Liao, S., & Tse, D. T. (2016). External ophthalmomyiasis due to *Dermatobia hominis* masquerading as orbital cellulitis. *Ophthalmic Plastic & Reconstructive Surgery, 32*(2), e113–e116.
16. Anane, S., & Hssine, L. B. (2010). La myiase conjonctivale humaine à *Oestrus ovis* dans le sud tunisien [Conjonctival human myiasis by *Oestrus ovis* in southern Tunisia]. *Bulletin de la Société de Pathologie Exotique, 103*(4), 299–304. (In French)
17. Armas-Herrera, G. L., Arévalo-Arévalo, L. F., & Alemán-Infante, J. (2018). Oftalmomiasis causada por Oestrus sp. en la selva peruana: A propósito de un caso. *Acta Médica Peruana, 35*(3), 229–232.
18. Arslan, F., Mete, B., Oztürk, R., & Samasti, M. (2010). External ophthalmomyiasis caused by *Oestrus ovis* in Istanbul. *Tropical Doctor, 40*(3), 186–187.
19. Ashenhurst, M., & Pietucha, S. (2004). Management of ophthalmomyiasis externa: Case report. *Canadian Journal of Ophthalmology, 39*(3), 285–287.
20. Balamurugan, R., Gupta, P. C., Dhingra, D., & Ram, J. (2020). External ophthalmomyiasis by *Oestrus ovis* larvae. *QJM: An International Journal of Medicine, 113*(10), 751.
21. Bali, J., Gupta, Y. K., Chowdhury, B., Nayyar, B., Gupta, M. M., & Thakur, R. (2007). Ophthalmomyiasis: A rare cause of short duration pre-septal cellulitis in a healthy non-compromised adult. *Singapore Medical Journal, 48*(10), 969–971.
22. Basmaciyan, L., Gabrielle, P. H., Valot, S., Sautour, M., Buisson, J. C., Creuzot-Garcher, C., & Dalle, F. (2018). *Oestrus ovis* external ophthalmomyiasis: A case report in Burgundy France. *BMC Ophthalmology, 18*, 335.
23. Bazaliński, D., Kózka, M., Karnas, M., & Więch, P. (2019). Effectiveness of chronic wound debridement with the use of larvae of *Lucilia sericata*. *Journal of Clinical Medicine, 8*(11), 1845).
24. Beltrán, M. F., Torres, G. V., Segami, H. S., & Náquira, C. V. (2006). Miasis ocular por Oestrus ovis. *Revista Peruana de Medicina Experimental y Salud Pública, 23*(2), 70–72.
25. Beristain, X., Alkorta, M., Egaña, L., Lacasta, A., & Cilla, G. (2001). Nasopharyngeal myasis by third stage larvae of Oestrus ovis. *Enfermedades Infecciosas y Microbiología Clínica, 19*(2), 86–87.
26. Bernhardt, V., Finkelmeier, F., Verhoff, M. A., & Amendt, J. (2019). Myiasis in humans—A global case report evaluation and literature analysis. *Parasitology Research, 118*(1), 389–397.
27. Berrozpe-Villabona, C., Avalos-Franco, N., Aguilar-Munoa, S., Bañeros-Rojas, P., Castellar-Cerpa, J., & Diaz-Valle, D. (2015). External ophthalmomyiasis: A case report from Spain. *Journal Français d'Ophtalmologie, 38*, e219–e220.

28. Bonzon, L., Toga, I., Piarroux, M., & Piarroux, R. (2015). Clustered cases of *Oestrus ovis* ophthalmomyiasis after 3-week festival, Marseille, France, 2013. *Emerging Infectious Diseases, 21*(2), 375–377.

29. Caça, I., Satar, A., Unlü, K., Sakalar, Y. B., & Ari, S. (2006). External ophthalmomyiasis infestation. *Japanese Journal of Ophthalmology, 50*(2), 176–177.

30. Calıskan, S., Ugurbaş, S. C., & Sağdık, M. (2014). Ophthalmomyiasis externa: Three cases caused by *Oestrus ovis* larvae in Turkey. *Tropical Doctor, 44*(4), 230–232.

31. Can, F. K., Alay, H., & Çinici, E. (2020). Unusual case: Ophthalmomyiasis. *Revista da Sociedade Brasileira de Medicina Tropical, 54*, e20200110.

32. Carrillo, I., Zarratea, L., Suárez, M. J., Izquierdo, C., Garde, A., & Bengoa, A. (2013). External ophthalmomyiasis: A case series. *International Ophthalmology, 33*(2), 167–169.

33. Cepeda-Palacios, R., & Scholl, P. J. (2000). Factors affecting the larvipositional activity of *Oestrus ovis* gravid females (Diptera: Oestridae). *Veterinary Parasitology, 91*(1–2), 93–105.

34. Chakraborti, C., Mukhopadhya, U., Mondal, M., Giri, D., & Khan, M. (2011). Ophthalmomyiasis in humans. *Nepal Journal of Ophthalmology, 3*(2), 193–195.

35. Choi, W., Kim, G. E., Park, S. H., Shin, S. E., Park, J. H., & Yoon, K. C. (2015). First report of external ophthalmomyiasis caused by *Lucilia sericata* Meigen in a healthy patient without predisposing risk factors. *Parasitology International, 64*(3), 281–283.

36. Choudhary, P., Rathore, M. K., Dwivedi, P., Lakhtakia, S., Chalisgaonkar, C., & Dwivedi, A. (2013). Red eye: rule out ophthalmomyiasis too. *Indian Journal of Ophthalmology, 61*(6), 293–295.

37. Couto Jr, A. S., Marcos, A. A. A., Barros, G. S. S., & Moraes, G. N. (2018). External ophthalmomyiasis. *Revista Brasileira de Oftalmologia, 77*(4), 219–221.

38. Cucera, A., Watzel, C., & Lang, G. K. (2009). Ophthalmomyiasis externa durch *Oestrus ovis* der Schafs- und Ziegenbremse [Ophthalmomyiasis externa due to *Oestrus ovis* a sheep botfly]. *Klinische Monatsblätter für Augenheilkunde, 226*(2), 189–190.

39. D'Assumpcao, C., Bugas, A., Heidari, A., Sofinski, S., & McPheeters, R. A. (2019). A case and review of ophthalmomyiasis caused by *Oestrus ovis* in the central valley of California, United States. *Journal of Investigative Medicine High Impact Case Reports, 7*, 2324709619835852.

40. Dadaci, Z., Saracligil, B., & Macin, S. (2020). External ophthalmomyiasis caused by *Oestrus ovis. Selcuk Medical Journal, 36*(1), 51–53.

41. Dar, M. S., Amer, M. B., Dar, F. K., & Papazotos, V. (1980). Ophthalmomyiasis caused by the sheep nasal bot, *Oestrus ovis* (Oestridae) larvae, in the Benghazi area of Eastern Libya. *Transactions of the Royal Society of Tropical Medicine and Hygiene, 74*(3), 303–306.

42. Delshad, E., Rubin, A. I., Almeida, L., & Niedt, G. W. (2008). Cuterebra cutaneous myiasis: Case report and world literature review. *International Journal of Dermatology, 47*(4), 363–366.

43. Denion, E., Dalens, P. H., Couppié, P., Aznar, C., Sainte-Marie, D., Carme, B., Petitbon, J., & Pradinaud, R. (2004). External ophthalmomyiasis caused by *Dermatobia hominis*. A retrospective study of nine cases and a review of the literature. *Acta Ophthalmologica Scandinavica, 82*(5), 576–584.

44. Dinçer, Ş. (1997). Ińsan ve hayvanlarda myiasis. In A. Özcel & N. Daldal (Eds.), *Parazitoloji'de Arthropod Hastalıkları ve Vektörler* (pp. 169–234). Türkiye Parazitoloji Derneǵi, Yayın No: 13; Ege Üniversitesi Basımevi.

45. Dokur, M., Eroglu, F., Ipek, D. N., & Ulutasdemir, N. (2015). Two different myiasis cases in southeast of Turkey: Ophthalmomyiasis and cutaneous myiasis. *Parasitology Research, 114*(8), 2767–2770. https://doi.org/10.1007/s00436-015-4476-7.

46. Dono, M., Bertonati, M. R., Poggi, R., Teneggi, E., Maddalo, F., Via, F., Orlandi, R., Maroli, M., Roncella, S., & Fedeli, F. (2005). Three cases of ophthalmomyiasis externa by sheep botfly *Oestrus ovis* in Italy. *New Microbiolog, 28*(4), 365–368. PMID: 16425634.

47. Dorchies, P. (1997). Comparative physiopathology of *Oestrus ovis* myiasis in man and animals. *Bulletin de l'Académie Nationale de Médecine, 181*(4), 673–684.

48. Dunbar, J., Cooper, B., Hodgetts, T., Yskandar, H., van Thiel, P., Whelan, S., Taylor, J., & Woods, D. R. (2008). An outbreak of human external ophthalmomyiasis due to *Oestrus ovis* in southern Afghanistan. *Clinical Infectious Diseases, 46*(9), e124–e126. https://doi.org/10.1086/587993.

49. Dutta Majumder, P., Jeswani, P., Jeyathilakan, N., & Biswas, J. (2019). External ophthalmomyiasis due to *Oestrus ovis*. *Indian Journal of Ophthalmology, 67*(3), 404–405. https://doi.org/10.4103/ijo.IJO_1254_18.

50. Emborsky, M. E., & Faden, H. (2002). Ophthalmomyiasis in a child. *Pediatric Infectious Disease Journal, 21*(1), 82–83.

51. Eyigör, H., Dost, T., Dayanir, V., Başak, S., & Eren, H. (2008). A case of nasoophthalmic myiasis. *Turkish Journal of Ear Nose Throat, 18*(5), 371–373.

52. Farias, L. A. B. G., Teixeira, M. J., & Pires Neto, R. D. J. (2020). Palpebral myiasis due *Cochliomyia macellaria* in an alcoholic patient. *Revista da Sociedade Brasileira de Medicina Tropical, 54*, e20200168. https://doi.org/10.1590/0037-8682-0168-2020.

53. Francesconi, F., & Lupi, O. (2012). Myiasis. *Clinical Microbiology Reviews, 25*(1), 79–105. https://doi.org/10.1128/CMR.00010-11.

54. Fries, F. N., Pattmöller, M., Seitz, B., Berger, F., Kampen, H., Szentmáry, N., & Becker, S. L. (2018). Ophthalmomyiasis externa due to *Oestrus ovis* in a traveler returning from Greece. *Travel Medicine and Infectious Disease, 23*, 101–102. https://doi.org/10.1016/j.tmaid.2018.03.002.

55. Garcia-Guerrero, J., Garza-Quiñones, J., Reza-Caballero, J., & González-Treviño, J. (2014). External ophthalmomyiasis by *Oestrus ovis* treated with tobacco: Clinical case report and medical literature review. *Medicina Universitaria, 16*(64), 181–183.

56. Gautam, N., Tomar, M., Thakur, C., & Kanga, A. (2019). Ophthalmomyiasis caused by *Oestrus ovis*. *Journal of Microbiology & Infectious Diseases, 9*(4), 161–163. https://doi.org/10.5799/jmid.644986.

57. Gholamhossein, Y., & Behrouz, H. (2013). External ophthalmomyiasis presenting to an emergency department: Corneal findings as a sign of *Oestrus ovis*. *Korean Journal of Ophthalmology, 27*(5), 341–344. https://doi.org/10.3341/kjo.2013.27.5.341.

58. Graffi, S., Peretz, A., Wilamowski, A., Schnur, H., Akad, F., & Naftali, M. (2013). External ophthalmomyiasis caused by a rare infesting larva, *Sarcophaga argyrostoma*. *Case Reports in Ophthalmological Medicine, 2013*, 850865. https://doi.org/10.1155/2013/850865.

59. Gregory, A. R., Schatz, S., & Laubach, H. (2004). Ophthalmomyiasis caused by the sheep bot fly *Oestrus ovis* in northern Iraq. *Optometry and Vision Science, 81*(8), 586–590. https://doi.org/10.1097/01.opx.0000144791.82459.4f.

60. Gültekin, K., Babat, S. Ö., Polat, E., & Dirim Erdoğan, D. (2022). External ophthalmomyiasis cases in Şırnak. *Turkiye Parazitoloji Dergisi, 46*(3), 163–165. https://doi.org/10.4274/tpd.galenos.2022.24918.

61. Gupta, A. K., Patel, A. P., Nathwani, Y. P., Kyada, G. C., & Kikani, K. (2020). Unilateral acute conjunctivitis caused by *Oestrus ovis* larva: A rare case report from Western India. *Journal of Clinical Ophthalmology and Research, 8*(3), 117–119. https://doi.org/10.4103/jcor.jcor_63_20.

62. Gupta, P. C., Ram, J., Faisal, T. T., Agarwal, A., Khurana, S., & Prasad, A. (2018). Ocular myiasis. *Journal of Ophthalmic and Vision Research, 13*(3), 361–362. https://doi.org/10.4103/jovr.jovr_170_17.

63. Hakan, U., Akyol, İ., Veysel, M., Lokman, C., & Akkaş, Ö. (2014). *Oestrus ovis* (sheep bot fly), external ophthalmomyiasis: A case report (*Oestrus ovis* (sheep bot fly), Ophtalmomyiasis externa: A case report). *Muş Alparslan Üniversitesi Fen Bilimleri Dergisi, 2*, 231–235.

64. Hartmannová, L., Mach, R., Záruba, R., & Pavlovský, M. (2020). External ophthalmomyiasis caused by *Oestrus ovis* (a case report). *Česká a Slovenská Oftalmologie, 76*(3), 130–134.

65. Hazratian, T., Dolatkhah, A., Akbarzadeh, K., Khosravi, M., & Ghasemikhah, R. (2020). A review of human myiasis in Iran with an emphasis on reported cases. *Malaysian Journal of Medical and Health Sciences, 16*(1), 269–274.

66. Hira, P. R., Hajj, B., al-Ali, F., & Hall, M. J. (1993). Ophthalmomyiasis in Kuwait: First report of infections due to the larvae of *Oestrus ovis* before and after the Gulf conflict. *Journal of Tropical Medicine and Hygiene, 96*(4), 241–244.

67. Hope, F. W. (1840). On insects and their larvae occasionally found in the human body. *Transactions of the Royal Entomological Society of London, 2*, 256–271.

68. Hoyer, P., Williams, R. R., Lopez, M., & Cabada, M. M. (2016). Human nasal myiasis caused by *Oestrus ovis* in the Highlands of Cusco, Peru: Report of a case and review of the literature. *Case Reports in Infectious Diseases, 2016*, 2456735. https://doi.org/10.1155/2016/2456735.

69. Huynh, N., Dolan, B., Lee, S., Whitcher, J. P., & Stanley, J. (2005). Management of phaeniciatic ophthalmomyiasis externa. *British Journal of Ophthalmology, 89*(10), 1377–1378. https://doi.org/10.1136/bjo.2005.075937.

70. Ibáñez, N. A., Rodríguez, A. E. H., Ruiz, A. M. A., & Rodríguez, P. A. (2018). Miasis ocular: El misterio es microscópico. *Revista Clínica de Medicina de Familia, 11*(3), 166–168.

71. Ijaz, L., Rao, R. Q., Imran, A., Mazhar, U., & Zaman, S. (2008). Ocular myiasis. *Pakistan Journal of Ophthalmology, 24*(3), 151–153.

72. Istek, Ş. (2014). Ophthalmomyiasis externa from Hakkari, the southeast border of Turkey. *BMJ Case Reports, 2014*, bcr2013201226. https://doi.org/10.1136/bcr-2013-201226.

73. Jenkins, K. S., & Layton, C. J. (2018). External ophthalmomyiasis caused by *Oestrus ovis*. *Clinical and Experimental Ophthalmology, 46*(3), 300–301. https://doi.org/10.1111/ceo.13116.

74. Jenzeri, S., Ammari, W., Attia, S., Zaouali, S., Babba, H., Messaoud, R., & Khairallah, M. (2009). External ophthalmomyiasis manifesting with keratouveitis. *International Ophthalmology, 29*(6), 533–535. https://doi.org/10.1007/s10792-009-9305-5.

75. Jiang, Y., Rengan, A., Matz, J., & Krakauer, M. (2020). Concurrent ophthalmomyiasis externa and aural myiasis: A case report in an urban hospital in the United States. *American Journal of Ophthalmology Case Reports, 17*, 100590. https://doi.org/10.1016/j.ajoc.2019.100590.

76. Jordan, V., & Mowatt, L. (2019). Ophthalmomyiasis externa due to sheep nasal botfly in rural Jamaica. *Tropical Doctor, 49*(1), 48–49. https://doi.org/10.1177/0049475518816820.

77. Joshi, K., Sindal, D. K., Pawar, V., & Pawar, S. (2013). Uniocular external ophthalmomyiasis due to *Oestrus ovis*: Two cases on two consecutive days. *International Journal of Recent Trends in Science and Technology, 7*(2), 89–90.

78. Kalezić, T., Stojković, M., Vuković, I., Spasić, R., Andjelković, M., Stanojlović, S., & Džamić, A. (2014). Human external ophthalmomyiasis caused by *Lucilia sericata* Meigen (Diptera: Calliphoridae)—A green bottle fly. *Journal of Infection in Developing Countries, 8*(7), 925–928. https://doi.org/10.3855/jidc.3860.

79. Kemmanu, V., Mahendradas, P., D'Souza, P. E., Yadav, N. K., & Shetty, B. (2009). Unilateral acute conjunctivitis due to ophthalmomyiasis externa caused by larva of *Oestrus ovis*. *Journal of Pediatric Ophthalmology and Strabismus, 46*(6), 380–381. https://doi.org/10.3928/01913913-20091117-12.

80. Keyt, F. T. (1900). A Case of "Beef Worm" (*Dermatobia Noxialis*) in the Orbit. *British Medical Journal, 1*, 316.

81. Khataminia, G., Aghajanzadeh, R., Vazirianzadeh, B., & Rahdar, M. (2011). Orbital myiasis. *Journal of Ophthalmic and Vision Research, 6*(3), 199–203.

82. Khurana, S., Biswal, M., Bhatti, H. S., Pandav, S. S., Gupta, A., Chatterjee, S. S., Lyngdoh, W. V., & Malla, N. (2010). Ophthalmomyiasis: Three cases from North India. *Indian Journal of Medical Microbiology, 28*(3), 257–261. https://doi.org/10.4103/0255-0857.66486.

83. Kuk, S., Yildirim, S., Ozden, M., Erensoy, A., & Saki, C. E. (2009). Ophthalmomyiasis is not only a problem for rural regions of Eastern Anatolia of Turkey. *Medical Science Monitor, 15*, CS166–CS168. https://doi.org/10.12659/msm.883647.

84. Kunduracı, M. S., Kutlutürk, I., Tanındı Duman, G., & Polat, E. (2020). Ophthalmomyiasis externa: A case report. *Turkiye Parazitoloji Dergisi, 44*(4), 261–263. https://doi.org/10.4274/tpd.galenos.2020.87035.

85. Kuria, S. K., & Oyedeji, A. O. (2020). Human myiasis cases originating and reported in Africa for the last two decades (1998–2018): A review. *Acta Tropica, 210*, 105590. https://doi.org/10.1016/j.actatropica.2020.105590.

86. Levett, P. N., Brooker, L., Reifer, C., Prussia, P. R., & Eberhard, M. L. (2004). Human external ophthalmomyiasis occurring in Barbados. *West Indian Medical Journal, 53*(3), 198–200.

87. Maharjan, N., Jamarkattel, A., & Prasad, B. N. (2021). External ophthalmomyiasis by *Oestrus ovis*: Two case reports from Nepal. *Journal of Lumbini Medical College, 9*(1), 4.

88. Mamani-Quispe, P., & Moreno-Loaiza, O. (2019). Oftalmomiasis por *Oestrus ovis* en un área urbana al sur del Perú [*Oestrus ovis* ophthalmomyiasis at an urban area in Southern Peru]. *Revista Chilena de Infectología, 36*(3), 384–386. https://doi.org/10.4067/s0716-10182019000300384.

89. Manimegalai, K. (2010). Studies on the mosquito populations from Coimbatore, Tamil Nadu, India. *Journal of Threatened Taxa, 2*(8), 961–969. https://doi.org/10.11609/jott.o2380.961-9.

90. Martínez-Rojano, H., Huerta, H., Hernández-Triana, L. M., Ruiz Pérez, E. F., & Sámano, R. (2020). Nosocomial myiasis caused by *Lucilia sericata* (Diptera: Calliphoridae) in a

pediatric patient in Mexico. *Case Reports in Infectious Diseases, 2020*, 1285459. https://doi.org/10.1155/2020/1285459.

91. Martínez-Rojano, H., Noguez, J. C., & Huerta, H. (2018). Nosocomial myiasis caused by *Lucilia sericata* (Diptera: Calliphoridae) and neonatal myiasis by *Sarcophaga* spp. (Diptera: Sarcophagidae) in Mexico. *Case Reports in Infectious Diseases, 2018*, 5067569. https://doi.org/10.1155/2018/5067569.
92. Masoudi, M., & Hosseini, K. (2004). External ophthalmomyiasis caused by sheep botfly (*Oestrus ovis*) larva: A report of 8 cases. *Archives of Iranian Medicine, 7*(2), 136–139.
93. Mishra, A. V., Gjerde, H., Mailman, T., & Archibald, C. (2020). Ocular myiasis secondary to *Dermatobia hominis*. *Canadian Journal of Ophthalmology, 55*, e139–e140. https://doi.org/10.1016/j.jcjo.2020.04.006.
94. Misra, S., Misra, N., & Reddy, B. (2008). External ophthalmomyiasis by *Oestrus ovis*: An unknown endemic eye disease in rural parts of Central India. *Tropical Doctor, 38*(2), 120–122. https://doi.org/10.1258/td.2007.060231.
95. Miura, M., Hayasaka, S., Yamada, T., Hayasaka, Y., & Kamimura, K. (2005). Ophthalmomyiasis caused by larvae of *Boettcherisca Peregrina*. *Japanese Journal of Ophthalmology, 49*(2), 177–179. https://doi.org/10.1007/s10384-004-0163-4.
96. Murga, H. (2014). Caso de miasis ocular por presencia de larvas de *Oestrus ovis* en paciente humano. *Revista Tecnología Ciencia Salud, 1*, 11–15.
97. Naimer, S. A. (2015). Images in emergency medicine. Man, with pain in left eye. Ophthalmomyiasis from the sheep nasal bot fly, *Oestrus ovis*. *Annals of Emergency Medicine, 65*(6), e7–e8. https://doi.org/10.1016/j.annemergmed.2015.01.020.
98. Naimer, S. A., & Mumcuoglu, K. Y. (2014). Diagnosis of ophthalmomyiasis externa by dermatoscopy. *Dermatology Practical & Conceptual, 4*(2), 85–87. https://doi.org/10.5826/dpc.0402a17.
99. Narayanan, S., & Jayaprakash, K. (1991). Incidence of ocular myiasis due to infection with the larva of *Oestrus ovis* (Oestridae Diptera). *Indian Journal of Ophthalmology, 39*(4), 176–178.
100. Naujokaitis, T., Khoramnia, R., Auffarth, G. U., & Augustin, V. A. (2022). Entlarvt: In Deutschland erworbene ophthalmomyiasis externa. *Ophthalmologie, 120*(1), 76–78.
101. Nene, A. S., Mishra, A., & Dhand, P. (2015). Ocular myiasis caused by *Chrysomya bezziana*—A case report. *Clinical Ophthalmology, 9*, 423–427. https://doi.org/10.2147/opth.s74218.
102. Norouzi, R., Manochehri, A., & Zarrin, S. (2017). External Ophthalmomyiasis Caused by *Lucilia sericata* (Diptera: Calliphoridae) Larva. *Iranian Journal of Parasitology, 12*(3), 466–469.
103. Otranto, D., Traversa, D., & Giangaspero, A. (2004). Le miasi da Oestridae: Diagnosi sierologica e molecolare [Myiasis caused by Oestridae: Serological and molecular diagnosis]. *Parassitologia, 46*(2), 169–172.
104. Özyol, P., Özyol, E., & Sankur, F. (2016). External ophthalmomyiasis: A case series and review of ophthalmomyiasis in Turkey. *International Ophthalmology, 36*(6), 887–891. https://doi.org/10.1007/s10792-016-0255-3.
105. Pal, N., & Majhi, B. (2016). Unilateral conjunctivitis of unique etiology: A case report from Eastern India. *Journal of Natural Science, Biology, and Medicine, 7*(1), 104–106. https://doi.org/10.4103/0976-9668.175030.

106. Panadero-Fontán, R., & Otranto, D. (2015). Arthropods affecting the human eye. *Veterinary Parasitology, 208*(1, 2), 84–93. https://doi.org/10.1016/j.vetpar.2014.12.006.

107. Pandey, A., Madan, M., Asthana, A. K., Das, A., Kumar, S., & Jain, K. (2009). External ophthalmomyiasis caused by *Oestrus ovis*: A rare case report from India. *Korean Journal of Parasitology, 47*(1), 57–59. https://doi.org/10.3347/kjp.2009.47.1.57.

108. Parikh, V., Biswas, J., Vaijayanthi, K., Das, D., & Raval, V. (2011). Bilateral ocular myiasis interna caused by botfly (*Oestrus ovis*): A case report. *Ocular Immunology and Inflammation, 19*(6), 444–447. https://doi.org/10.3109/09273948.2011.618303.

109. Parola, P., Socolovschi, C., Jeanjean, L., Bitam, I., Fournier, P. E., Sotto, A., Labauge, P., & Raoult, D. (2008). Warmer weather linked to tick attack and emergence of severe rickettsioses. *PLOS Neglected Tropical Diseases, 2*(11), e338. https://doi.org/10.1371/journal.pntd.0000338.

110. Pather, S., Botha, L. M., Hale, M. J., & Jena-Stuart, S. (2013). Ophthalmomyiasis externa: Case report of the clinicopathologic features. *International Journal of Ophthalmic Pathology, 2*(1).

111. Price, K. M., Murchison, A. P., Bernardino, C. R., Kang, S. J., & Grossniklaus, H. E. (2007). Ophthalmomyiasis externa caused by *Dermatobia hominis* in Florida. *British Journal of Ophthalmology, 91*(5), 695. https://doi.org/10.1136/bjo.2006.105460.

112. Pupić-Bakrač, A., Pupić-Bakrač, J., Škara Kolega, M., & Beck, R. (2020). Human ophthalmomyiasis caused by *Oestrus ovis*-first report from Croatia and review on cases from Mediterranean countries. *Parasitology Research, 119*(2), 783–793. https://doi.org/10.1007/s00436-019-06513-6.

113. Raina, U. K., Gupta, M., Kumar, V., Ghosh, B., Sood, R., & Bodh, S. A. (2009). Orbital myiasis in a case of invasive basal cell carcinoma. *Oman Journal of Ophthalmology, 2*(1), 41–42.

114. Ramírez-Miranda, A., González-Gomar, A., & Muñoz-Salas, S. (2011). External ophthalmomyiasis due to sheep botfly *Oestrus ovis* Larvae. *Vision Pan-America, 10*, 58–59.

115. Ranjan, R., & Jain, A. (2014). External ophthalmomyiasis. *Oman Journal of Ophthalmology, 7*(3), 160. https://doi.org/10.4103/0974-620X.142594.

116. Rao, S., Radhakrishnasetty, N., Chadalavada, H., & Hiremath, C. (2018). External ophthalmomyiasis by *Oestrus ovis*: A case report from Davangere. *Journal of Laboratory Physicians, 10*(1), 116–117. https://doi.org/10.4103/JLP.JLP_156_17.

117. Richard, Y., Castel, T., Bois, B., Cuccia, C., Marteau, R., Rossi, A., Thévenin, D., & Toussaint, H. (2014). Évolution des températures observées en Bourgogne (1961–2011) [Evolution of observed temperatures in Burgundy (1961–2011)]. *Bourgogne Nature, 19*, 110–117.

118. Rivasi, F., Campi, L., Cavallini, G. M., & Pampiglione, S. (2009). External ophthalmomyiasis by *Oestrus ovis* larvae diagnosed in a Papanicolaou-stained conjunctival smear. *Cytopathology, 20*(5), 340–342. https://doi.org/10.1111/j.1365-2303.2008.00589.x.

119. Rizvi, S. W., Akram, S. M., Ashraf, H., & Siddiqui, M. A. (2016). Extreme Ophthalmomyiasis externa with simultaneous facial and scalp involvement. *Nepal Journal of Ophthalmology, 8*(1), 95–96. https://doi.org/10.3126/nepjoph.v8i1.15001.

120. Sante Fernández, L., Hernández-Porto, M., Tinguaro, V., & Lecuona Fernández, M. (2017). Ophthalmomyiasis and nasal myiasis by *Oestrus ovis* in a patient from the Canary Islands with uncommon epidemiological characteristics. *Enfermedades Infecciosas y Microbiología Clínica, 35*(8), 461–462. https://doi.org/10.1016/j.eimc.2016.07.004.

121. Sen, M., Das, D., Sharma, M., Mittal, V., & Rahul, S. (2017). External ophthalmomyiasis: Case reports of two cases associated with agrarian practices. *Journal of Bacteriology & Mycology, 5*(2), 356–358.

122. Sen, P., Mohan, A., Jain, S., Shah, C., & Jain, E. (2020). External ophthalmomyiasis in a neonate masquerading as an orbital cellulitis. *Indian Journal of Ophthalmology, 68*(5), 900, 901. https://doi.org/10.4103/ijo.ijo_1444_19.

123. Serra Moltó, A., Molina Martín, J. C., Mengual Verdú, E., & Hueso Abancens, J. R. (2018). External ophthalmomyiasis due to Dermatobia hominis. A case report. *Archivos de la Sociedad Española de Oftalmología, 93*, 402–405.

124. Sevgili, M., Saki, C. E., & Ozkutlu, Z. (2004). External myiasis in the Sanliurfa province: The distribution of flies. *Acta Parasitologica Turcica, 28*, 150–153.

125. Shankar, M. K., Diddapur, S. K., Nadagir, S. D., & Kota, S. G. (2012). Ophthalmomyiasis externa caused by *Oestrus ovis*. *Journal of Laboratory Physicians, 4*, 43, 44.

126. Sharma, K. (2018). Ophthalmomyiasis externa: A case report from Alkharj, Saudi Arabia. *Saudi Journal of Ophthalmology*, 32, 250–252.

127. Sigauke, E., Beebe, W. E., Gander, R. M., Cavuoti, D., & Southern, P. M. (2003). Case report: Ophthalmomyiasis externa in Dallas County, Texas. *American Journal of Tropical Medicine and Hygiene, 68*, 46–47.

128. Singh, A., & Singh, Z. (2015). Incidence of myiasis among humans—A review. *Parasitology Research, 114*, 3183–3199.

129. Singh, A., Rajwadkar, V., & Aggarwal, I. (2022). External ophthalmomyiasis due to *Oestrus ovis* a rare case series. *Ophthalmology Journal, 7*, 51–54.

130. Singh, P. K., Prakash, P., Singh, S., Singh, M., Shekhawat, S. S., Vyas, C., & Bhargav, G. (2012). Ophthalmomyiasis externa caused by Muscae fly larva in deserts of the Thar. *Ocular Immunology and Inflammation, 20*, 145–147.

131. Smillie, I., Gubbi, P. K., & Cocks, H. C. (2010). Nasal and ophthalmomyiasis: Case report. *Journal of Laryngology and Otology, 124*, 934–935.

132. Solomon, M., Lachish, T., & Schwartz, E. (2016). Cutaneous myiasis. *Current Infectious Disease Reports, 18*, 28.

133. Sreejith, R. S., Reddy, A. K., Ganeshpuri, S. S., & Garg, P. (2010). *Oestrus ovis* ophthalmomyiasis with keratitis. *Indian Journal of Medical Microbiology, 28*, 399–402.

134. Stacey, M. J., & Blanch, R. J. (2008). A case of external ophthalmomyiasis in a deployed U.K. soldier. *Journal of the Royal Army Medical Corps, 154*, 60–62.

135. Sucilathangam, G., Meenakshisundaram, A., Hariramasubramanian, S., Anandhi, D., Palaniappan, N., & Anna, T. (2013). External ophthalmomyiasis which was caused by sheep botfly (*Oestrus ovis*) larva: a report of 10 cases. *Journal of Clinical and Diagnostic Research, 7*, 539–542.

136. Sudhir, S., Shweta, R. S., Umar, F., Shewtank, G., & Imran, A. (2018). Ophthalmomyiasis externa: Two cases identified in a tertiary care center, North India. *JOJ Case Studies, 8*, 555744.

137. Sundu, C., Dinç, E., Kurtuluş, U. C., & Yıldırım, Ö. (2015). Ophthalmomyiasis externa: A report of three cases. *Turkish Journal of Ophthalmology, 45*, 220–222.

138. Tabuenca-Del Barrio, L., Mozo-Cuadrado, M., Zubicoa-Eneriz, A., & Plaza-Ramos, P. (2018). Ocular external myiasis. A series of cases due to larvae *Oestrus ovis* in Navarra, Spain. *Archivos de la Sociedad Española de Oftalmología, 93*, 567–570.

139. Tamponi, C., Pasini, C., Ahmed, F., Dessì, G., Contu, E., Porcu, F., & Scala, A. (2022). External ophthalmomyiasis by *Oestrus ovis* in tourists visiting Italy. Report of three cases and a literature review. *Travel Medicine and Infectious Disease, 46*, 102279.

140. Taormina, Y. A., Gannon, C., Nguyen, J., Rhodes, J., Foxworth, M., Koch, W., & Dodson, K. (2013). Cuterebral ophthalmomyiasis externa presenting as preseptal cellulitis. *Eplasty*, 13, ic40.

141. Taylor, M. A. (2012). Emerging parasitic diseases of sheep. *Veterinary Parasitology, 189*, 2–7.

142. Thabit, A. M., Ayman, S. M., & Mohammad, Y. H. (2008). Ophthalmomyiasis externa in Jordan. *Journal of the Royal Medical Services, 15*, 35–40.

143. Thakur, K., Singh, G., Chuahan, S., & Sood, A. (2009). Vidi, vini, vinci: External ophthalmomyiasis infection that occurred, and was diagnosed and treated in a single day: A rare case report. *Oman Journal of Ophthalmology, 2*, 130–132.

144. Tomy, R. M., & Prabhu, P. B. (2013). Ophthalmomyiasis externa by *Musca domestica* in a case of orbital metastasis. *Indian Journal of Ophthalmology, 61*, 671–673.

145. Usta, G., Karslioglu, M. Z., & Adanir, R. (2015). Differential diagnosis and proper approach for ophthalmomyiasis externa: An experience of 12 patients. *European Research Journal, 1*, 50–54.

146. Velev, V., & Mikov, O. (2018). Ophthalmomyiasis caused by larvae of the parasite *Oestrus ovis*. *QJM: An International Journal of Medicine, 111*, 727–728.

147. Verma, S., & Gupta, S. (2012). Ocular manifestations due to *Paederus sabaeus* (*econda*). *Medical Journal Armed Forces India, 68*, 245–248.

148. Verstrynge, K., & Foets, B. (2004). External ophthalmomyiasis: A case report. *Bulletin de la Société Belge d'Ophtalmologie, 294*, 67–71.

149. Vijayalekshmi, S., & Shukla, H. (2013). Unilateral acute conjunctivitis due to *Oestrus ovis* in a veterinary doctor. *Journal of Natural Science, Biology, and Medicine, 4*, 228–230.

150. Villeda, S., Rodríguez, M. E., & Bonilla, C. E. (2017). External ophthalmomyiasis in pediatrics: Case report. *Archives of Medicine, 13*, 6.

151. Vogt, R., Holzmann, T., & Jägle, H. (2015). Ophthalmomyiasis externa [Ophthalmomyiasis externa]. *Der Ophthalmologe, 112*, 61–63.

152. Wakamatsu, T. H., & Pierre-Filho, P. T. (2006). Ophthalmomyiasis externa caused by *Dermatobia hominis*: A successful treatment with oral ivermectin. *Eye, 20*, 1088–1090.

153. Weinand, F. S., & Bauer, C. (2001). Autochthon in deutschland erworbene ophthalmomyiasis externa: Kasuistik und Literaturübersicht [Ophthalmomyiasis externa acquired in Germany: Case report and review of the literature]. *Ophthalmologica, 215*, 383–386. (In German)

154. Yar, K., Özcan, A. A., & Koltaş, İ. S. (2011). Oftalmomiyazis eksterna: Olgu sunumları [External ophthalmomyiasis: Case reports]. *Türkiye Parazitoloji Dergisi, 35*, 224–226.

155. Zammarchi, L., Giorni, A., Gabrielli, S., Strohmeyer, M., Cancrini, G., & Bartoloni, A. (2014). Human oestriasis acquired in florence and review on human myiasis in Italy. *Parasitology Research, 113*, 2379–2385.

156. Zayani, A., Chaabouni, M., Gouiaa, R., Ben Hadj Hamida, F., & Fki, J. (1989). Myiases conjonctivales. A propos de 23 cas dans le Sahel tunisien [Conjunctival myiasis. 23 cases in the Tunisian Sahel]. *Archives de l'Institut Pasteur de Tunis, 66*, 289–292. (In French)

157. Zhang, A., Nie, Q., & Song, J. (2018). External ophthalmomyiasis caused by *Oestrus ovis* in east China. *Tropical Doctor, 48*, 169–171. https://doi.org/10.1177/0049475518766206.

158. Zhou, X., Kambalame, D. M., Zhou, S., Guo, X., Xia, D., Yang, Y., & Yuen, M. (2019). Human *Chrysomya bezziana* myiasis: A systematic review. *PLoS Neglected Tropical Diseases, 13*(12), e0007391. https://doi.org/10.1371/journal.pntd.0007391.

Chapter

3

ENHANCING COMMUNITY AND PUBLIC HEALTH THROUGH NUTRITIONAL STRATEGIES

Contents

Introduction

Public Health Nutrition (PHN) is a specialized field that focuses on the intersection of community health and nutrition, aiming to apply the principles of nutrition science to improve the well-being of populations. This area of study and practice encompasses a broad range of activities designed to enhance the health status of communities through dietary interventions, policy implementation, and research initiatives. PHN professionals work to address nutritional issues at the population level, promoting healthy eating habits, preventing nutrition-related diseases, and ensuring equitable access to nutritious food.

An example of PHN in action is the development and implementation of programs aimed at increasing vaccination rates to prevent the spread of infectious diseases. Public health authorities might coordinate mass vaccination campaigns, utilizing media outlets to raise awareness and educate the community about the importance of immunization. Similarly, PHN initiatives often involve promoting public awareness about the benefits of good nutrition and the availability of health services, which might include organizing community health fairs or distributing educational materials on healthy eating. PHN also plays a critical role in ensuring food security and access to health services for all community members, particularly vulnerable populations such as children and pregnant women. Programs like school meal initiatives or maternal nutrition programs are examples of how PHN can support the nutritional needs of specific groups, thereby contributing to the overall health and resilience of the community.

Furthermore, PHN practitioners are involved in emergency preparedness, planning for and responding to health crises such as natural disasters, pandemics, or bioterrorism threats. This might involve setting up emergency nutrition assistance programs or coordinating with other agencies to ensure the continuation of essential health and nutrition services during crises.

Inspection and regulation of public facilities, including restaurants, public pools, and healthcare institutions, are other critical components of PHN. These activities help to maintain high standards of hygiene and safety, preventing the outbreak of foodborne illnesses and other health hazards.

At its core, PHN aims to create environments that support healthy lifestyles and choices. Through initiatives like nutrition education programs, individuals and families are empowered to make informed food choices, leading to improved health outcomes. For instance, teaching people to incorporate more fruits, vegetables, and whole grains into their diets can have a profound impact on public health by reducing the prevalence of obesity and chronic diseases.

Nutrition assistance programs are another key element of PHN, providing access to healthy foods for those in need. These programs can be particularly effective when combined with policy changes, such as requiring the availability of healthy food options in workplace cafeterias or improving the infrastructure to support physical activity in communities.

PHN is a multifaceted field that leverages the collective knowledge of nutrition, public health policy, and community engagement to foster environments where healthy choices are accessible and encouraged, ultimately aiming to improve the nutritional status and health of entire populations. This chapter focuses on the critical role nutrition plays in the overall health and well-being of populations. It explores the interplay between nutrition and public health issues, highlighting how dietary habits influence the prevalence of chronic diseases.

Orientation and Directional Terms

Term	Definition	Illustration
Public Health	The science and practice of protecting and improving the health of communities through education, policy making, and research for disease and injury prevention.	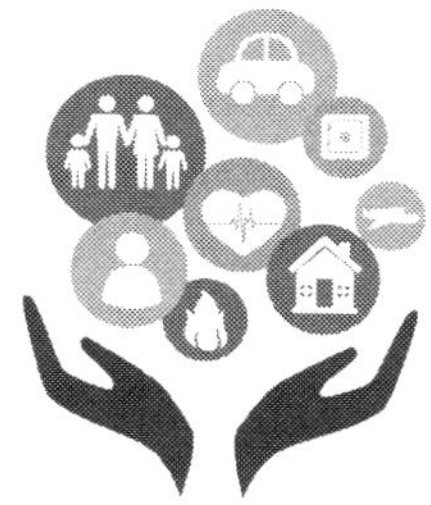
Nutritional Epidemiology	The study of the relationship between dietary intake and the incidence, distribution, and control of diseases within populations.	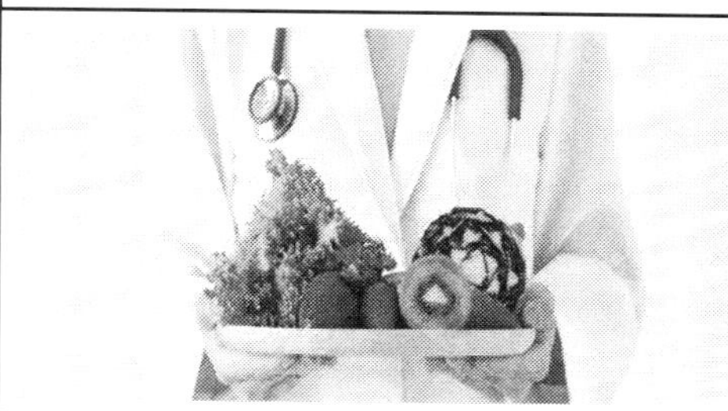
Public Health Workforce	The group of professionals involved in the practice of public health, including roles in epidemiology, health education, health promotion, and policy development.	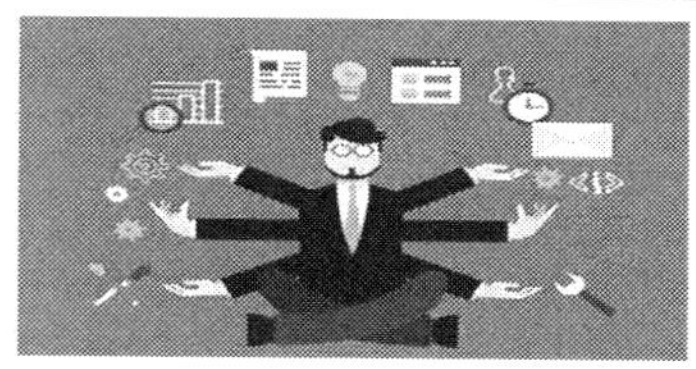
Non-Communicable Diseases	Diseases that are not caused by infectious agents and are generally long-lasting, such as heart disease, stroke, cancer, and diabetes.	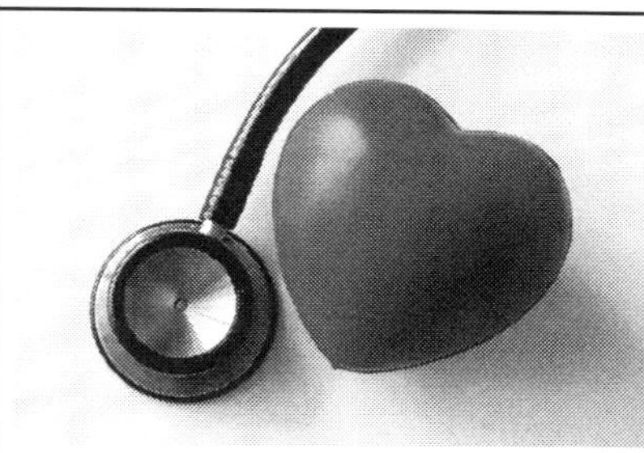

3.1. Public Health Concept

Public health involves many issues and fields, all of which deal with maintaining and promoting global health and healthcare for a community. Part of public health efforts may involve educational lectures and distributing information. Providing knowledge of preventable causes of death to citizens is a fundamental aspect as well (Figure 3.1).

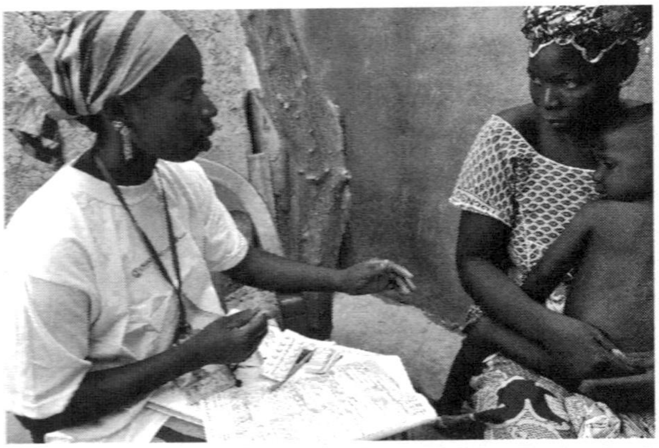

Figure 3.1. *Demonstration of public health.*

Source: By President's Malaria Initiative – Community Health Worker treats child, Public Domain, https://commons.wikimedia.org/w/index.php?curid=72085321.

Regarding the spread of infectious diseases within a community, public health authorities initiate efforts to prevent outbreaks. This might mean making adequate vaccinations available to immunize the public against the disease. Bringing about public awareness through press conferences and local news is another means.

Promoting good health by helping to ensure all citizens have access to nutritional food and medical care is another integral role of the healthcare system. By receiving proper nutrition and medical care, the public can safeguard against illness by strengthening immunity. Such programs may include pediatric nutritional support and prenatal care.

A career in public health may involve jobs in a variety of fields. Jobs may be available in environmental health. Environmental health experts may do water testing to ensure safety for the public, as well as food safety testing and regulation. Working in a laboratory or teaching in a classroom are other common health-related careers.

National and international health agencies have workers from various nations across the world. Their goals are generally to strengthen and improve public health strategies and form new enterprises.

Public health officials often hold special events to help raise awareness and funds for various projects. Grants that are provided by other organizations and corporations may be used for various projects. Conferences to discuss environmental issues and technological advances are another way to bring about awareness and initiate action.

Many communities in the United States have local public health agencies that administer state- and federally-funded health programs. One such program is the Women, Infants and Children (WIC) Program. Nursing services and dental clinics for children are among others.

The public health system must also be prepared for health-related emergencies. This may include natural disasters, man-made dangers, or chemical warfare. Being prepared for the threat of bioterrorism is a top priority.

One other responsibility of health departments is to inspect public facilities to ensure they maintain proper safety standards. These safety and health inspectors inspect public housing, shelters, nursing homes, and hospitals to name a few. Restaurants and public swimming pools are other public places that must be inspected regularly as well.

3.1.1. The Narrow Approach

The narrow approach focuses on disease prevention and cost containment, with health defined as the absence of disease. The underlying theory is that the way in which individuals live their lives (what they eat. what they do. whether they smoke or drink or engage in risky behavior) is the main cause of disease, and that the motivation to change behavior is based on reducing risk at an individual level. The evidence base comes from clinical and molecular epidemiology: research is undertaken that identifies differences in risk factors, and based on that information, advice is given to the public that if they change their behavior they will reduce their risk of developing the disease (cancer or heart disease, etc.). This approach links an individual's own behavior to the risk of disease. The burden of prevention and health promotion lies with the individual and it is seen as their responsibility to address their risk behavior. The approach is aimed at identifying immediate and obvious problems and addressing them now. The disadvantage of the narrow approach is that it may miss fundamental threats within society that may be outside the individual's control (basic and underlying causes such as the wider socioeconomic factors, education and access to services. environmental factors, and the overarching values in society).

3.1.2. The Broad Approach

The broad approach defines health as more than the absence of disease (Smith, 2001). It considers well-being in terms of mental and physical health and also includes a sense of having some control over your life. The approach links public health science with policy: the action and structures agreed by society aimed at improving and maintaining health (Jones et al., 2005). The underlying theoretical model is sociocultural: it focuses on the wider environment and seeks to understand the factors that enable individuals to make healthy choices, or inhibit them (Brown, 2008). The motivating concern is about addressing the underlying socio-structural factors such as poverty, global issues and structures at a local, regional, national and international level that affect health (Black et al., 2010). The evidence base for a broad approach comes from epidemiology as well as other approaches more suitable to exploring the socio-structural context (White, 2013). The broad approach takes a more long-term view of causes and solutions, addressing structural issues in society that make it more difficult for individuals to make optimal choices. The disadvantage of a broad approach is that because the approach is so broad it may never address the key rate limiting steps in a timely manner (Green, 2015).

The broad public health approach has been taken up and developed by UNICEF into a conceptual model. The UNICEF model is now widely used, at least in research and development in developing countries (UNICEF, 2010). This conceptual model acknowledges that while the immediate causes of undemubition may be a lack of food often coupled with a high burden of infection, the provision of adequate education and healthcare has an important impact on health. The provision of these underlying factors is determined by basic causes such as the resources that are available in a society, and decisions about how these resources will be used. The model acknowledges that dealing only with the immediate causes will never lead to long-term improvements, which are dependent on the societal view as to how resources will be used and distributed in society to maximize the health and wellbeing of all members of society (UNICEF, 2010).

These arguments do not apply only to developing countries; how governments prioritize the use of taxation is a function of the underlying values of the society (as expressed through the election of governments that reflect the popular view): for example, the balance of spending priorities between education, health and defense, or priorities for agricultural policies that subsidize farmers but not manufacturing industry. Policy decisions as to the priorities on spending are complex and reflect a balance of tensions and pressures that often pull in different directions. Policy will be discussed in more detail later in this chapter. In reality, in most countries there is a recognition that a narrow (individual and immediate cause-oriented) approach needs to be balanced with addressing, at least to some extent, the basic and underlying (broad) causes.

Most governments acknowledge that there are differences in health outcomes in different sectors of society and that state resources should be used to try to redress these differences. The food supply is regulated in all countries, even if the regulation is restricted to issues of food safety. Many of the first efforts in public health were about developing regulations to protect the public against the adulteration of staple foods. It has always been recognized that freedom of choice does not operate in a vacuum. Many countries have regulations about the accuracy of information contained in labels. There are few countries where the government does not intervene in the food supply to some extent, either through legislation to recommend the fortification of foods or to subsidize the production of some foods such as in the Common Agricultural Policy in Europe and fanning subsidies in the USA and elsewhere. In developing a public health perspective it is important to balance the narrow with the broad. Striking the right balance is difficult and influenced by philosophical and political considerations. As a public health nutritionist, when trying to solve a local or national problem, it is important that both the narrow and broader determinants of behavior are considered and that it is not assumed that knowledge and individual choice are all that matters. Recently the UK Faculty of Public Health has agreed on the key concepts that underpin public health. These reiterate to some extent the debate about broad versus narrow approaches to public health. The key issues are population approaches to promoting and protecting health and well-being. They also highlight the importance of information (UK Faculty of Public Health, 2019).

3.2. Aims of Public Health Nutrition

Public health nutritionists integrate the knowledge, skills, and experiences fundamental to all public health disciplines and apply this integrated knowledge to alleviate diet-related health problems among diverse population groups (Basiotis et al., 2000). Employment often includes health departments, federal and private food assistance programs, worksite health promotion programs, nutrition advocacy organizations, health centers, and schools (Basiotis et al., 2000). An understanding of human nutrition is important to maximize the health of individuals in a diverse society that faces nutrition-related diseases of both deficiency and excess (Krebs-Smith et al., 1997). A complete understanding of human nutrition is built on knowledge of its fundamental biological and biochemical bases (Krebs-Smith et al., 1997). It also involves an understanding of societal, psychological, cultural, and behavioral influences that affect food consumption, and therefore, human well-being (Story et al., 2008). Public health nutrition advances knowledge regarding the role of nutrition in disease prevention and health promotion and applies this knowledge to planning, managing, delivering, and evaluating nutrition services and programs (Story et al., 2008) (Figure 3.2).

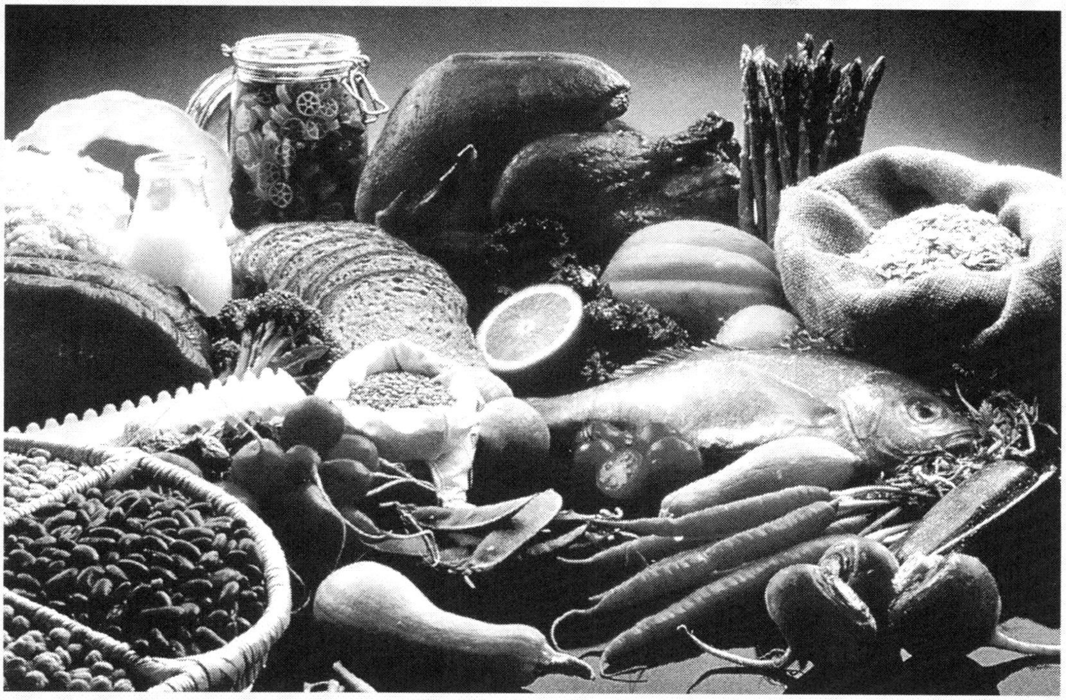

Figure 3.2. *Role of nutrition in public health.*

Source: By Unknown author – This image was released by the National Cancer Institute, an agency part of the National Institutes of Health, with the ID 2397 (image) (next)., Public Domain, https://commons.wikimedia.org/w/index.php?curid=10531946.

The MPH major in public health nutrition trains students to integrate the knowledge, skills, and experience fundamental to all public health disciplines and to apply this integrated knowledge to alleviate diet-related health problems among diverse population groups. The program is designed to train professionals to assume leadership positions in assessing community-nutrition needs and in planning, directing and evaluating the nutrition component of health-promotion and disease-prevention efforts. Graduates of the program will be expected to participate in policy analysis, and program development, and to design and manage population-based community-wide interventions as part of large-scale public health programs.

- Identify and assess diet-related health problems of under-nutrition and over-nutrition among diverse population groups
- Identify the social, cultural, economic, environmental and institutional factors that contribute to the risks of under-nutrition and over-nutrition among diverse populations
- Develop educational and other population-based intervention strategies to improve food security
- Develop policies to reduce barriers to food insecurity and to improve the food choices and nutritional status of diverse populations

- Describe techniques to guide consumers in the selection of food and nutritionally adequate diets
- Communicate nutrition-related issues skillfully, utilizing different media in varied settings
- Apply the principles of management to community nutrition programs
- Participate in advocacy efforts to improve the nutritional status of various populations
- Monitor and recommend public policies to protect and promote the nutritional status and health of diverse populations
- Contribute to the body of nutrition knowledge through active research of an applied nature

The Public Health Nutrition concentration trains individuals to promote health and reduce the risk of chronic diseases and obesity through educational and environmental approaches to improved nutrition and physical activity.

The goals of the Public Health Nutrition concentration are to prepare health and nutrition professionals to:

- Identify and assess diet-related health problems—of both undernutrition and overnutrition—among diverse population groups in the United States and internationally;
- Identify the social, cultural, economic, environmental, and institutional factors that contribute to the risk of undernutrition and overnutrition among populations;
- Demonstrate the linkages between agriculture, food, nutrition, and public health;
- Develop educational, institutional, and other population-based intervention strategies to improve food security and reduce obesity;
- Develop policies to reduce barriers to food insecurity and to improve the food and activity choices and nutritional status of diverse population groups;
- Promote policies to ensure the safe production, distribution, and consumption of food;
- Develop effective strategies for advocating for improved nutrition and physical activity among diverse population groups; and
- Apply population-based research findings to the development and implementation of nutrition policies and programs in the United States and internationally.

Public health nutrition is about applying knowledge to the solution of nutrition-related health problems (Smith, 2005). Often when confronted with a problem, people do not know where to start, become lost in the details, and sometimes miss the obvious and simple critical steps that will really make a difference (Jones et al., 2010).

If nutrition is only thought of as the supply side of this balance, this is likely to lead to a misunderstanding of the key rate-limiting steps that link good nutrition to wellbeing (Brown & Patel, 2013). It is also important to consider the social as well as the biological context within which individuals live and interact in society (Garcia et al., 2018).

While it is beyond the scope of this text to cover all aspects of whole-body integrated metabolism, some understanding of the underlying mechanisms that link diet and style of living to health is required to understand whether the lifestyle changes that are being suggested to improve health make sense biologically (White & Lee, 2016). Inevitably, good nutrition-related health is about understanding the relationships between the biological and sociological context within which individuals live and interact in society (Smith, 2005).

Where food supply is limited, there is a clear biological imperative to obtain enough to eat; where supply is in excess, social imperatives that restrain or limit behavior come into play (Brown & Patel, 2013). In all societies, especially those in transition, there is a complex mix of problems of overnutrition and undernutrition occurring in close proximity (Garcia et al., 2018). The job of the public health nutritionist is to try to understand this complexity and to provide guidance as to what is best for most people (Jones et al., 2010).

3.2.1. Primary Prevention

Primary prevention is concerned with preventing the onset of disease; it aims to reduce the incidence of disease. It involves interventions that are applied before there is any evidence of disease or injury. Examples include protection against the effects of a disease agent, as with vaccination. It can also include changes to behaviors such as cigarette smoking or diet. The strategy is to remove causative risk factors (risk reduction), which protects health and so overlaps with health promotion. Primary prevention may be aimed at individuals or at whole communities. Individual approaches (encouraging your patient to stop smoking) have the advantages that the clinician's personal contact should be motivational; the message can be tailored to the patient, and you can support him in actually deciding to stop. But the limitation is that your advice does not tackle the underlying forces driving his behavior in the first place or the context in which his behavior occurs (his friends may continue to smoke). Therefore, a community or population approach (e.g., via mass media advertising, increasing taxes, or banning smoking in public places) tries to change risk factors in the whole population. It is more radical and may produce cultural and contextual changes that may support individual efforts. Examples of primary prevention include smoking cessation, preserving good nutritional status, physical fitness, immunization, improving roads, or fluoridation of the water supply as a way to prevent dental caries. These are the roles of health promotion and public health. A successful primary prevention program requires that we know at least one modifiable risk factor, and have a way to modify it (Figure 3.3).

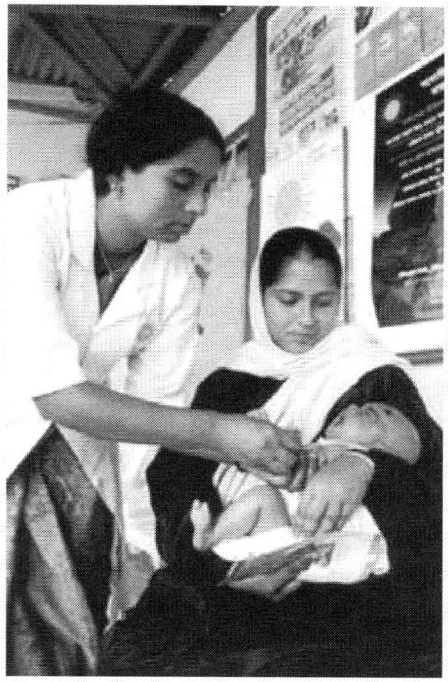

Figure 3.3. *Primary prevention helps people to avoid developing certain health problems.*

Source: Public Domain, https://commons.wikimedia.org/w/index.php?curid=1023.

Primary prevention refers to the actions people take that help them avoid developing certain health problems. These problems can include diseases, sicknesses, injuries or conditions that are not beneficial to the body.

These actions are the first type of preventive behaviors that are conducted before the problems occur. They not only save people from experiencing illnesses but help them to save time and money in health care. The aim of primary prevention is to reduce, control or eliminate the sources of work-related mental health problems. Thus, primary prevention strives to reduce the negative impacts of organizational risk factors on individuals. This type of intervention directly affects the work environment or work situation and, by that very fact, the organization as well as management and work practices. The following main prevention strategies are suggested:

Examples of Primary Prevention Strategies	
Hold Regular Team Meetings	Team meetings provide an opportunity for discussion and thus to improve relations between employees and with their superior. They are also an occasion to recognize the work accomplished and efforts made. In addition, they provide an opportunity to recall and clarify each person's roles and tasks, thus helping to reduce role conflicts and ambiguity.
Conduct an Annual Evaluation of Employees' Contribution	The evaluation of staff can be an occasion to clarify the roles, responsibilities and powers of each person, thus decreasing the risks of role conflicts. It is also an opportunity to clearly define different expectations and to establish precise goals and objectives that reflect these expectations, thus reducing the risk of confusion and ambiguity.
Encourage a Participative Management Style	The organization can decentralize the decision-making process and increase the level of participation of workers in decisions. This approach can have a positive impact on workers' sense of belonging to the organization.
Recognize Work Accomplished	The recognition of workers' and managers' accomplishments is an important way to foster a healthy psychological balance. This recognition must be shown daily through simple and meaningful gestures.
Include Workers in Planning Their Career Progress	The organization can provide workers with the tools to identify their strengths, weaknesses, interests and career goals. In this way, they will be better equipped to manage their career progress.
Establish Flexible Work Schedules	The organization can give workers more discretionary power over the management of their work time. This will make it easier for them to reconcile their personal life and work life.

Improve Physical Working Conditions	Wherever possible, the organization can reduce to a minimum noise and heat levels, assess lighting, number of workers in a given space, supplies and equipment used, etc. These factors influence the work climate and environment and can, as a consequence, increase the comfort of individuals and their work performance.

Before primary prevention is carried out, certain information about the person needs to be identified. Risk factors are the traits people possess or the behaviors they choose to practice that increase the chance of them getting a specific condition. Although there are some risk factors a person cannot control, such as their age, gender and family history, there are some behaviors they can control.

Let us first look at some risk factors that cannot be controlled:

- Older adults are at risk of breaking a hip bone when they fall.
- Men are at a higher risk of getting high blood pressure than women.
- Daughters of mothers with breast cancer are at risk of getting it too.

Now look at some examples of risk factors that can be controlled:

- Decreased physical activity contributes to the risk of childhood obesity
- Unprotected sex practices increase the risks of getting sexually transmitted diseases
- People who use tobacco products are at a higher risk of developing certain cancers

3.2.2. Nutritional Epidemiology

Nutritional epidemiology is one of the younger disciplines in epidemiology. This may be partially due to the difficulties in measuring diet as an exposure. Diet and physical activity are arguably the most difficult exposures to assess in observational research and are plagued by considerable measurement error. We all eat, we all eat many different foods, we tend to forget rather quickly what we ate, and we often do not know the ingredients of the dishes we consume. Hence we are all exposed, and the variation may be more subtle than with other, more distinct exposures such as smoking or use of hormone replacement therapy. Few people maintain extreme diets; thus assessing diets within fairly homogeneous populations makes it difficult to detect associations between dietary patterns (or particular foods and nutrients) and health or disease due to the lack of sufficient variation.

The quality and quantity of the food supply is a key determinant of human health and world development. Aspects of food production, safety testing and distribution are critically important to public health, international trade, and economic development. Guidelines for the food and nutrient consumption of individuals and groups are developed by various scientific bodies in various parts of the world, with myriad nutritional and international health and welfare policy implications. For example, in the United States, the Food and Nutrition Board of the National Academy of Sciences periodically conducts a nutrient by nutrient review of the literature to update such dietary reference indices as estimated average requirement, recommended daily allowances, adequate intake, and upper levels. Much of this work focuses on the intakes needed to avoid deficiency diseases, specific to age and sex, but there is also a developing emphasis on nutrient intakes that may reduce the risk of prominent chronic condition. More generally the topic of nutrient and food consumption patterns that may reduce chronic disease risk has been a substantial epidemiologic research focus for the past few decades, with selected cancers and cardiovascular diseases receiving the most attention. While diet and disease prevention hypotheses have often arisen from population comparisons or animal experimentation, the testing of hypotheses has almost uniformly centered on traditional epidemiologic case-control and cohort study designs. However, following a quarter century of extensive investigation rather few consistent diet and chronic disease associations have emerged from these studies, and associations that have emerged have tended not to be supported by randomized controlled intervention trials in the few instances where pertinent RCT's have been conducted. Hence, one is obliged to think that either the dietary elements or patterns that have been studied are not particularly important determinants of chronic disease risk, or that the study methods that are being employed may not be able to reliably identify important associations.

There are a number of reasons for thinking that diet and nutrition, presumably in conjunction with physical activity, may have a major role in determining the risks of a broad range of chronic diseases. For example:

- The pattern of consumption of macronutrients is related to establishing chronic disease risk factors.
    - Fat intake by degree of saturation relates strongly to blood cholesterol, a strong risk factor for coronary heart disease.
    - Energy consumption, and energy balance, relate to obesity and various aspects of body mass and shape, which in turn relate to the risk of many chronic diseases including prominent cancers, vascular diseases, diabetes and fractures.
- Controlled feeding experiments, mostly over the past 60 years, have revealed many strong diet and disease associations in inbred strains of laboratory animals.
    - Some of the most impressive observations have concerned the risk reduction that follows from energy restriction. However, both macronutrient distribution and micronutrient content of the diet can be important.
- International variations in disease rates and trends over time in national disease rates often correlate strongly with national dietary consumption patterns.
    - Good information is available on chronic disease rates for various populations worldwide. For example the Cancer Incidence in Five Continents series coordinated by the International Agency for Research on Cancer is comprehensive with good quality control. Many human cancers have tenfold or greater variations in incidence around the world, and cancer incidence patterns in many countries

Epidemiology is the study of the etiology of illness and related phenomena in human populations. Nutritional epidemiology, a branch of epidemiology, socks to unfold the causal relationship between aspects of the diet and occurrence of human illness. Historically, nutritional epidemiology was concerned mainly with nutritional deficiency diseases where a gross deficiency in a particular food or nutrient caused an untoward condition to occur. It was the observation that consumption of lemons and oranges prevented the occurrence of scurvy among sailors on British ships, and this has led to the discovery of vitamin C deficiency as a cause of scurvy. In recent years, the focus of nutritional epidemiology has shifted from nutritional deficiency syndromes to the dietary determinants of chronic diseases such as heart disease and cancer. The underlying premise in contemporary nutritional epidemiology is that a person's long-term habitual diet has an impact on the occurrence of chronic disease. However, because the etiology of chronic diseases is a great deal more complex than that of deficiency syndromes, this shill in focus has indeed presented immense challenges. Whereas the occurrence of a deficiency syndrome typically has a single cause (deficiency in a food or nutrient item), the risk of a chronic disease not only can be attributed to numerous causal factors, including genetic, environmental, personal lifestyle (e.g., smoking. drinking, physical exercise) as well as dietary, but also the factors exert varying effects with complex Interactions on disease occurrence (Figure 3.4).

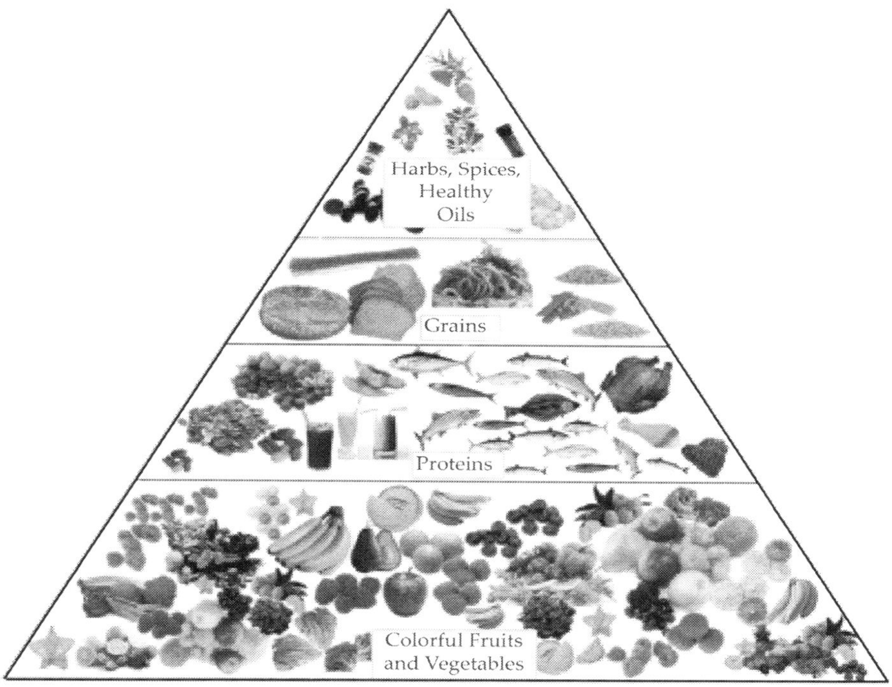

Figure 3.4. *An overview of nutritional epidemiology.*

Source: By Spmallare – Own work, CC BY 3.0, https://commons.wikimedia.org/w/index.php?curid=9953034.

Moreover, a person's diet is made up of a myriad of dietary components all of which tend to be correlated with each other, and some of which may increase the risk of disease while others may have a protective effect. Whereas a deficiency syndrome has a short latent period of exposure to a single cause (the time interval between onset of deficiency and onset of disease), many chronic diseases have latent periods of exposure that are protracted and ill-defined. Because humans are exposed to most dietary factors for their entire lives, there is no clear standard for comparison. Unlike a deficiency syndrome, where the exposure variable can be categorized as "not deficient" or "deficient," the degree of risk for a chronic disease attributed to most dietary factors varies on a continuum. Also choosing the most relevant time (person's age) at which to begin measuring diet relative to disease onset (the reference period) is difficult and subjective because the reference period is seldom known and may vary not only from one disease to another but also among persons. Additionally, diet can at any time affect the disease process, and its effects may vary over time. The greatest challenge of all which confronts the nutritional epidemiology of chronic diseases is how to measure accurately and precisely a person's long-term diet. Clearly, these factors make it difficult to attribute the occurrence of a chronic disease to any single food or nutrient item, and consequently, any observed relationship between a food or nutrient item and chronic disease must be interpreted with care and replicated in multiple studies. Notwithstanding, nutritional epidemiology has made important contributions to our knowledge regarding the influence of diet on the etiology of human diseases.

3.2.2.1. Hypothesis Development

Nutrition and chronic disease hypotheses have frequently been generated by animal experimentation or by the comparison of disease rates among populations having differing dietary habits. Another source of hypotheses is analytic epidemiologic studies themselves. For example, dietary assessment in a cohort study context typically leads to individual consumption estimates for a lengthy list of foods, and hence to consumption estimates for various nutrients through the use of nutrient databases that provide estimates of the nutrient content of foods. Hence a single cohort study can potentially examine a large number of food and nutrient associations with a large number of diseases, given sufficient size and study duration, potentially yielding many nutritional epidemiology leads.

Each of these study design and data sources has important limitations, even for hypothesis development. Animal experiments are excellent for motivating this research area, but the disease experience of inbred strains may have unclear relevance to human health, and the dietary contrasts that may be necessary to control experimental costs and logistics (e.g., 25–50% energy restriction) may not be practical for free living humans. On the other hand, pertinent animal models for a given dietary prevention hypothesis could yield much insight into mechanisms and hence contribute to hypothesis strengthening and refinement. Population comparisons and time trend analyzes, as they are typically conducted, suffer from a limited ability to control for both dietary and non-dietary confounding. The readily available nutrient and food supply (disappearance) data, even though objective, are rather crude. For example, these data are not age or sex-specific, and they are restricted to per capita averages which do not allow estimation of the consumption distribution of foods or nutrients within each population group. There is potential for migrant studies to contribute substantially to hypothesis identifications and development.

3.3. Public Health and Health Promotion

Health promotion is a behavioral social science that draws from the biological, environmental, psychological, physical and medical sciences to promote health and prevent disease, disability and premature death through education-driven voluntary behavior change activities. Health promotion is the development of individual, group, institutional, community and systemic strategies to improve health knowledge, attitudes, skills and behavior. The purpose of health promotion is to positively influence the health behavior of individuals and communities as well as the living and working conditions that influence their health (Figure 3.5).

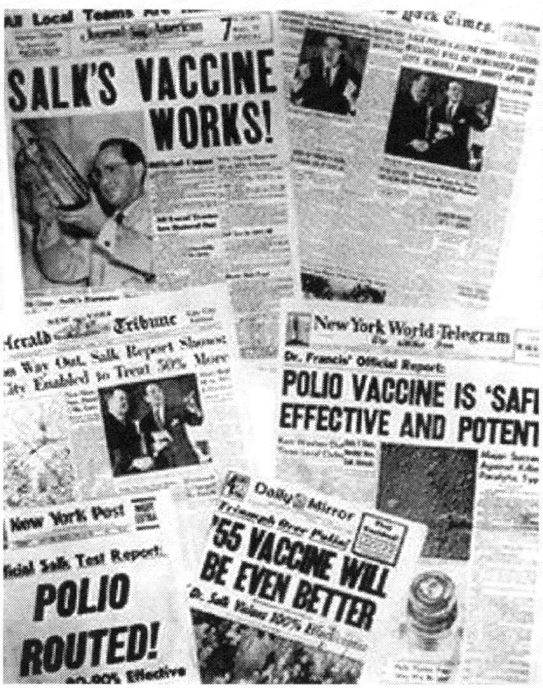
SALK'S VACCINE WORKS!
New York World-Telegram
POLIO VACCINE IS 'SAFI
EFFECTIVE AND POTENT
New York Post
POLIO ROUTED!
Daily Mirror
'55 VACCINE WILL BE EVEN BETTER

Figure 3.5. *Public health promotion activities.*

Source: By March of Dimes – March of Dimes, Public Domain, https://commons.wikimedia.org/w/index.php?curid=6204033.

Public health is defined as "the science and art of preventing disease prolonging life, and promoting health and efficiency through organized community efforts, so organizing these benefits as to enable every citizen to realize his/her birthright of health and longevity?" It has been viewed as the scientific diagnosis and treatment of the community. In this vision, the community, instead of the individual, is seen as the patient. When the focus is on the community, patterns and processes begin to emerge and combine to form a unified whole. Using this approach avoids focusing on risks and diseases; instead, the focus is on the community's strengths and resilience. Community strengths can be physiological, psychological, social, or spiritual. They include such factors as education, coping skills, support systems, knowledge, communication skills, nutrition, coherent belief systems, fitness, ability to develop a supportive environment, and self-care skills.' Increasing nutrition knowledge can reduce medical care costs and improve the quality of life. The negative consequences of nutrition related problems include malnutrition and chronic health conditions such as obesity, cardiovascular disease, cancer, and diabetes mellitus. In addition, these conditions contribute significantly to the world's burden of morbidity, incapacity, and mortality, despite the tremendous amount of biological knowledge accumulated over the years." The WHO estimated that prevention of the major nutrition-related risk factors (cigarette smoking, inactivity, poor dietary habits. and alcohol abuse) could translate into a gain of 5 years of disability-free life expectancy. A community and public health nutrition approach will make it possible to reverse the course of major nutrition problems." Dietetic professionals can take the lead in prevention programming because their training as counselors and educators provides skills that make them important members of the public health profession.

Public health nutrition was developed in the United States in response to societal events and changes in the following situations:

- Infant mortality
- Access to healthcare
- Epidemics of communicable disease
- Poor hygiene and sanitation
- Malnutrition
- Agriculture and food production (in response to changes in food production)
- Economic depression, wars, and civil rights
- Aging of the population
- Behavior-related problems/lifestyle (poor dietary practices. alcohol abuse, inactivity, and cigarette smoking)
- Chronic diseases (obesity, heart disease, diabetes mellitus, mental health, cancer, osteoporosis, and hypertension)
- Poverty and immigration
- Preschool/afterschool child care and school-based meals

Public health has been defined as the 'science and art of preventing disease, prolonging life, and promoting health through the organized efforts of society? As an activity, public health is concerned with health improvement, health service improvement and health protection. As a discipline, public health draws from many other disciplines including epidemiology, biostatistics, health service administration, environmental health, behavioral health, health economics, policy studies and occupational health. As a profession, public health has regulating and accrediting bodies, and processes for selecting and training people who wish to become public health specialists. There is a clear overlap between public health and health promotion but they are not identical. Within public health, there are many sub-specialties and very few public health specialists could claim to be competent in all aspects of public health. Health promotion is most sensibly seen as one of the many elements of public health. Most public health specialists could not claim to be competent in the specialty of health promotion.

3.3.1. The Public Health Workforce

The former Chief Medical Officer (CMO) recognized three groups in the public health workforce:

- Public health specialists, those who work at a strategic or management level managing change and leading public health programs, and who have a common core of knowledge, skills and experience acquired from postgraduate public health qualifications. They may come from a variety of professional backgrounds.
- Public health practitioners, professionals who spend a major part or all of their time in public health practice. These include most health promotion specialists as well as health visitors, many environmental health officers and community development workers. They have in-depth knowledge and skills in their specific areas and are a vital part of the workforce.
- Wider public health workforce, these include the many professionals who have a role in health improvement and reducing inequalities. They include health service managers, healthcare professionals, teachers, social workers and local government staff.

The use of the word specialist in this classification is confusing since most health promotion specialists are classed as public health practitioners rather than public health specialists. Health promotion is one of several 'defined' sub-specialisms open to public health specialists but the majority of public health specialists are qualified as 'general' public health specialists.

3.3.2. Health Promotion

Health promotion is another major concept that is important to community and public health nutrition. Health promotion can be defined as the process of enabling people to increase control over the determinants of good health and subsequently improve their health. Two strategies that can be used to design a health promotion campaign to reduce risk are presented in Table 3.1.

Table 3.1. Design of a Health Promotion Campaign

	Concept	**Benefit**	**Example**
Population	Instruction is directed at the entire population (national, local community, schools, and neighborhoods) with messages and programs aimed at reducing behavioral risk factors, such as poor eating habits or physical inactivity	Members of the community may lower their risk by a small percentage, thereby reducing new cases of chronic health conditions and mortality.	A nutritionist changing the eating patterns of families and advocating for fluoridation of the water supply—rather than screening all postmenopausal women for bone loss or hiring dentists to treat every child and adolescent—may reduce the risk of osteoporosis and dental decay
			Instruction about reducing sodium intake may reduce a population's mean systolic blood pressure by 3%, which will decrease the number of people in the high-risk group by 25% if high risk for systolic blood pressure is considered to begin at 140 mmHg.
			If excess body weight is 92/kg/202 pounds, reducing the populations mean weight by 1kg/2.2 pounds (about 1%) will cut the number of overweight people by 25%.
			Instruction could be provided to engage in regular physical activity and reduce excess calorie consumption

			If everyone is encouraged to consume high calcium and/or low-fat food products and then food industries develop and market these food products, this will subsequently prevent osteoporosis and obesity
			The Fruits & Veggies—More Matters campaign is an example of a population approach to health promotion
Individual	The nutritionist focuses on identifying individuals at risk, and the intervention is directed specifically at these "high risk individuals.	This method may be more beneficial when the risk conditions are highly restricted, such as with preschool children who were exposed to foods containing lead.	Intervention could be limited to persons with family histories of heart disease, and these people could be taught about reducing fat intake and increasing physical activities to reduce the potential of experiencing heart disease.
			Nutrition intervention could be limited to the children of adult alcoholics, individuals with a family history of diabetes, and low-income pregnant women participating in the Special Supplemental Nutrition Program for Women, Infants, and Children (WIC), which may translate to risk reduction.

3.2.2.1. Advantages

Population Approach:

- The population approach may instigate a behavior change that may become the norm and create conditions that make it easier for any individual to change. For example, if everyone is urged to reduce their fat and saturated fat intake, this increases the incentive for the food industry to develop and market products that are low in fat and/or saturated fat, such as low-fat milk, which makes it easier to adopt a low-fat diet.
- The population approach is likely to save more lives and prevent more illness than the individual approach when the risk factors are widely diffused throughout the community.

Individual Approach:

- Using the individual approach, people at high risk are specifically targeted, and the intervention is provided on time. More attention is given to ensuring that individuals with chronic disease are following necessary, strict dietary programs.
- Using the individual approach reduces the costs associated with screening an entire population and releases health professionals to attend to the community's other healthcare needs.

3.2.2.2. Disadvantages

Population Approach:

- This approach requires mass change and may not be needed by the entire population.
- It may not be cost-effective and may inconvenience people.

Individual Approach:

- With the individual approach, screening may not be universal and thus some high-risk individuals may not be identified.

3.3.3. Knowledge and Skills of Public Health and Community Nutritionists

In most instances, a community or public health nutritionist must be a member of an interdisciplinary team to provide an effective nutrition program. An interdisciplinary team is a collaboration among personnel representing different disciplines of public health workers (nurses, social workers, physicians, daycare workers, dietitians, and dietetic technicians).

They use various approaches to diagnose and address public or community issues, including:

- Utilizing interventions that promote health and prevent communicable or chronic diseases by managing or controlling the community's environment.
- Channeling funds and energy to problems that affect the lives of the largest numbers of people in a community.
- Seeking out unserved or underserved populations (due to income, age, ethnicity, heredity, or lifestyle) and those who are vulnerable to disease, hunger, or malnutrition.
- Collaborating with the public, consumers, community leaders, legislators, policymakers, administrators, and health and human service professionals to assess and respond to community needs and consumer demands.
- Monitoring the public or community's health in relation to public health objectives, and continuously addressing current and future needs.
- Planning, organizing, managing, directing, coordinating, and evaluating the nutrition component of health agency services.

For community nutritionists to accomplish these actions, they need to acquire normal and clinical nutrition knowledge and be skilled in educating the public regarding changes in eating behavior. The minimum education requirements for a community nutritionist include a bachelor's degree in foods and nutrition or dietetics from an accredited college or university and a Master of Public Health degree with a major in nutrition or a Master of Science degree in applied human nutrition with a minor in public health or community health. Some community nutrition positions require certification as a Registered Dietitian (RD) and/or an advanced degree in nutrition. Academic training includes knowledge of biostatistics and skill in collecting, analyzing, and reporting demographic, health, and food nutrition data. The community nutritionist must understand the epidemiology of health and disease patterns in the population as well as trends of diseases over a long period of time. She or he must be knowledgeable about the principles of health education, program planning, program evaluation, community organization, management, and marketing and policy formation. Marketing skills are very important because they help nutritionists know how to convey effective nutrition messages using a variety of media formats for their audiences.

Community nutritionists must keep current with advances in research and food and nutrition sciences, and changing practices in public health service. In some situations, Dietetic Technicians, Registered (DTRs) are employed in the food service area, clinical settings, and community settings. They may assist the community nutritionist/Registered Dietitian in determining the community's nutritional needs and in providing community nutrition programs and services. At a minimum, DTRs must have an associate's degree from an approved educational program. After that, they must successfully complete a national examination administered by the Commission on Dietetic Registration (CDR). Both community and public health nutritionists provide a wide variety of nutrition services through government and non-government agencies at the local, state, national, and international levels. In most cases, the activities require multitasking roles such as blood pressure screening, diet counseling, and medical nutrition therapy. At the international level, duties may include education on sanitation, water purification, and gardening.

3.3.4. Relationship between Eating Behaviors and Chronic Diseases

The area of eating behavior and chronic disease, the relationship between eating behaviors and chronic diseases is significant and impacts individuals and communities greatly. It is important to note that dietary factors overlap with other problems and apply to many of the health conditions.

Nutrition and Health, government agencies, and nonprofit health and scientific organizations have provided comprehensive analyzes of the relationship among diet, lifestyle, and major chronic diseases. Health conditions such as coronary heart disease, stroke, cancer, and diabetes are still the leading causes of death and disability.

In addition to dietary intake, many other factors contribute to chronic diseases, such as genetic factors and lifestyle factors (e.g., cigarette smoking). Medical geneticists working on the Human Genome, a major international initiative to decipher the 3-billion-unit code of DNA in the 80,000 to 100,000 genes found in humans, have already identified genes associated with many chronic diseases, such as breast, colon, and prostate cancers; severe obesity; and diabetes.

The public health approach to prevention understands that the reduction of risk for individuals with average risk profiles might be small or negligible. However, high-risk persons need special attention through primary, secondary, and tertiary preventions. Although it may not eliminate a disease for people who are genetically inclined to it, good primary prevention strategies could reduce the severity of the disease (WHO, 2020).

3.3.4.1. Reducing Risk Through Prevention

Prevention is important in public health as well as community nutrition practice. The three important parts of prevention are personal, community-based, and systems-based. Each part has a different role and focus. Establishing an overall effective community nutrition practice involves correctly using and combining each part

- Personal prevention involves people at the individual level; for instance, educating and supporting a breastfeeding mother to promote the health of her infant.
- Community-based prevention targets groups; for example, public campaigns for low-fat diets to decrease the incidences of obesity and/or heart disease.
- Systems-based prevention deals with changing policies and laws in order to achieve the objectives of prevention practice; for example, laws regarding childhood immunization, food labels, food safety, and sanitation.

One part of systems-based prevention deals with socioeconomic status, which affects health through environmental or behavioral factors. The socioeconomic model hypothesizes that poor families do not have the economic, social, or community resources needed to be in good health. For instance, poverty affects children's well-being by influencing health and nutrition, the home environment, and neighborhood conditions.

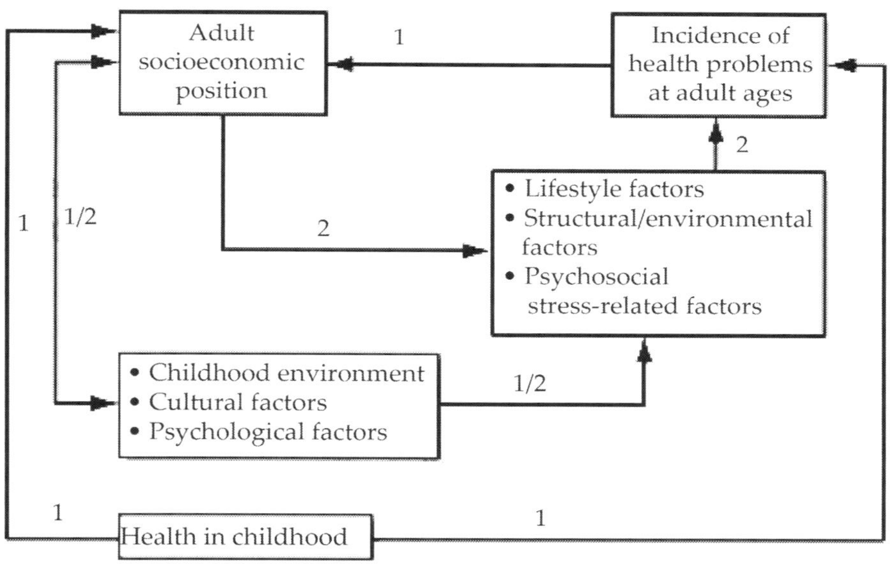

Figure 3.6. *Selective and causative factors involved in the development of health inequalities in society.*

Source: *De Henauw, S., Matthys, C., & De Backer, G. (2003). Socio-Economic status, nutrition and health. Archives of Public Health, 61, 15–31.*

The combined effects of poverty provide the foundation for a cycle of poverty and hopelessness among family members, who in turn engage in risky health behaviors, such as substance abuse, smoking, and poor dietary habits that can result in obesity and nutrition-related chronic diseases.

Socioeconomic models have been used to develop policies and disease prevention strategies, such as the Mackenbach model, which can be used as a basis for developing policies and intervention strategies. The Mackenbach model is presented in Figure 3.6. Mackenbach proposed that the link between socioeconomic status and health-related problems is triggered and maintained by two processes (selective and causative) that are active during different periods of life.

The selective process is represented by childhood health, which determines adult health as well as socioeconomic position. The causative process represents three groups of risk factors (lifestyle, structural/environmental, and psychosocial stress-related factors), which are intermediaries between socioeconomic position and health problems. The model also acknowledges that childhood environment and cultural and psychological factors contribute to inequalities in health through both selection and causation. Health inequalities become self-perpetuating through a cycle of inadequate childhood health, adult socioeconomic position, and incidence of health problems at adult ages.

3.4. Nutrition Related Non-Communicable Diseases

Non-communicable diseases (NCDs), also known as chronic diseases, are not passed from person to person. They are of long duration and generally slow progression. The 4 main types of non-communicable diseases are cardiovascular diseases (like heart attacks and stroke), cancers, chronic respiratory diseases (such as chronic obstructed pulmonary disease and asthma) and diabetes. These diseases are driven by forces that include aging, rapid unplanned urbanization, and the globalization of unhealthy lifestyles. For example, globalization of unhealthy lifestyles like unhealthy diets may show up in individuals as raised blood pressure, increased blood glucose, elevated blood lipids, and obesity. These are called 'intermediate risk factors' which can lead to cardiovascular disease, a NCD (Figure 3.7).

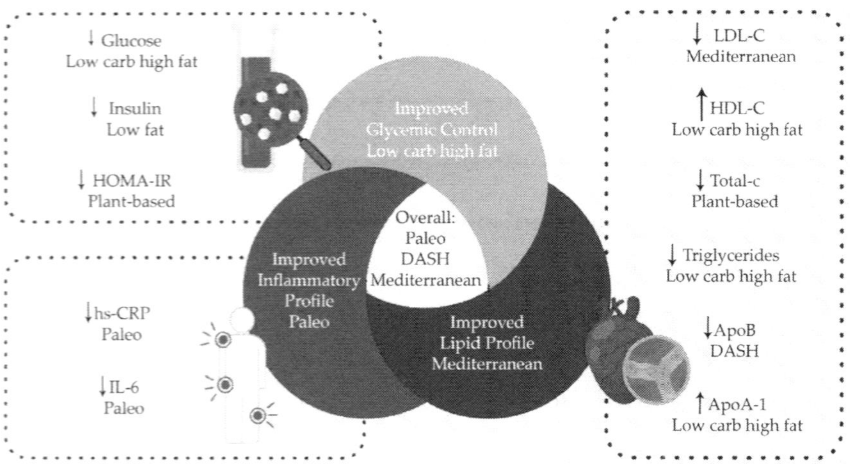

Figure 3.7. *Dietary patterns and non-communicable disease biomarkers.*

Source: *Liang S, Mijatovic J, Li A, Koemel N, Nasir R, Toniutti C, Bell-Anderson K, Skilton M, & O'Leary F. (2023). Dietary patterns and non-communicable disease biomarkers: A network meta-analysis and nutritional geometry approach. Nutrients, 15(1), 76. https://doi.org/10.3390/nu15010076.*

To lessen the impact of NCDs on individuals and society, a comprehensive approach is needed that requires all sectors, including health, finance, foreign affairs, education, agriculture, planning and others, to work together to reduce the risks associated with NCDs, as well as promote the interventions to prevent and control them (WHO, 2020). An important way to reduce NCDs is to focus on lessening the risk factors associated with these diseases. Low-cost solutions exist to reduce the common modifiable risk factors (mainly tobacco use, unhealthy diet and physical inactivity, and the harmful use of alcohol) and map the epidemic of NCDs and their risk factors (WHO, 2020). Other ways to reduce NCDs are high impact essential NCD interventions that can be delivered through a primary health-care approach to strengthen early detection and timely treatment (WHO, 2020).

Evidence shows that such interventions are excellent economic investments because, if applied to patients early, can reduce the need for more expensive treatment. These measures can be implemented at various resource levels. The greatest impact can be achieved by creating healthy public policies that promote NCD prevention and control and reorienting health systems to address the needs of people with such diseases. Lower-income countries generally have a lower capacity for the prevention and control of non-communicable diseases. High-income countries are nearly 4 times more likely to have NCD services covered by health insurance than low-income countries. Countries with inadequate health insurance coverage are unlikely to provide universal access to essential NCD interventions (WHO, 2020). A non-communicable disease (NCD) is a medical condition or disease that is non-infectious or non-transmissible. NCDs can refer to chronic diseases which last for long periods of time and progress slowly. Sometimes, NCDs result in rapid deaths such as seen in certain diseases such as autoimmune diseases, heart diseases, stroke, cancers, diabetes, chronic kidney disease, osteoporosis, Alzheimer's disease, cataracts, and others. While sometimes (incorrectly) referred to as synonymous with "chronic diseases," NCDs are distinguished only by their non-infectious cause, not necessarily by their duration. Some chronic diseases of long duration, such as HIV/AIDS, are caused by infections. Chronic diseases require chronic care management as do all diseases that are slow to develop and of long duration. NCDs are the leading cause of death globally. In 2012 they caused 68% of all deaths (38 million) up from 60% in 2000. About half were under age 70 and half were women. Risk factors such as a person's background, lifestyle and environment increase the likelihood of certain NCDs. Every year, at least 5 million people die because of tobacco use and about 2.8 million die from being overweight. High cholesterol accounts for roughly 2.6 million deaths and 7.5 million die because of high blood pressure. It is increasingly recognized that developing countries are undergoing an epidemiologic transition similar to that which occurred in industrialized countries. While infectious diseases are still the main cause of morbidity and mortality, there is a marked increase in chronic non-communicable diseases, particularly in the most advanced developing countries, and these diseases are expected to take the lead in a decade or two. Most of these diseases, above all coronary heart diseases, stroke and diabetes, are related to diet and lifestyles, for example, tobacco and alcohol consumption. As a matter of fact, these societies are also facing a growing epidemic of overweight and obesity, due to the frequent energetic imbalance between energy-dense food consumption and reduced daily physical expenditure. This health transition, favored by demographic changes towards aging populations, is occurring at an increased pace in urban societies widely exposed to the modernization of lifestyle, sedentary occupation, and to lipid- and sugar-rich food, often poor in fiber and micronutrients. Increased world access to cheaper vegetable oil is thought to have triggered this accelerated and generalized trend, though animal food, rich in saturated fat, and imported or locally-made industrialized food also play a role. While increased national and household incomes facilitate the initial change, as the transition advances poor people progressively become the main victims, as has been observed in the more advanced developing countries. Metabolic imprinting due to intra-uterine and infant malnutrition, which are still common in these societies, is also thought to play a significant role in the increase in the expression of insulin resistance, obesity and chronic diseases when these children are exposed to abundant food and modern lifestyle, later in life. Treatment and secondary prevention of nutrition-related chronic diseases and associated disabilities have an ever-rising cost in industrialized countries, which is far beyond the means of the still fragile economies of developing countries. This double burden of infectious diseases and undernutrition that still exist, and of non-communicable diseases and over nutrition represents a threat to the frequently unprepared healthcare services in developing countries. There is a clear need to focus health policies on the prevention of chronic diseases through primary healthcare services, the use of mass media for communication and education about healthy nutrition and lifestyle, and the adaptation of public policies. Nutritionists must also adapt to this changing nutritional situation which may result in apparently contradictory nutritional status findings within societies if not even within households.

3.4.1. Demographics

Demographics are the study of a population based on factors such as age, race, sex, and economic status, level of education, income level and employment, among others. Demographics are used by governments, corporations and non-government organizations to learn more about a population's characteristics for many purposes. With the aging of populations in developing countries, there is both a demographic and an epidemiological transition that affects the impact of chronic degenerative diseases on the health status of the populations. A demographic transition takes place in countries where there are effective programs of disease control that allow for survival during the early years of childhood and adolescence. This results in an increase in life expectancy which places larger proportions of the population in the age range (60 years and older) in which chronic degenerative diseases become the major determinants of health status. Epidemiological transition in diseases may also be brought about by shifts in social and economic patterns which favor detrimental changes in risk factors for the chronic degenerative diseases. Such changes may include health-related behavior which augments dietary consumption of fats and alcohol, increases obesity, increases smoking and decreases physical activity. Such changes in risk-factor levels increase the prevalence of chronic degenerative diseases which manifest themselves at later ages, and for which early preventive actions could be cost-effective. In order to illustrate the impact of both demographic and risk-factor effects, analyzes are made of the impact of increases in life expectancy on cause-specific mortality in both developing and developed countries. It is shown that there is great similarity in the effect of major non-communicable diseases on the life expectancy of adults in both developed and developing countries. The major differences are seen to be in the proportions of deaths expected from such diseases as cancer, diabetes, heart disease, stroke and cirrhosis; but not in the distribution of age at death which is the better measure of disease impact. Demographic analyzes, computing indirect estimates of mortality, also demonstrate that there are currently more chronic disease deaths in developing than in developed countries and that as the expectation of life increases in developing countries, the global chronic disease burden will be greatly concentrated in the developing countries. Analyzes of risk-factor reduction by feasible intervention strategies, e.g., smoking cessation campaigns, treatment of high blood pressure, using relationships between risk factors and diseases established in longitudinal studies carried out in developed countries, point out that the effect of risk-factor control in long-living populations can be hidden by the dependency of risk factors and various related causes of death, e.g., smoking has an impact on lung cancer, ischemic heart disease and emphysema, but at different ages. However, this demographic change has led to an epidemiological transition. The predominance of infectious diseases is shifting to non-communicable or chronic diseases. Non-communicable diseases (NCDs) include a range of chronic conditions, including cancer, diabetes, cardiovascular disease, hypertension, as well as Alzheimer's and other dementias. They are commonly thought of as "diseases of affluence." But in reality, four-fifths of deaths from NCDs are in low- and middle-income countries and older people in developing countries are particularly at risk (WHO, 2020).

3.4.2. Prevention and Control of Non-Communicable Diseases

Control, in the broadest sense, of non-communicable diseases (NCD), amongst them diseases of the cardiovascular system, cancer, diabetes mellitus, mental disorders, and many other determinants of chronic ill health, has become an integral and important part of health services in many countries. Control of NCD consists of a series of measures based on present knowledge of prevention, detection, diagnosis, treatment, after-care, and rehabilitation aimed at reducing significantly the number of new cases, increasing the number of cures, and reducing the invalidism and premature death due to NCD.

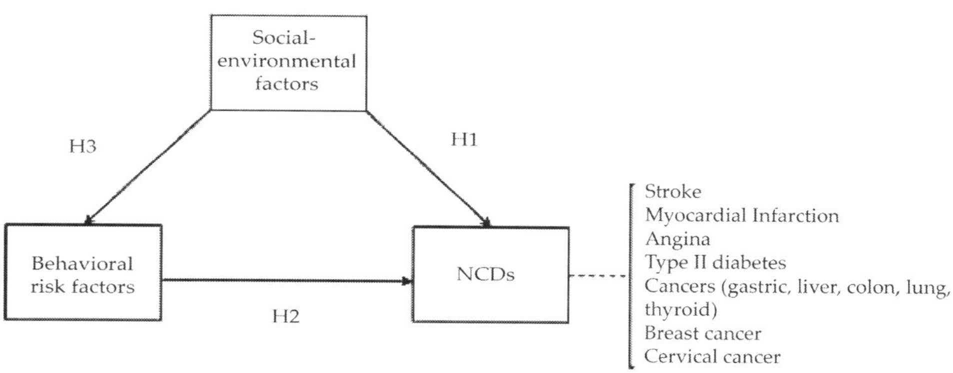

Figure 3.8. *The prevention and control of noncommunicable diseases.*

Source: Jeong NJ, Park E, & Del Pobil AP. (2021). Effects of behavioral risk factors and social-environmental factors on non-communicable diseases in South Korea: a national survey approach. International Journal of Environmental Research and Public Health, 18(2),612. https://doi.org/10.3390/ijerph18020612.

An NCD could be defined as a set of chronic diseases of major public health importance such as cardiovascular diseases (CVD), cancer, diabetes mellitus, lung diseases such as asthma and chronic obstructive pulmonary disease, chronic lesions of bone and joints, mental disorders and many others, the development of which is influenced by one or more common risk factors of an endogenous or environmental nature including frequent involvement of genetic components and which are not known to be caused by infectious agents. However, recent discoveries have demonstrated that the latter plays a much greater role in the origin of certain diseases than was thought and the borderline between infectious diseases and NCD is in many instances no longer distinct (Figure 3.8).

The magnitude and significance of the control of NCD are obvious from the observation that at least four of the ten most common causes of death worldwide during the 1990s were ischemic heart disease, cerebrovascular disease, chronic obstructive pulmonary disease, and cancer. Since 1950, most countries worldwide have experienced increased life expectancy at birth and have entered the phase of epidemiological transition from a disease pattern dominated by infectious diseases to one characterized by NCD such as cardiovascular conditions, cancer, injuries, and diabetes. For countries in epidemiological transition, most of which belong to the developing world, it would not be feasible to replicate the process that many industrialized countries have undergone in an attempt to control NCD: building curative healthcare infrastructure first and adding parallel services aimed at prevention at a later stage. An integrated approach that relies on preventive measures, curative interventions, and social care is needed to solve problems of effective control of NCD that could offer effective services at an acceptable cost. Leading representatives of the medical profession, international and national nongovernmental organizations (NGOs) dealing with problems of disease control, and the World Health Organization (WHO) have often warned about the rise in NCDs and their causes, the unpreparedness of most governments and communities, and the insufficiency of health policy actions undertaken so far. There is unequivocal evidence that much of the burden for which NCDs are responsible can be reduced. Therefore, the need for an integrated approach to their prevention and control is no longer challenged. Since 1950, many observational studies, controlled trials, and intervention projects have shown the causal association of certain risk factors with NCD as well as the effects of preventive programs. Support from community health programs is an essential component of an integrated approach to the control of NCD. Health promotion and the reduction of major risk factors for chronic diseases by broader public health actions and by integrating preventive measures within functions of health services could be the basis for the development of the long-term plan for control of NCD. Within the NCD control agenda, there are some major issues, such as the role of government and the private sector, inequalities in access to health services, health research, and sustainable development, that require special consideration due to the characteristics of NCD that are closely related to economic, social, cultural, political, and environmental dimensions of human communities.

3.4.3. Developmental and Nutrition Transition

The nutrition transition theory concerns the broad changes in the pattern of the human diet that have occurred across time and space. The nutrition transition is described by five stages: food gathering, famine, receding famine, degenerative diseases, and behavioral change toward a healthy, balanced diet. Currently, the vast majority of the world's people remain in pattern (receding famine) or pattern (degenerative diseases). They are either emerging from under nutrition because of a lack of calories or certain nutrients or they are engaged in a modern form of malnutrition consisting of too many calories from unhealthy sources. The modern diet pattern is high in oils, sugars, animal products, fat, cholesterol, sweeteners, and processed and prepared foods. The results of this transition are the diminishment of famine and the diseases that accompany it, which have plagued humankind for most of our existence. Unfortunately, this is complemented by the rapid growth of nutrition-related non-communicable diseases (NR-NCDs). The most obvious of these is obesity, but it also includes diabetes, cardiovascular disease, cancer, and the metabolic syndrome.

The transition to this new diet has already occurred throughout the developed world and is occurring in developing nations at an alarming speed. However, the shift between eating patterns remains incomplete, and many places face both the diseases of undernutrition and malnutrition, the so-called double burden. The negative outcomes of these two patterns are exacerbated among the world's poor; both the poor portions of the developed world and the poor nations of the developing world. This topic is one that overlaps with many academic fields, including medicine, nutrition, public health, epidemiology, and demography. The nutrition transition is spatially heterogeneous; a slum household in a city may be in stage 2 of the transition, while a nearby luxury home may be in stage. Geography and geographical methods sensitive to spatial scale are therefore critical. Since much of the research on this topic is in public health, there is a great opportunity for geographers to become more active in solving existing nutrition paradoxes (WHO, 2020).

Two historic processes of change precede or occur simultaneously with the nutrition transition. One is the demographic transition: the shift from a pattern of high fertility and high mortality to one of low fertility and low mortality (typical of modern industrialized countries). Even more directly relevant is the epidemiologic transition, first described by Omron: the shift from a pattern of prevalent infectious diseases associated with malnutrition, periodic famine, and poor environmental sanitation to a pattern of prevalent chronic and degenerative diseases associated with urban-industrial lifestyles. Interpretations of the demographic and epidemiologic transition share a focus with the nutrition transition on how populations move from one pattern to the next.

Large shifts have occurred in dietary and physical activity patterns. These changes are reflected in nutritional outcomes, including changes in average stature and body composition. Modern societies seem to be converging on a diet high in saturated fat, sugar, and refined foods and low in fiber, often termed the "Western diet." Many see this dietary pattern to be associated with high levels of chronic and degenerative diseases and reduced disability-free time. These three relations are presented in Figure 3.9.

Human diet, activity patterns, and nutritional status have undergone a sequence of major shifts, defined as broad patterns of food use and their corresponding nutrition-related diseases. Over the past three centuries, the pace of dietary and activity change appears to have accelerated in varying degrees in different regions of the world. Moreover, dietary and activity changes parallel major changes in health status as well as major demographic and socioeconomic changes. Obesity emerges early in these shifts, as does the age and level of morbidity and mortality. We can think of five broad nutrition patterns. They are not restricted to particular time periods of human history.

For convenience, the patterns are outlined as historical conditions/events; early patterns are not restricted to the periods in which they first arose but continue to characterize certain geographic and socioeconomic subpopulations.

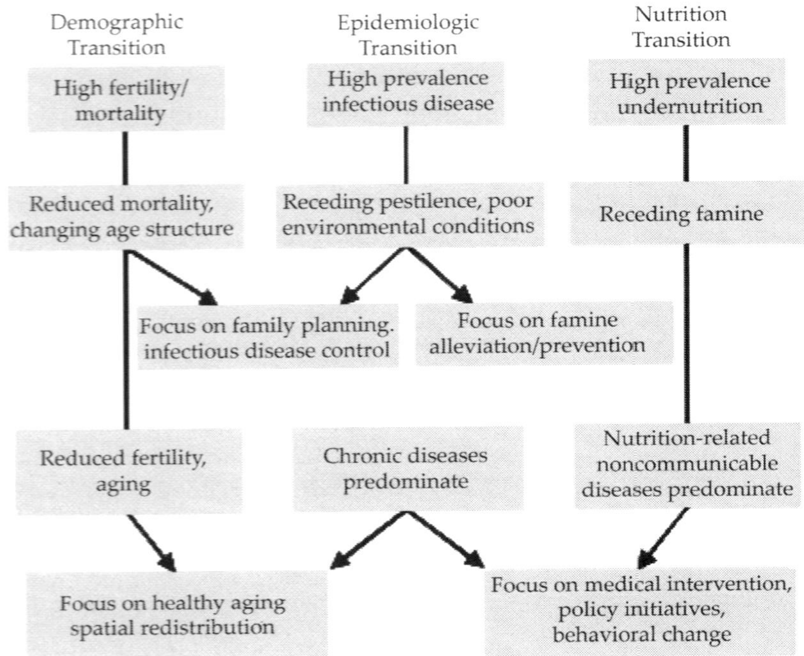

Figure 3.9. *Stages of health, nutrition and demographic change.*

Source: http://www.cpc.unc.edu/.

- **Pattern 1: Collecting Food:** This diet, which characterizes hunter-gatherer populations, is high in carbohydrates and fiber and low in fat, especially saturated fat. The proportion of polyunsaturated fat in meat from wild animals is significantly higher than that from modern domesticated animals. Activity patterns are very high and obesity among hunter-gatherer societies is rare. Note that much of the research on hunter-gatherers is based on modern hunter-gatherers, as there is much less evidence on pre-historic people.
- **Pattern 2: Famine:** While the variety of food becomes much less diverse, changes in diet vary across cultures and periods of acute scarcity. Dietary changes are hypothesized to be associated with nutritional stress and a reduction in stature (estimated by some at about 4 inches). During the later phases of this pattern, social stratification intensifies, and dietary variation increases according to gender and social status. The pattern of famine (as with each of the patterns) has varied over time and space. Some civilizations are more successful than others in alleviating famine and chronic hunger, at least for their more privileged citizens. The types of physical activities change but there is little change in activity levels during this period.

- **Pattern 3: Receding Famine:** The consumption of fruits, vegetables, and animal protein increases, and starchy staples become less important in the diet. Many earlier civilizations made great progress in reducing chronic hunger and famine, but only in the last third of the last millennium have these changes become widespread, leading to marked shifts in diet. However, famines continued well into the 18th century in portions of Europe, and today they remain common in some regions of the world. Activity patterns start to shift and inactivity and leisure become part of the lives of more people.
- **Pattern 4: Nutrition-Related Non-communicable Disease (NR-NCD):** In most high-income societies (and increasingly in portions of low-income societies) a diet high in total fat, cholesterol, sugar, and other refined carbohydrates and low in polyunsaturated fatty acids and fiber is often accompanied by an increasingly sedentary life. The result is an increased prevalence of obesity that leads to degenerative diseases characterized in Omran's final epidemiologic stage.

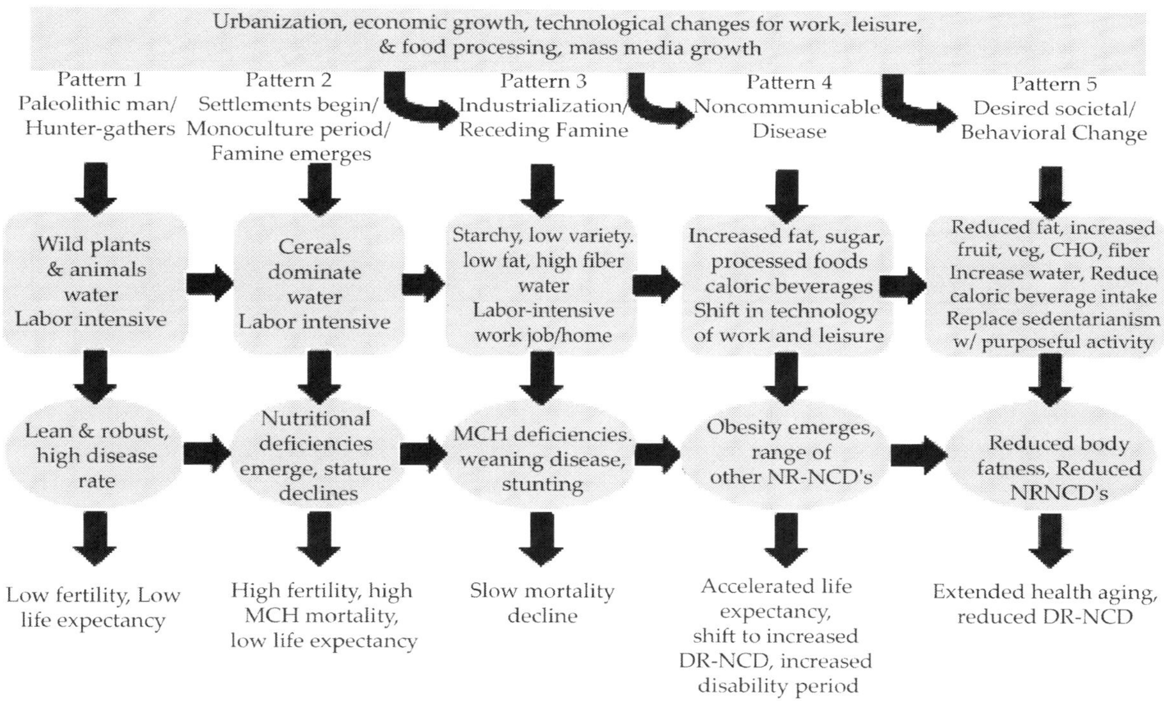

Figure 3.10. *Stages of the nutrition transition.*

Source: http://www.cpc.unc.edu/.

- **Pattern 5: Behavioral Change:** A new dietary pattern appears to be emerging as a result of changes in diet, evidently associated with the desire to prevent or delay degenerative diseases and prolong health. These changes, which are instituted in some countries by consumers and in others by government policy, may be found to constitute a large-scale transition in dietary structure and body composition. If such a new dietary pattern takes hold, it may be very important in enhancing successful aging, i.e., postponing infirmity and increasing the disability-free life span. Our focus is increasingly on patterns 3, 4, and 5, in particular on the rapid shift in much of the world's low- and moderate-income countries from the stage of receding famine to NR-NCD. Figure 3.10 presents this focus. The concern about this period is so great that the term the nutrition transition is synonymous, for many, with the shift from Pattern 3 to 4.

3.4.4. Nutrition Impact on Chronic Diseases

Chronic non-communicable diseases are rapidly increasing in importance as a global public health problem. An emerging epidemic of non-communicable diseases is closely related to lengthening life expectancy in developed and many developing countries, profound and frequently unhealthy changes in lifestyles, and adverse physical and social environments. By the end of the twentieth century, non-communicable diseases were estimated to have contributed to more than 60% of deaths in the world and almost half of the global burden of disease. The problem is universal and low- and middle-income countries suffer the severe and growing impact of non-communicable diseases, which creates tremendous difficulties for public health services in areas where human and technical resources are extremely limited.

Chronic non-communicable diseases now pose the greatest threat to health in both industrialized and developing countries. Health or epidemiological transition results in the changing pattern of health by which poor countries inherit the problems of the rich, and leads to the "double burden" of disease in the developing world because of the continuing weight of endemic infectious diseases. There is an important commonality to the risk factors for non-communicable diseases and many of these risk factors are preventable. At the same time, most chronic non-communicable diseases cannot be easily cured and almost every instance carries a burden of expensive and long-term treatment and, frequently, a supportive social environment of care. Therefore, a realistic response is demanded for the feasible and effective control of non-communicable diseases. Emphasis must be placed on preventing the premature onset of non-communicable diseases, delaying their development in later life, reducing the suffering they cause, and providing social and medical rehabilitation for those they disable. Addressing the major risk factors should be given the highest priority. Risk factors related to lifestyle, such as tobacco smoking, heavy alcohol consumption, inappropriate diet, and inadequate physical activity, are to some extent within the control of well-informed individuals. Therefore, health education as an essential component of any comprehensive program for the control of non-communicable diseases cannot be overestimated. However, the individual has little control over numerous other risk factors, such as the effects of poverty, poor reproductive and maternal health, genetic predisposition, occupational hazards, unhealthy living, and stressful conditions. It is clear that an integrated approach to the prevention and clinical management of non-communicable diseases should be provided at individual, community, and national levels. Until recently, most interventions have been medical, conducted through traditional disease-specific vertical programs. Integrated packages of disease-specific interventions must now be developed that incorporate primary and secondary prevention, timely detection, diagnosis, treatment, and rehabilitation for the most prevalent chronic non-communicable diseases. This demands a new relationship in which specialists, experts, and policymakers in various fields look beyond their own professional boundaries and requires broad partnerships of different social sectors (WHO, 2020).

3.4.5. Nutritional Management and Prevention Strategies

Nutritional management of patients in a rehabilitation setting often involves dealing with patients on a nutritional spectrum ranging from debilitated individuals who are undernourished to patients who have been admitted for complications of obesity. Nutritional care and therapy form an integral part of the management of patients with disease. Nutritional deficiencies result from reduced oral intake, malabsorption, medication side effects and systemic inflammation due to active disease. Enteral nutrition has a role in support for the malnourished patient, as well as in primary therapy to induce and maintain remission. The use of parenteral nutrition in disease is mainly limited to the preoperative setting or for patients with intestinal failure but does not offer any additional advantage over disease control. Dietary modifications, including elimination–reintroduction diets and a low fermentable, oligosaccharides, disaccharides, monosaccharide and polyols diet may improve symptoms but there are currently no data to suggest that these approaches have any role in the induction or maintenance of remission.

3.4.5.1. Nutrition Support

- **Oral Nutritional Supplementation:** For patients with CD who are malnourished, or at risk of malnutrition, oral nutritional supplements (ONS) can be well tolerated, allowing individuals to meet their nutritional requirements with resultant improvements in anthropometry. European Society for Clinical Nutrition and Metabolism (ESPEN) guidelines recommend up to 600 kcal/day in the form of ONS, suggesting this to be beneficial.
- **Enteral Tube Feeding for Nutritional Support:** If daily nutritional requirements are not adequately met by oral intake, alternative routes such as enteral tube feeding can be used in patients to achieve target intake. In a group of growth-retarded adolescents with CD, nocturnal tube feeding of 1–1.5 liters of non-elemental feed improved weight gain and growth. Continuous feeds are preferred to bolus regimes due to the reduced risk of complications. For patients requiring long-term enteral tube feeding, gastrostomy insertion is well tolerated in children and adults with CD.
- **Parenteral Nutrition:** There is no evidence that PN provides any benefit over EN as primary therapy for CD (or UC). PN is only indicated for nutritional support in patients with CD if nutrition cannot be optimized using oral or enteral routes alone. Examples may include intestinal failure (IF) due to short bowel syndrome resulting from multiple bowel resections or associated with high output stomas or fistulas. It is important that most patients should be

allowed to continue oral intake if possible, despite the use of PN. In practice, a mixture of oral, enteral and parenteral routes may be used together to achieve the best nutritional status.

- **Preoperative Parenteral Nutrition:** PN may be used to improve nutritional status before bowel surgery to improve postoperative outcomes in the malnourished patient when the oral or enteral route cannot be used. ESPEN guidelines do not give any other specific guidance for the perioperative patient with CD, except to state use of PN should be considered as for any surgical patient.
- **Postoperative Parenteral Nutrition:** Postoperative PN is principally required for patients who develop IF, defined as 'obstruction, dysmotility, surgical resection, congenital defect or disease associated loss of absorption, characterized by the inability to maintain protein energy, fluid, electrolyte or micronutrient balance.'

IF has been classified into three types. Type 1 IF is transient and occurs in patients who develop a postoperative ileus and may require short-term intravenous nutrition, although this is often not needed. Type 2 IF describes patients with complex diseases, often with septic, metabolic and nutritional complications, for which a multidisciplinary approach is essential, using the 'SNAP' algorithm (treat Sepsis, support Nutrition, demonstrate Anatomy and Plan future management). These patients may require long periods of PN, often in specialist centers or at home. Type 3 IF includes patients with more stable disease on long-term home PN, who may be candidates for intestinal transplantation (Figure 3.11).

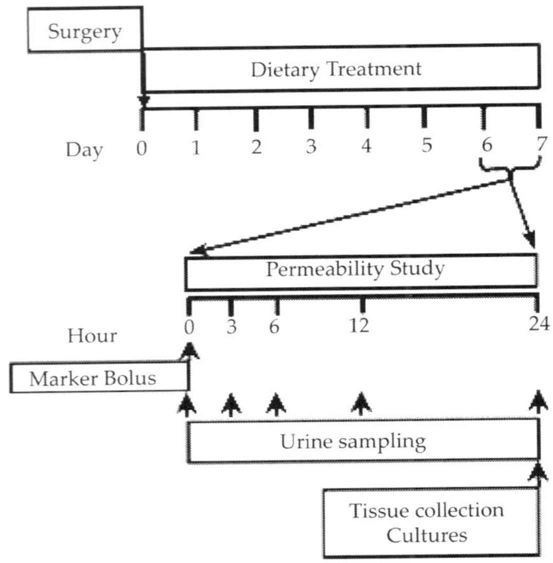

Figure 3.11. *Postoperative PN.*

Source: http://d3n1qfjutz9qb9.cloudfront.net/content/ajpgi/285/6/G1162/F1.large.jpg.

3.4.5.2. Enteral Nutrition as Primary Therapy

There is evidence to suggest that EN can induce and maintain remission in children and adults with CD but not with UC. Though corticosteroids are often used in adults to induce remission, it is important to recognize that these medications carry significant risks and do not necessarily lead to mucosal healing. EN is often used as first-line therapy to induce remission in children, not least because this approach is associated with growth and minimal side effects compared with steroids and may be associated with mucosal healing, although this has not been confirmed. By contrast, EN may be underused as a primary therapeutic option in adults, partly due to compliance issues.

3.4.5.2.1. Induction of Remission: Enteral Nutrition

Initial data suggesting a role for EN came from a small uncontrolled study of 13 patients who received an elemental diet to improve nutritional status prior to surgery. While weight gain and improved nutrition parameters were observed, there also appeared to be an anti-inflammatory effect. A further small series of patients with protein-calorie malnutrition due to extensive small bowel Crohn's demonstrated similar results with reduced protein and lymphocyte loss from the gut.

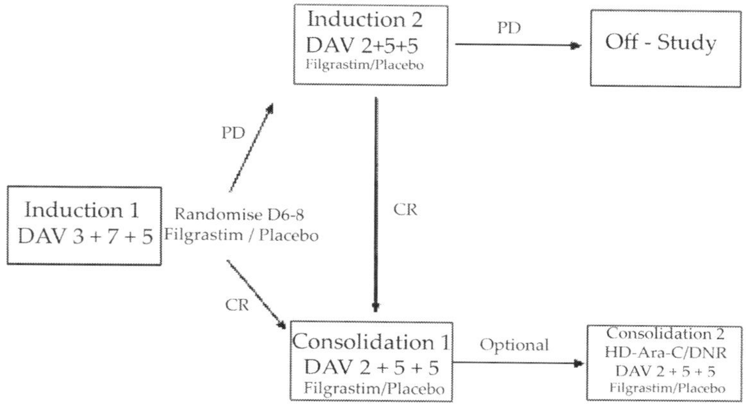

Source: http://www.bloodjournal.org/.

Since then, there have been multiple trials and meta-analyzes evaluating the role of EN as primary therapy in CD, but often with small numbers and heterogeneous groups of patients. With these caveats in mind, the most recent meta-analysis has demonstrated a significant benefit of steroids over EN for inducing remission in CD (OR 0.36, 95% CI 0.23–0.56, with a number needed to treat 4). When only data for 'higher quality' studies were assessed (based on randomization, blinding and description of withdrawals and dropouts), there was no significant difference between steroids and EN. However, this finding should be interpreted with caution due to the low numbers of patients and the heterogeneous nature of the studies included. Indeed, EN should be considered in appropriate patients. The challenge, however, is to know who these are: there are no trials comparing EN versus placebo; it is unclear how long exclusive EN is needed; and data are very heterogeneous with regards to response related to disease distribution (Figure 3.12).

EN as primary therapy has been evaluated in various formulations, including elemental and polymeric feeds. Elemental feeds consist of nutrition in its simplest form, for example, single amino acids, as opposed to oligopeptide 'semi-elemental' or full protein polymeric feeds. Elemental feeds were originally designed by the National Aeronautics and Space Administration (NASA) as easily digestible, water-soluble foods that produced smaller fecal bulk when consumed in space. There is clear evidence that elemental feeds have a primary anti-inflammatory effect in CD, with evidence of improved intestinal permeability, reduced inflammatory cytokine production and mucosal healing, although only when given exclusively. Various theories have been proposed as to how these benefits are rendered, but a definitive answer is lacking.

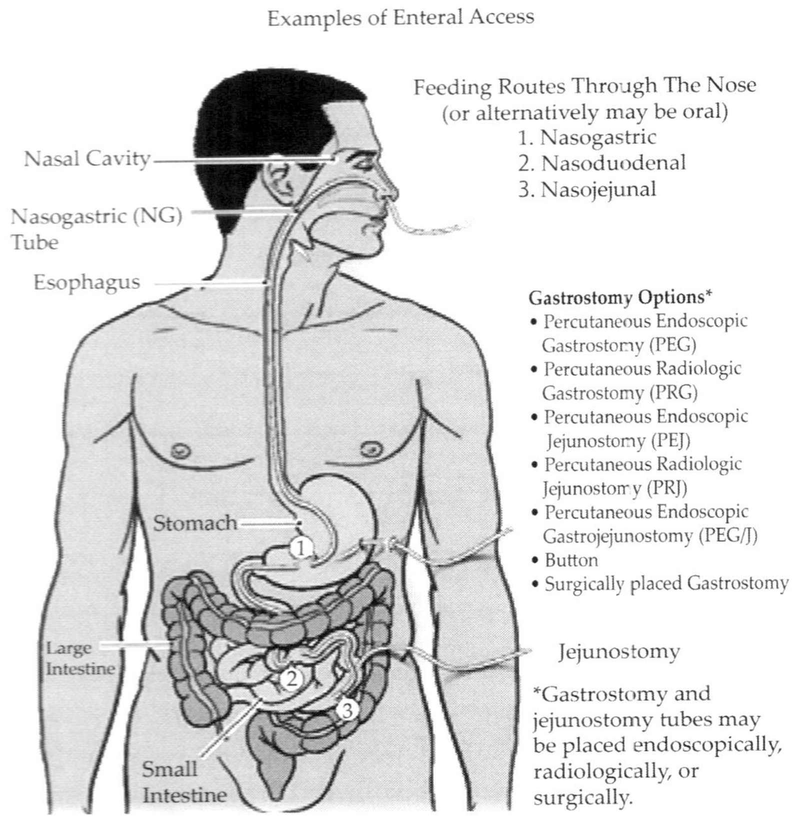

Figure 3.12. *Enteral access.*

Source: *http://patients.gi.org/.*

The most popular theory was that elemental diets had a reduced antigenic load to the inflamed bowel compared with full protein feeds. However, this may not be the case because polymeric feeds have since been found to be equally efficacious. In addition, because polymeric feeds are more palatable than elemental feeds, the former tend to be used first line. It has been further suggested that the anti-inflammatory properties of enteral feeds relate to their fat content, with emerging evidence that lower-fat feeds are more efficacious. Indeed modification of various dietary components, such as reducing long-chain triglyceride content or enrichment with fish oils have been evaluated but studies are small and results equivocal. For example, subgroup analysis in a Cochrane review of six studies did not demonstrate a statistically significant difference in remission rates between low and high long-chain triglyceride feeding formulae.

3.4.5.2.2. Maintenance of Remission: Enteral Nutrition

While induction of remission can be achieved with EN, the use of exclusive EN for longer-term disease maintenance is more challenging due to compliance issues. Uncontrolled, prospective data have suggested maintenance of CD can be prolonged by the addition of EN to an unrestricted normal diet. These lent support to retrospective data in children and adolescents, demonstrating prolonged remission (and also improved growth) if patients received nocturnal nasogastric feeding. There have only been two randomized controlled trials assessing EN as maintenance therapy in CD. The first of these gave 33 patients with steroid-dependent CD (two failed attempts to wean steroids) either an elemental or a polymeric diet to make up 30–50% of their requirements. Response was defined as the successful withdrawal of steroids without a CDAI increase of more than 100 points to a score greater than 200 and avoidance of surgery; this was achieved in 14 of the 27 patients who tolerated the feed. Subsequently, an open-label extension allowed the 14 'responders' to choose whether or not to remain on enteral supplements. Of the seven patients who chose to return to an unrestricted diet, all relapsed within 4 months, requiring further steroids, whereas six of the seven patients who continued on enteral supplements remained in remission at 24 months.

As with induction of remission, the identification of factors that predict which patients will respond would facilitate a targeted approach. A retrospective study of 145 patients in remission, with two-thirds receiving maintenance EN, identified penetrating CD (RR 3.89; 95% CI 1.58–9.62), colonic involvement (RR 3.10; 95% CI 1.39–6.90) and history of surgery (RR 2.48; 95% CI 1.16–5.33) to be factors that predicted recurrence. Recurrence rates were high (42/98 EN group versus 29/47 normal diet; $p = 0.047$), and it is difficult to assess the applicability of these data since remission was induced with PN and the only other therapy used was 5-aminosalicylic acid drugs.

While there are no studies comparing EN with immune-modulators for CD maintenance, one study has looked at the effect of using EN as an adjunct to biological therapy. EN provided at approximately half of the daily energy requirement over 56 weeks, in addition to infliximab maintenance therapy, did not alter clinical remission rates, which may not be an unexpected finding given that EN tends to be used in relatively mild disease, whereas infliximab is used in patients with CD at higher risk of relapse.

Postoperative recurrence rates of CD are high, with symptomatic recurrence rates of 20% and endoscopic recurrence rates of 73% of patients within 1 year following surgery. A prospective, non-randomized trial studied recurrence in 40 patients with CD after either ileal or ileocolonic resection, using EN (versus normal diet) for disease maintenance. Maintenance of EN over 12 months was associated with reduced clinical (5% versus 35%, $p = 0.048$) and endoscopic (30% versus 70%, $p = 0.027$) recurrence compared with the non-EN group. Notably, all 20 patients with EN completed this study, which represents an unusually low dropout rate, likely reflecting patient selection preoperatively.

Concerns have also arisen as to whether long-term EN for CD maintenance may impair quality of life because of the restrictive nature of the dietary intervention or the need for repeated nasogastric tube intubations. Tagaki et al. found no difference in quality of life (as measured by the short IBD questionnaire) in patients maintained on EN versus those who continued a normal diet. Furthermore, multivariate analysis demonstrated EN to be independently associated with improvement of health-related quality of life in patients with CD with a disease duration of over 10 years (WHO, 2020).

A Closer Look

Nutritionist

A nutritionist is a health professional specializing in the science of nutrition, working to promote healthy eating habits and overall well-being. They analyze the dietary needs of individuals and communities, providing personalized guidance to help clients achieve their health goals. This role requires a deep understanding of how different foods affect the body, knowledge of nutritional values, and awareness of the latest dietary trends and research.

Nutritionists work in various settings, including hospitals, schools, private practices, and public health organizations. In clinical environments, they often collaborate with other healthcare providers to develop comprehensive care plans for patients with medical conditions like diabetes, heart disease, or obesity. In community settings, they might design and implement nutrition education programs to address public health issues, such as malnutrition or obesity epidemics. Additionally, nutritionists may work in research, contributing to scientific studies that explore the links between diet, health, and disease.

The primary goal of a nutritionist is to foster a healthy relationship with food. They educate clients on balanced diets, portion control, and mindful eating practices. By assessing factors like age, gender, activity level, and health status, nutritionists tailor dietary recommendations to meet the unique needs of each person. They also address psychological aspects of eating, recognizing the emotional and behavioral components that influence dietary choices.

Professional nutritionists must stay current with ongoing research and evolving guidelines in nutrition science. They often pursue continuous education and certification to ensure their advice is evidence-based and aligned with current standards. Communication skills are essential, as they must convey complex nutritional information in an accessible and motivating manner.

Therefore, a nutritionist plays a crucial role in preventive healthcare, empowering individuals to make informed dietary decisions that enhance their quality of life. Their expertise not only contributes to the management of chronic diseases but also promotes lifelong health and wellness through informed and balanced nutrition.

Summary

This chapter focuses on the critical role nutrition plays in the overall health and well-being of populations. It explores the interplay between nutrition and public health issues, highlighting how dietary habits influence the prevalence of chronic diseases, such as obesity, diabetes, heart disease, and certain cancers. The chapter discusses strategies for improving nutritional status across diverse communities, including policy development, nutritional education programs, and interventions designed to increase access to healthy foods. It also examines the importance of surveillance and research in identifying nutritional deficiencies and guiding public health initiatives. Through a comprehensive approach that involves stakeholders at all levels, the chapter emphasizes the need for integrated efforts to address the complex challenges of ensuring adequate nutrition for all, thus contributing to the prevention of disease and the promotion of health at a population level.

References

1. Blencowe H, Krasevec J, de Onis M, Black RE, An X, Stevens GA, Borghi E, Hayashi C, Estevez D, Cegolon L, Shiekh S, Ponce Hardy V, Lawn JE, Cousens S. National, regional, and worldwide estimates of low birthweight in 2015, with trends from 2000: a systematic analysis. Lancet Glob Health. 2019;7(7):e849–60.
2. FAO, IFAD, UNICEF, WFP and WHO. In brief to the state of food security and nutrition in the world 2022. Repurposing food and agricultural policies to make healthy diets more affordable. Rome: FAO; 2022. https://doi.org/10.4060/cc0640en.
3. FAO/WHO. Second International Conference on Nutrition. Conference Outcome Document. Rome: Framework for Action; 2014. https://www.who.int/news-room/events/detail/2014/11/19/default-calendar/fao-who-second-international-conference-onnutrition-(icn2).
4. GBD 2017 Diet Collaborators. Health effects of dietary risks in 195 countries, 1990–2017: a systematic analysis for the Global Burden of Disease Study 2017. Lancet. 2019;393:1958–72.
5. Headey D, Heidkamp R, Osendarp S, Ruel M, Scott N, Black R, Shekar M, Bouis H, Flory A, Haddad L, Walker N. Standing together for nutrition consortium. Impacts of COVID-19 on childhood malnutrition and nutrition-related mortality. Lancet. 2020;396(10250):519–21.
6. Popkin BM, Corvalan C, Grummer-Strawn LM. Dynamics of the double burden of malnutrition and the changing nutrition reality. Lancet. 2020;395(10217):65–74.
7. WHO. Comprehensive implementation plan on maternal, infant and young child nutrition. Geneva; 2014. https://www.who.int/publications/i/item/WHO-NMH-NHD-14.1.
8. WHO. Essential nutrition actions: mainstreaming nutrition through the life-course. Geneva; 2019. https://www.who.int/publications/i/item/9789241515856.
9. WHO. Food systems delivering better health: executive summary. Geneva; 2021. https://www.who.int/publications/i/item/9789240031814.

Chapter

EMPOWERING WOMEN'S HEALTH: UNDERSTANDING, CARE, AND WELLNESS ACROSS THE LIFESPAN

4

Contents

Introduction

The society does not prioritize the health of women, even though it is critical to their overall well-being. It is important to give priority to the health concerns that are relevant to women. This provides a guarantee that they will receive the care and support that they require to lead lives that are not only healthy but also happy. Biological and hormonal differences between men and women, which can influence their health, are the reason why women's health is so important (Peters et al., 2016). These differences can have an impact on the health of both men and women (Figure 4.1).

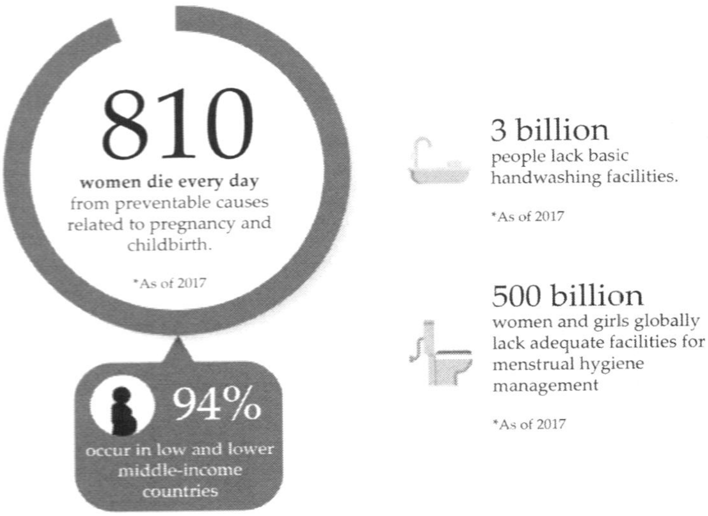
810
women die every day
from preventable causes related to pregnancy and childbirth.
*As of 2017
94%
occur in low and lower middle-income countries
3 billion
people lack basic handwashing facilities.
*As of 2017
500 billion
women and girls globally lack adequate facilities for menstrual hygiene management
*As of 2017

Figure 4.1. *Illustration of perinatal health framework for women.*

Source: By UN Women – https://interactive.unwomen.org/multimedia/explainer/covid19/en/index.html, CC BY-SA 3.0 igo, https://commons.wikimedia.org/w/index.php?curid=91557664.

Women are more susceptible to specific reproductive health issues, such as

- Menstrual disorders.
- Complications during pregnancy
- Symptoms associated with menopause

These conditions typically require specialized medical care and attention in order to effectively manage and prevent long-term health consequences. This is particularly true in the case of chronic conditions.

In addition, women are more likely to suffer from certain chronic conditions, such as osteoporosis, autoimmune diseases, and mental health disorders. Also included in this category are mental health disorders.

These conditions can have a significant impact on the overall well-being and quality of life of women if they are not administered treatment or managed properly. The occurrence of this circumstance can take place in a great number of different scenarios. It is within our power to assist them in leading lives that are both healthier and more satisfying by actively addressing the health problems that they are experiencing. In addition, it is of the utmost importance to make certain that they are available with the resources and assistance that they require (Peters et al., 2016). When it comes to women's health, the influence of social determinants on health outcomes is an essential component that must not be overlooked. Certain aspects of a woman's social environment have the potential to have an effect on both her physical and mental illnesses. This includes the following items:

- Economic standing and social standing
- The degree of education attained
- The availability of medical care
- Societal norms and standards

The likelihood of women experiencing unfavorable health outcomes is increased when they are confronted with obstacles to gaining access to healthcare or when they reside in environments that are not conducive to achieving optimal health. We have the potential to make a significant contribution to the improvement of women's health and well-being if we make it a priority to address the social factors that have an impact on health and if we work toward the establishment of healthcare systems that are equitable and comprehensive. In addition to the biological and social factors that have an effect on women's health, it is of the utmost importance to recognize the impact that women's mental health has on their overall satisfaction with life. The prevalence of mental health conditions such as anxiety, depression, and eating disorders is significantly higher among women than it is among men. With regard to the likelihood of experiencing these conditions, females have a higher probability. In addition to having a negative impact on a woman's overall quality of life, these conditions can significantly hinder her ability to function in her day-to-day life. According to Peters et al. (2016), if we make mental healthcare a priority and make sure that women have access to mental health services, we will be able to assist them in effectively managing their symptoms and improving their overall well-being.

Orientation and Directional Terms

Term	Definition	
Menstrual Disorders	Conditions that affect the regularity, duration, and flow of menstruation, such as heavy bleeding (menorrhagia), painful periods (dysmenorrhea), or irregular cycles.	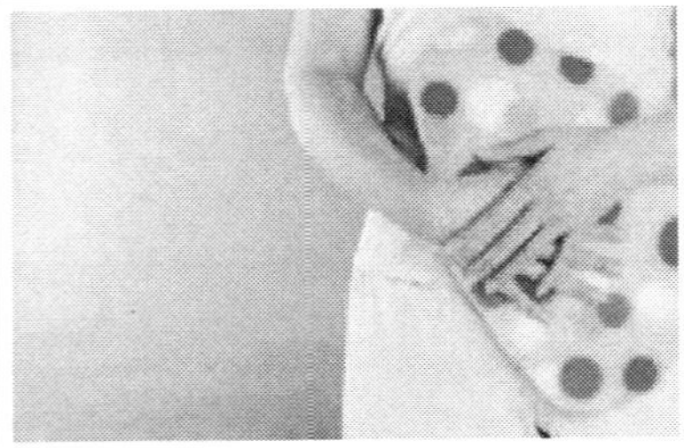
Stigma	A mark of disgrace or disapproval associated with a particular circumstance, quality, or person, often leading to discrimination and social exclusion.	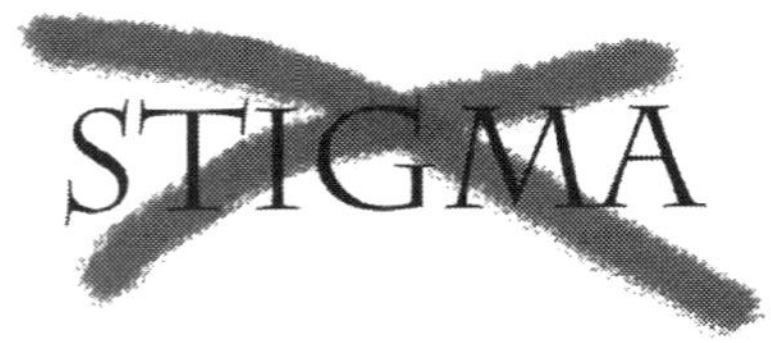
Reproductive Health	A state of complete physical, mental, and social well-being in all matters related to the reproductive system and its functions, including the ability to reproduce, and the access to appropriate healthcare services.	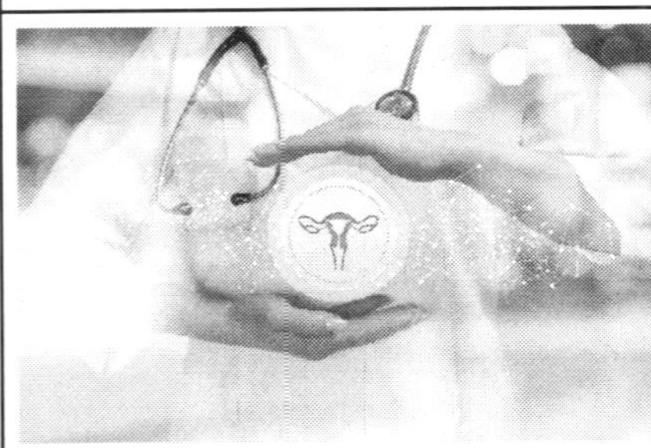
Menopause	The natural biological process marking the end of a woman's menstrual cycles, usually occurring in the late 40s to early 50s, characterized by the cessation of menstruation and a decrease in estrogen levels.	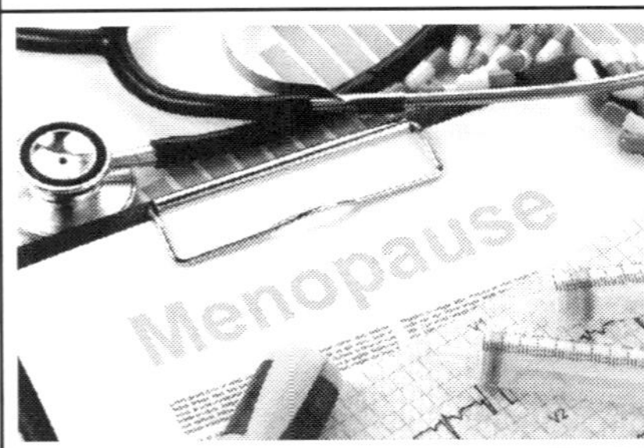
Gender-Based Violence	Harmful acts directed at an individual based on their gender, which can include physical, sexual, emotional, or psychological abuse and coercion, often rooted in unequal power dynamics and gender discrimination.	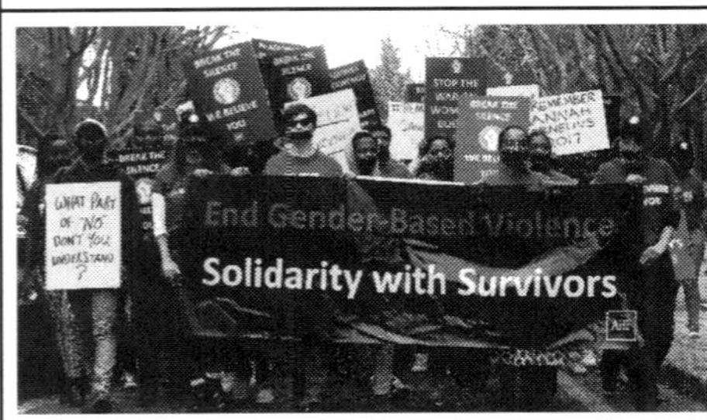

4.1. Physical Well-Being of Women

When it comes to women's overall health and quality of life, females' physical well-being is an essential component to consider. It incorporates a wide range of components, including the following:

- Wellness in sexual and reproductive areas
- Health of the cardiovascular system
- State of the skeleton
- Psychological health and wellness

As a result of the fact that women frequently face distinct obstacles and limitations when it comes to obtaining high-quality healthcare, the issue of women's physical health has been the subject of extensive discussion and disagreement throughout the course of history.

Ensure that women's reproductive health is a priority. Menstruation, pregnancy, childbirth, and menopause are all biological processes that fall under this category. A woman's reproductive health has an impact on her overall well-being as well as the quality of life she leads through her lifetime. For women to be able to maintain their health and make educated decisions about their bodies, they must have access to reproductive healthcare, which includes both methods of birth control and family planning (Inhorn, 2006). It is impossible to overstate the significance of maintaining a healthy cardiovascular system in women. Contrary to popular belief, heart disease is the leading cause of death among women around the world. Women are more likely to die from heart disease than men because they receive less timely and appropriate medical care. This is the reason why women have higher mortality rates. It is of the utmost importance for women to be aware of the factors that put them at risk for cardiovascular disease and to take preventative measures, such as consuming a healthy diet, engaging in regular physical activity, and avoiding smoking. It is essential for women to maintain the health of their bones to maintain their physical well-being. When compared to men, women have a greater likelihood of developing osteoporosis during their lifetime. Because of many factors, including the following, women have a higher risk of developing osteoporosis than men do:

- Increases and decreases in hormone levels
- The consumption of calcium in insufficient amounts
- An insufficient amount of participation in activities that require one to support their own body weight
- It is important for women to make their bone health a priority by ensuring that they consume an adequate amount of calcium and vitamin D, engaging in weight-bearing exercises, and undergoing bone density screenings regularly.

There is a strong correlation between the mental and physical well-being of women of all ages. The likelihood of women experiencing mental health disorders, such as anxiety and depression, is significantly higher than that of men on average. As a result of the negative perception that is associated with mental health issues, women may be dissuaded from seeking assistance and obtaining the necessary treatment. Women have a responsibility to make their mental health a top priority and to actively seek assistance when it is required. This may include:

- Pharmaceuticals for treatment
- routines for one's own self-care
- the presence of social support networks.

4.2. Women's Mental Health and Well-Being

It is vital that women's mental health and well-being are not overlooked. Support and resources are needed because women's mental health issues are unique. Women's mental health can be affected by the following factors:

- Social expectations and pressures
- Multiple roles, such as caregiver, professional, and homemaker, can cause stress and overwhelm for women who often balance them
- Discrimination and gender-based violence
- Lifelong hormonal changes
- Menstruation, pregnancy, and menopause.

It's important for women to be aware of these changes and to seek support if needed. Women are more likely to experience mental health disorders like depression and anxiety. It is important for women to be able to identify these disorders and seek mental health treatment if necessary. By addressing mental health issues early, women can improve their health and quality of life (Inhorn, 2006).

4.2.1. Stigma and Issues Surrounding Women's Mental Health

When it comes to seeking support for mental health, women frequently face a unique set of challenges and prejudices. However, mental health is essential to overall well-being. The stigma associated with mental health can discourage women from seeking treatment, which can have negative effects on their health and quality of life. Social expectations and stereotypes can lead to feelings of shame and inadequacy, both of which have a negative impact on the mental health of women. It is traditional for women to fulfill the roles of caregivers, homemakers, and successful professionals while also maintaining a flawless appearance and demeanor. It is common to view seeking assistance for mental health as a sign of weakness, although this pressure can cause feelings of being overwhelmed and anxious. In addition, women who seek treatment for mental health may experience bias within the healthcare system. According to studies, medical professionals are less likely to take the symptoms of mental illness in women seriously, which subsequently delays the diagnosis and treatment of these conditions. The absence of validation can make feelings of isolation and hopelessness even more severe. Violence and trauma that are based on gender can also have an impact on the mental health of women. Abuse of any kind, including sexual assault, domestic violence, and other forms, is more likely to occur to women, which can have a negative impact on their mental health. Many women may not receive the necessary support to recover from traumatic experiences, which can result in post-traumatic stress disorder (PTSD), depression, and anxiety. It may be more difficult for women to receive mental healthcare due to the intersectionality of gender, race, sexuality, and socioeconomic status on their part. It may be difficult for marginalized women to receive treatment due to factors such as a lack of insurance, language barriers, and stigma associated with mental health. These inequalities can result in women from these communities receiving care that is below acceptable standards or none at all, which in turn leads to worse health outcomes (Inhorn, 2006).

4.2.2. Women's Mental Health Conditions and Symptoms

Understanding women's mental health conditions and symptoms is crucial.

- **Depression:** Depression can severely impact a woman's life. Depression can cause;
  - Sadness
  - Hopelessness
  - Worthlessness
  - Changes in sleep, appetite, and energy.

Women are more likely than men to develop depression, which can be caused by hormonal changes, genetics, and life events.

- **Anxiety:** Anxiety is another common female mental health issue. Anxiety can cause:
  - Excessive worry
  - Restlessness
  - Irritability
  - Muscle tension
  - Concentration problems.

Women are more likely than men to develop anxiety disorders, which can be caused by stress, trauma, and genetics.

- **Perinatal Depression:** Perinatal depression, also called postpartum depression, occurs during or after pregnancy. Perinatal depression can cause:
  - Sadness
  - Guilt
  - Worthlessness
  - Changes in appetite, sleep, and energy.

Perinatal depression can harm both mother and child, so women with symptoms should seek help.

- **Eating Disorders:** Eating disorders are serious mental illnesses that affect eating, thinking, and emotions. Anorexia, bulimia, and binge-eating are examples. Eating disorders can cause:
  - Severe food restriction
  - Binge eating
  - Vomiting
  - Laxative use
  - Body image issues.

These conditions can cause serious physical and mental health issues if untreated.

- **Body Dysmorphic Disorder:** A psychological condition called body dysmorphic disorder involves obsessing over perceived appearance flaws. This can cause;
  - Compulsive grooming
  - Reassurance seeking
  - Social avoidance.

Body dysmorphic disorder causes significant distress and daily functioning impairment.

- **Bipolar Disorder:** It causes:
  - Extreme mood swings from manic episodes of high energy
  - Euphoria to depressive episodes of sadness and hopelessness.

Women with Bipolar Disorder may have more severe and frequent mood swings than men, disrupting their daily lives and relationships.

- **Borderline Personality:** Borderline Personality Disorder causes mood, behavior, and relationship instability. Women with BPD may have intense emotions, impulsivity, and a distorted self-image. They may struggle to manage their emotions and form stable relationships, which can affect their health.
- **Substance Abuse:** Substance Abuse is a pattern of harmful use of substances, such as drugs or alcohol that leads to negative consequences. Women with substance abuse may use drugs to manage mental health issues like depression or anxiety. Substance abuse can worsen mental health symptoms and cause a cycle of addiction and illness (Inhorn, 2006).

4.3. Reproductive Health

When we talk about women's reproductive health, we are referring to the full and complete health of their reproductive systems. Examples of these are:

- Wellness of the body
- Health of the mind
- Well-being of the mind

It encompasses a wide range of issues, such as menstruation, pregnancy, childbirth, and menopause, among others.

The menstrual cycle is of critical importance to the reproductive health of women. Regular menstruation is a natural process that involves the shedding of the lining of the uterus monthly. In addition to being an essential component of fertility, it is a natural part of the reproductive cycle of a woman. On the other hand, some women may suffer from menstrual disorders, which can have a negative impact on their quality of life. These disorders include menstrual cramps that are severe or periods that are irregular. If a woman experiences any abnormal symptoms during her menstrual cycle, it is significant for her to seek the advice of a medical professional (Lobo, 2013).

An additional significant component of women's reproductive health is the experience of pregnancy. Even though pregnancy is a one-of-a-kind and life-changing experience for women, it also comes with its own set of difficulties that they must overcome. Therefore, it is essential for women to take care of their physical and emotional health throughout their pregnancies in order to guarantee a healthy outcome for both them and their unborn child. It is essential to receive prenatal care in order to accurately monitor the progression of the pregnancy and address any potential complications that may arise. It is imperative that this always includes checking in with healthcare providers regularly (Figure 4.2).

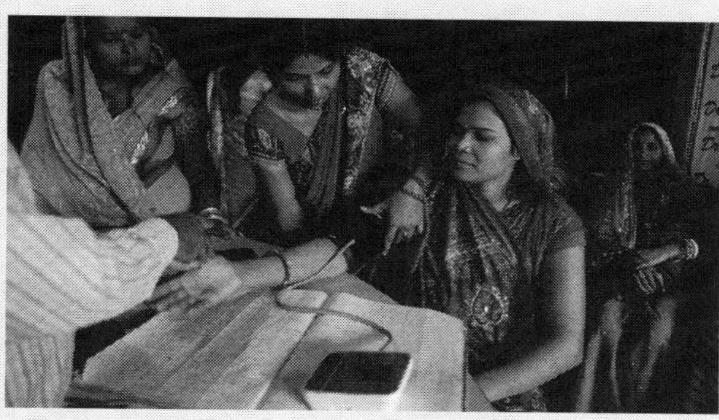

Figure 4.2. *Integrated women's health camp to ensure access to sexual and reproductive health services.*

Source: https://www.who.int/images/default-source/departments/reproductive-health/family-planning/india-2.jpg?sfvrsn=e5a28642_3.

The birth of a child is another significant event that occurs in the reproductive health of women. It is essential for women to have access to appropriate medical care and support during labor and delivery because the process of giving birth can be physically and emotionally taxing. Giving birth can be a challenging experience for women. As a result of the fact that complications during childbirth can have severe repercussions for both the mother and the baby, it is essential for medical professionals to be ready to deal with any emergencies that may occur (Lobo, 2013). A woman's reproductive cycle comes to an end when she reaches the menopause stage. It is characterized by the cessation of menstruation and typically affects women who are toward the end of their forties or the beginning of their fifties. The menopause is associated with a variety of symptoms, including but not limited to:

- hot flashes
- Changes in mood
- An assortment of symptoms, including sleep disturbances

Having these symptoms can have an effect on the quality of life of a woman. For women to effectively manage their symptoms during this transitional period, it is essential for them to seek support and guidance from healthcare providers.

4.3.1. Common Reproductive Health Concerns for Women

Reproductive health is a crucial aspect of overall well-being for women, as it encompasses a range of issues related to the reproductive system. Women can take control of their health and make informed decisions about their bodies by understanding and addressing these concerns (Lobo, 2013).

- **Endometriosis:** Endometriosis is a condition in which tissue similar to the lining of the uterus grows outside of the uterus.
  - This tissue can cause pain, heavy periods, and infertility
  - It affects about 1 in 10 women of reproductive age.
  - The exact cause of endometriosis is unknown, but it is believed to be related to hormonal imbalances and genetics.
  - Treatment options include pain medication, hormonal therapy, and surgery.
- **Uterine Fibroids:** Uterine fibroids are noncancerous growths in the uterus that can cause heavy periods, pelvic pain, and pressure on the bladder or rectum.
  - They are very common, affecting up to 70% of women by the age of 50.
  - The exact cause of uterine

fibroids is unknown, but they are believed to be influenced by hormones and genetics.
  - Treatment options include medication, hormonal therapy, and surgery.

- **Gynecological Cancer:** Gynecological cancer refers to cancers that affect the female reproductive system, including ovarian, cervical, uterine, vaginal, and vulvar cancer.
  - These cancers can be caused by a variety of factors, including genetic mutations, HPV infection, and hormonal imbalances.
  - Symptoms of gynecologic cancer can vary depending on the type of cancer, but may include abnormal bleeding, pelvic pain, and changes in bowel or bladder habits.
  - Treatment options for gynecologic cancer include surgery, chemotherapy, and radiation therapy.
- **Polycystic Ovary Syndrome:** Polycystic Ovary Syndrome (PCOS) is a hormonal disorder that affects women of reproductive age.
  - It is characterized by enlarged ovaries with small cysts on the outer edges.
  - Symptoms of PCOS include irregular periods, excess hair growth, acne, and weight gain.
  - PCOS can also lead to infertility and an increased risk of developing other health problems such as diabetes and heart disease.
- **Interstitial Cystitis:** Interstitial Cystitis is a chronic bladder condition that causes pain and pressure in the pelvic area.
  - Women with Interstitial Cystitis may experience frequent urination, urgency, and discomfort during intercourse.
  - The exact cause of this condition is unknown, but it is believed to be related to inflammation of the bladder lining.
  - Treatment for Interstitial Cystitis may include dietary changes, physical therapy, and medication to help manage symptoms.
- **HIV/AIDS:** HIV/AIDS is a sexually transmitted infection caused by the human immunodeficiency virus (HIV).
  - Women are at risk of contracting HIV through unprotected sex, sharing needles, or from mother to child during pregnancy, childbirth, or breastfeeding.
  - HIV weakens the immune system, making it difficult for the body to fight off infections and diseases.
  - Without proper treatment, HIV can progress to AIDS, which is a more advanced stage of the infection.
  - Early detection and treatment of HIV are crucial in preventing the progression of the disease and improving the quality of life for women living with HIV/AIDS.

- **Sexually Transmitted Diseases (STDs):** Sexually transmitted diseases (STDs) are infections that are spread through sexual contact. They can be caused by bacteria, viruses, or parasites. The table shows some common STDs and their characteristics.

Common STDs	Characteristics
Chlamydia	This is one of the most common STDs in the United States, with over 1.7 million cases reported in 2017. It is caused by the bacterium *Chlamydia trachomatis* and can be easily cured with antibiotics if detected early. If left untreated, chlamydia can lead to serious health problems such as pelvic inflammatory disease (PID) and infertility.
Gonorrhea	This STD is caused by the bacterium *Neisseria gonorrhoeae*. Like chlamydia, gonorrhea can be cured with antibiotics, but if left untreated, it can also lead to PID and infertility.
Syphilis	Caused by the bacterium *Treponema pallidum*. It can be cured with antibiotics If left untreated, it can progress to more serious stages that can affect the heart, brain, and other organs.
Genital herpes	This is a common viral infection caused by the herpes simplex virus (HSV). There is no cure for genital herpes, but antiviral medications can help to manage symptoms and reduce the risk of transmission to sexual partners.
Human papillomavirus (HPV)	This is a group of viruses that can cause genital warts and cervical cancer. The HPV vaccine is available to help prevent infection with the most common types of HPV that can cause cancer.
HIV/AIDS	This is a sexually transmitted infection caused by the human immunodeficiency virus (HIV). It weakens the immune system, making it harder for the body to fight off infections and diseases. There is no cure for HIV/AIDS, but antiretroviral therapy can help to manage the infection and prevent it from progressing to AIDS.

- **Sexual Violence:** Sexual violence is also a significant reproductive health concern for women.
  - Sexual violence includes any unwanted sexual activity or behavior, such as rape, sexual assault, and sexual harassment.
  - It can have serious physical, emotional, and psychological consequences for survivors.
  - Sexual violence can lead to unintended pregnancies, sexually transmitted infections, and long-term mental health issues such as depression, anxiety, and post-traumatic stress disorder (PTSD).
  - Survivors of sexual violence may also experience feelings of shame, guilt, and self-blame, which can prevent them from seeking help and support.

In order to protect their reproductive health, it is essential for women to be aware of the dangers that are associated with sexually transmitted diseases and sexual violence, and to take measures to shield themselves from these dangers. As part of this, individuals should engage in safe sexual practices, undergo routine screenings for sexually transmitted diseases (STDs), and seek support and counseling if they have been victims of sexual violence (Lobo, 2013).

4.4. Preventive Care for Women

It is common practice to overlook the significance of women's health as a component of individuals' overall well-being. It is imperative that women make their health a top priority and commit to taking preventative measures to avoid getting sick or sickening themselves. The provision of preventive care is of critical importance in the process of preserving good health and addressing potential health problems before they escalate into more serious conditions.

Women receive preventive care, which includes a variety of services and screenings, intending to identify potential health issues at an earlier stage and foster overall wellness. This includes the following:

- Exams on a regular basis
- Cancer screenings for conditions such as breast cancer and cervical cancer
- The vaccinations
- Counseling on making healthy choices in one's lifestyle
- Women can improve their quality of life and lower their risk of developing chronic diseases if they maintain a current knowledge of preventive care and ensure that they are receiving it.

Preventive care for women should include regular screenings for breast cancer, which is one of the most important aspects of this type of care. Since breast cancer is the most prevalent form of cancer in females, early detection is absolutely necessary for effective treatment. Mammograms are the recommended screening for women beginning in their forties; however, the frequency of screenings may vary depending on the individual risk factors that are present. Through the practice of getting mammograms regularly, women can improve their chances of detecting breast cancer at an earlier stage, when treatment is most likely to be successful.

Cancer screening for the cervix is yet another important preventive care service for women. When performed on a regular basis, Pap smears can assist in the detection of abnormal cells in the cervix before they develop into cancer.

One more reason why young women should get the HPV vaccine is to protect themselves against the most prevalent strains of the virus that can lead to cervical cancer. In order to significantly lower their chances of developing cervical cancer, women can take preventative measures such as receiving the HPV vaccine and maintaining a current screening schedule for cervical cancer.

Not only does preventive care for women include screenings for cancer, but it also includes vaccinations to protect against infectious diseases. For women at different stages of their lives, it is recommended that they receive vaccinations such as the flu shot, the HPV vaccine, and the Tdap vaccine. Women can protect their health and help prevent serious illnesses by ensuring that they receive all of their vaccinations at the recommended intervals.

Women also benefit from counseling on how to make healthy lifestyle choices, which is another essential component of preventive care. It is possible for healthcare providers to provide advice on how to maintain a healthy diet, how to get regular exercise, how to manage stress, and how to avoid engaging in harmful behaviors such as smoking and drinking to excess. To improve their overall health and lower their risk of developing chronic diseases, women can improve their lifestyle choices and make positive lifestyle choices.

4.5. Access to Healthcare Services

It is of the utmost importance to ensure that women have access to healthcare services to guarantee that they receive the necessary care to maintain their health. Unfortunately, a significant number of women encounter obstacles when attempting to gain access to healthcare, which can have significant repercussions for the outcomes of their health.

The fact that women have medical requirements that are distinct from those of men is one of the primary reasons why women need to have access to healthcare services. Beginning with reproductive health and continuing through menopause, women face a wide range of health concerns that call for specialized medical attention. According to Messing and Stellman (2006), women face the possibility of not receiving the treatment and support they require in order to effectively manage these conditions if they do not have access to appropriate healthcare services.

To add insult to injury, having access to healthcare services is absolutely necessary in order to encourage preventive care among women. Preventative measures such as vaccinations, screenings, and checkups at regular intervals are all essential components of a healthy lifestyle. If, on the other hand, they do not have access to healthcare services, a significant number of women might not receive these preventive measures, which would put them at risk of developing serious health problems in the future.

Access to healthcare services is essential for addressing disparities in health outcomes among women. This is in addition to addressing the specific health needs of women and promoting preventive care which are both important aspects of health care. When it comes to gaining access to healthcare services, women who come from marginalized communities, such as women with low incomes and women of color, must frequently contend with additional obstacles. Due to these disparities, the health outcomes of these women may be worse than those of their counterparts who have more privileged financial circumstances.

It is not only a matter of fairness but also a matter of public health imperative to make sure that all women have access to treatment and medical care. According to Messing and Stellman (2006), if we make it easier for women to access healthcare services, we can contribute to the reduction of health disparities, the improvement of overall health outcomes, and the promotion of the well-being of women and the communities in which they live.

4.6. Nutrition and Fitness for Women

It is crucial for women to prioritize their health, as it not only affects their own well-being but also the well-being of their families. One of the key components of women's health is nutrition and exercise.

First and foremost, nutrition plays a vital role in women's health. A well-balanced diet that includes a variety of fruits, vegetables, whole grains, and lean proteins is essential for maintaining optimal health. Women have unique nutritional needs, especially during different stages of their lives such as pregnancy, menopause, or post-menopause. Women need to consume enough nutrients to support their bodily functions and prevent chronic diseases.

Additionally, regular exercise is crucial for women's health. Physical activity not only helps women maintain a healthy weight but also improves their cardiovascular health, strengthens their bones, and boosts their mental well-being. Exercise can also reduce the risk of developing chronic conditions such as heart disease, diabetes, and certain types of cancer. Women should aim to incorporate a mix of aerobic, strength training, and flexibility exercises into their routine to reap the full benefits of physical activity (Messing & Stellman, 2006).

4.7. Managing Chronic Conditions

Conditions that are chronic, such as heart disease, diabetes, and autoimmune disorders, can have a significant impact on the quality of life of a woman. For this reason, it is absolutely necessary for women to make their health a top priority and to take preventative measures to effectively manage these conditions.

The fact that women are frequently the primary caregivers in their families is one of the primary reasons why the health of women is of such critical importance. It can be difficult for them to fulfill their responsibility of ensuring the health and well-being of their loved ones if they do not take care of themselves. They play an essential part in this process. Women can ensure that they have the energy and strength to care for others if they allow themselves to prioritize their own health.

Furthermore, studies have shown that women are more likely than men to suffer from certain chronic conditions, such as osteoporosis and autoimmune disorders. Pain, disability, and a reduction in mobility are all symptoms that can result from these conditions, which can have a significant impact on the quality of life of a woman. According to Tannenbaum, Mayo, and Ducharme (2005), individuals who can effectively manage these conditions are able to lessen the severity of their symptoms and improve their overall well-being. It is necessary to take a multi-pronged approach to effectively manage chronic conditions. This approach should include regular medical checkups, medication management, lifestyle modifications, and emotional support. The development of a personalized treatment plan that takes into account the specific requirements and worries of women should be a collaborative effort between women and their healthcare providers. This may require them to make adjustments to their diet, their exercise routine, and their methods of stress management.

Women may also benefit from support groups, therapy, and other forms of emotional support in addition to the medical interventions that are generally available to them. Living with a chronic condition can be difficult, and it is essential for women to have a solid support system in place in order to cope with the challenges that they face. Women can gain valuable insights, advice, and encouragement by setting up connections with other people who are going through challenges that are comparable to their own.

The practice of self-care is an additional essential component of managing chronic conditions. Women need to prioritize activities that help them relax, reduce stress, and improve their overall well-being. Engaging in activities such as yoga, meditation, keeping a journal, or spending time in nature are examples of this. Women can better manage the demands of managing a chronic condition and recharge their batteries by taking time for themselves and allowing themselves to take care of themselves.

Additionally, it is essential for women to advocate for themselves and pay attention to their health. When they speak with their healthcare providers, they should feel as though they have the authority to ask questions, seek second opinions, and express their concerns. According to Tannenbaum, Mayo, and Ducharme (2005), women are frequently socialized to prioritize the needs of others as opposed to their own, despite the fact that it is essential for them to prioritize their own health and well-being.

4.8. Women's Health at Various Stages of Life

Over the course of their lives, women experience a variety of physical and hormonal shifts, each of which has the potential to significantly influence their overall health and well-being status. Women need to have an understanding of these changes and how they can impact their health at various developmental stages throughout their lives.

Women's Health in Different Life Stages		
Stage	**Experience**	**Care**
During Puberty	Girls experience the onset of menstruation and the development of secondary sexual characteristics. It is a crucial time for young women to learn about their reproductive health and how to take care of their bodies.	It is important for girls to have access to accurate information about puberty and menstruation so that they can make informed decisions about their health.

In Their Reproductive Years	Women may experience pregnancy, childbirth, and menopause.	Pregnancy is a unique and transformative experience that requires special care and attention. Women need to be aware of the importance of prenatal care, proper nutrition, and exercise during pregnancy to ensure the health of both themselves and their babies.
Childbirth	A woman has long-lasting effects on her health.	Having access to quality maternity care and support during labor and delivery. Should also be aware of the potential complications that can arise during childbirth and how to prevent or manage them.
Menopause	Typically occurs in their late 40s or early 50s. Women may experience symptoms such as hot flashes, mood swings, and changes in libido.	It is important for women to understand the physical and emotional changes that come with menopause and how to manage them effectively.
Elderly Women	They may be at higher risk for certain health conditions, such as osteoporosis, heart disease, and breast cancer.	It is crucial for women to prioritize their health and well-being as they get older by staying active, eating a balanced diet, and getting regular check-ups with their healthcare provider.

4.9. Gender-based Disparities in Women's Health

Women's health disparities must be addressed. Women, especially marginalized ones, face barriers to quality healthcare. This may be due to a lack of insurance, transportation, or local healthcare providers. Unfortunately, many women don't get the preventive care and screenings they need. Socioeconomic status also affects women's health. Poor women have worse health outcomes than wealthier women. Lack of access to healthy food, safe housing, and other health-promoting resources is to blame.

Women's health disparities may also be caused by healthcare system gender bias. Men are taken more seriously than women when reporting symptoms or seeking medical attention. Endometriosis and autoimmune diseases, which disproportionately affect women, can be delayed and poorly treated. Addressing women's health disparities requires a comprehensive approach that addresses their root causes. This includes increasing healthcare access, especially in underserved communities, and training healthcare providers to provide gender-sensitive care. Poverty and education must also be addressed to reduce women's health disparities. By addressing these root causes, we can create a more equitable healthcare system for all women, regardless of socioeconomic status.

4.10. Advocating for the Self-Care and Well-Being of Women

Self-care is a crucial aspect of one's overall state of being, and it holds particular significance for women who frequently prioritize the needs of others over their own. Amidst the rapid pace of modern life, it is essential to prioritize self-care to uphold one's physical, mental, and emotional well-being (Tannenbaum, Mayo, & Ducharme, 2005).

Women encounter distinct obstacles when it comes to taking care of themselves. Women frequently prioritize the needs of others over their own, whether it be managing work and family obligations, navigating societal expectations regarding appearance, or balancing various responsibilities. Nevertheless, self-care is not self-centered – in reality, women must give precedence to their own welfare in order to competently attend to others.

An essential element of self-care for women is the maintenance of their physical well-being. This encompasses engaging in regular physical activity, consuming a well-rounded and nutritious diet, obtaining sufficient rest, and maintaining proper hydration. Physical self-care encompasses the maintenance of one's appearance, which includes activities such as receiving regular haircuts, wearing attire that promotes a positive self-image, and adhering to proper hygiene practices.

Women must prioritize their mental and emotional well-being in addition to taking care of their physical health. This can entail establishing limits with others, implementing mindfulness and relaxation methods, seeking therapy or counseling as necessary, and participating in activities that provide happiness and satisfaction. Women should prioritize mental and emotional self-care alongside physical self-care, as it plays a crucial role in managing stress, anxiety, and other mental health concerns.

Self-care can also encompass allocating time for oneself and participating in activities that foster relaxation and revitalization. Some examples of self-care activities are reading, bathing, walking, meditating, and pursuing hobbies or creative interests. Carving out personal time is imperative for women, as it enables them to rejuvenate and replenish their energy, enabling them to effectively handle the responsibilities of their daily routines.

Incorporating self-care practices into daily life can be challenging, especially for women who are busy and have many responsibilities. However, it is important for women to make self-care a priority and to carve out time in their schedules for self-care activities. This may involve saying no to additional commitments, delegating tasks to others, or setting aside specific times each day for self-care.

4.10.1. What Is the Significance of Self-Care and Wellness for Women?

Self-care and wellness are essential components of sustaining a healthy and harmonious lifestyle, particularly for women. In the contemporary and high-pressure society we live in, women frequently encounter the challenge of managing numerous roles and obligations, encompassing their professional pursuits, familial duties, and social commitments. The persistent pressure can have a negative impact on their physical, mental, and emotional health, highlighting the importance for women to prioritize self-care and wellness (Tannenbaum, Mayo, & Ducharme, 2005) (Figure 4.3).

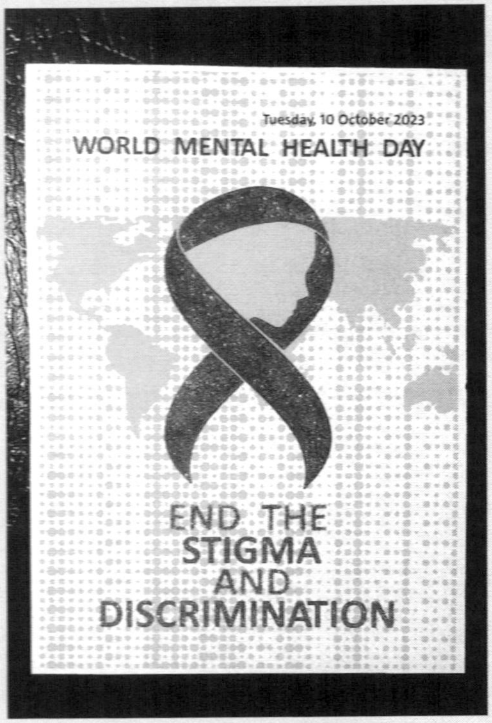
Tuesday, 10 October 2023
WORLD MENTAL HEALTH DAY
END THE STIGMA AND DISCRIMINATION

Figure 4.3. *Various forms of self-care is needed for long-term well-being.*

Source: By Dr Partha Sarathi Sahana – https://www.flickr.com/photos/ps_sahana/52992361185/, CC BY 2.0, https://commons.wikimedia.org/w/index.php?curid=133593636.

Women should prioritize self-care and wellness because they improve health. Proper nutrition, exercise, and rest can prevent heart disease, diabetes, and obesity. Self-care also boosts immunity and lowers chronic illness risk. Women live longer and healthier by prioritizing their health. Furthermore, self-care and wellness play a significant role in mental health. Women are more likely to experience stress, anxiety, and depression due to the pressures they face in their personal and professional lives. Engaging in self-care activities such as meditation, yoga, or journaling can help women manage their emotions and improve their mental well-being. Taking time to relax and unwind can also reduce feelings of overwhelm and burnout, allowing women to cope better with life's challenges.

In addition to physical and mental health benefits, self-care and wellness can also enhance women's relationships. When women take care of themselves, they are better able to show up for their loved ones and maintain healthy boundaries. By prioritizing their own needs and well-being, women can avoid feelings of resentment or burnout in their relationships. This, in turn, can lead to stronger and more fulfilling connections with others.

Self-care and wellness are also essential for personal growth and development. When women invest in themselves and prioritize their well-being, they can discover their strengths, passions, and purpose. Engaging in self-care activities that bring joy and fulfillment can boost self-esteem and confidence, empowering women to pursue their goals and dreams. By taking care of themselves, women can become more resilient, adaptable, and capable of overcoming obstacles in life (Tannenbaum, Mayo, & Ducharme, 2005).

Moreover, self-care and wellness can empower women to set boundaries and prioritize their needs. In a society that often expects women to be selfless and nurturing, practicing self-care can be a radical act of self-love and self-empowerment. By saying no to things that drain their energy and yes to activities that nourish their soul, women can reclaim their power and autonomy. This can lead to a greater sense of self-worth and fulfillment in all areas of life.

4.10.2. How Women Can Gain Power and Control Over Their Lives

Emphasizing the importance of self-care and wellness is essential for women to experience a sense of empowerment, both psychologically and physically. This can be accomplished by:

- **Engaging in the Deliberate Cultivation of Mindfulness and Self-Awareness:** Engaging in self-reflection and introspection allows women to gain insight into their own needs and establish clear boundaries. Developing self-awareness can result in making more informed choices and experiencing a heightened feeling of control.
- **Establishing Limits:** Women are frequently anticipated to fulfill the role of caregivers and prioritize the needs of others over their own. Nevertheless, it is crucial for women to give utmost importance to their own well-being and establish limits to safeguard their mental and emotional well-being. Asserting boundaries and articulating one's desires with clarity are essential measures in fostering personal empowerment through self-care.
- Engaging in Physical self-care involves consistently participating in physical exercise, consuming nutritious food, and obtaining sufficient sleep, which are crucial for preserving physical health and overall well-being. Engaging in proper self-care not only enhances physical well-being but also enhances self-assurance and self-worth. When women have a positive perception of their physical appearance, they are more inclined to experience a sense of empowerment in various areas of their lives.
- Women frequently encounter distinct obstacles that can have a negative impact on their mental well-being, including societal norms, gender disparities, and difficulties in balancing work and personal life. Engaging in self-care practices such as meditation, journaling, and therapy can assist women in effectively coping with stress, anxiety, and other mental health issues. By placing mental and emotional well-being as a top priority, women can develop the ability to bounce back from challenges and gain the confidence and strength to overcome them.

4.11. Women's Family Planning and Birth Control

Women need to have access to birth control and family planning in order to maintain their reproductive health. Women can make educated decisions regarding the timing of their childbearing and the number of children they wish to have as a result of these practices. Women can take charge of their reproductive choices and ensure that they are able to achieve the family size that they desire if they have access to methods of family planning and birth control (Seifer, Minkoff, & Merhi, 2015).

Family planning is the process of preventing or delaying pregnancy through the utilization of a variety of methods. Natural methods, such as monitoring ovulation, are examples of this type of method. Contraceptive pills, intrauterine devices (IUDs), condoms, and sterilization are examples of modern methods of contraception.

Because there is a variety of options available, women are able to select the approach that caters to their specific requirements and preferences the most effectively.

On the other hand, birth control is a term that specifically refers to all of the methods that are used to prevent pregnancy. Some examples of this are birth control pills and condoms, which are considered to be temporary methods. Surgical procedures, such as sterilization, are permanent.

It is possible for women to have a greater degree of control over their reproductive choices and to avoid unintended pregnancies with the assistance of birth control technologies.

To better prepare themselves physically and emotionally for pregnancy and childbirth, women can benefit from planning when they will have children. Women have a greater chance of receiving appropriate prenatal care and support when they plan their pregnancies, which ultimately leads to better outcomes for both the mother and the child. There are social and economic benefits associated with family planning and birth control, in addition to the health benefits. Women who plan their pregnancies have a greater chance of completing their education, finding employment, and being active members of society. It is possible for women to make choices that affect their lives and their futures, which can enhance their economic autonomy.

There is no assurance that individuals will always have access to family planning and birth control services, although these services offer numerous advantages. In many regions of the world, women often face obstacles that prevent them from gaining access to contraception, such as:

The absence of information: cultural taboos and a scarcity of resources.

Because of this, women and their families may experience unintended pregnancies, unsafe abortions, and other adverse health outcomes as a result of this situation.

To address these challenges, it is essential to raise awareness about family planning and birth control, as well as to make certain that women have access to a variety of contraceptive options. Here are some examples:

- The dissemination of information concerning reproductive health
- Education of medical professionals to enable them to provide family planning services
- Programs that provide contraception should receive more funding.

4.11.1. Alternative Methods of Birth Control for Women

Contraception serves the purpose of averting pregnancy by employing the following methods:

- Suppressing the release of eggs from the ovaries
- Preventing the process of fertilization
- Preventing the attachment of a fertilized egg

It empowers women to make well-informed decisions regarding their desired timing and intention of pregnancy. There are numerous contraceptive options available to women, each with its own advantages and disadvantages. It is crucial to provide women with information about these options so that they can make an informed decision that suits their specific needs and circumstances (Seifer, Minkoff, & Merhi, 2015).

4.11.2. Oral Contraceptives

Oral contraceptives, commonly referred to as birth control pills, are widely utilized by women globally as a highly favored method of contraception. Contraceptives function by releasing hormones, typically a blend of estrogen and progestin, into the body. This prevents ovulation, thickens cervical mucus to impede sperm, and thins the uterine lining to hinder the implantation of a fertilized egg (Figure 4.4).

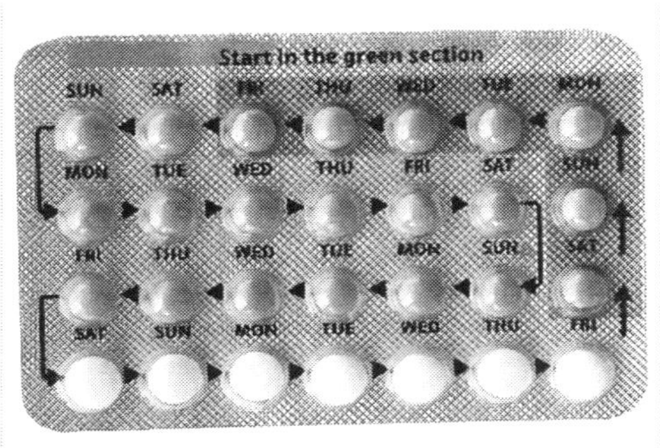

Figure 4.4. *Oral contraceptive pill.*

Source: By Tristanb at English Wikipedia - Self-photographed, CC BY-SA 3.0, https://commons.wikimedia.org/w/index.php?curid=116094.

There are two main types of oral contraceptives:

1. **Combination Pills:** They contain both estrogen and progestin and are taken daily for 21 days, followed by a week of placebo pills or no pills.
2. **Progestin-Only Pills:** they are also known as mini-pills, do not contain estrogen and must be taken at the same time every day without a break.

There are many advantages of oral contraceptives. These include;

- They are highly effective when used correctly. They have a failure rate of less than 1% with perfect use and around 9% with typical use. This makes them one of the most reliable forms of contraception available.
- They can help regulate menstrual cycles, reduce menstrual cramps, and make periods lighter and more predictable.
- They can also improve acne and reduce the risk of certain cancers, such as ovarian and endometrial cancer.

Oral contraceptives have risks and side effects like any medication. Nausea, breast tenderness, headaches, and breakthrough bleeding are common. Blood clots, stroke, and heart attack are more serious risks for women who smoke or have other risk factors. Before using oral contraceptives, women should discuss their medical history, lifestyle, and needs with a doctor. High blood pressure, diabetes, and blood clots may make oral contraceptives unsuitable for some women. Consider alternative contraceptives in such cases. Women must also know how to use oral contraceptives properly to maximize their efficacy. Missing a dose or taking it at different times can reduce the pill's efficacy. Antibiotics and anticonvulsants may interact with the pill, so women should be aware (Seifer, Minkoff, & Merhi, 2015). Newer oral contraceptives have different dosing schedules and hormone combinations. Extended-cycle pills allow women to have fewer periods per year by taking active pills for months. Continuous-dosing pills eliminate the placebo week, allowing women to skip periods. The progestin-only pill is another option for women who cannot take estrogen for medical reasons. It is less effective than combination pills, but it is still effective when taken correctly. There are also non-hormonal contraception options for women. Barrier methods like condoms, diaphragms, and cervical caps prevent pregnancy without hormones. IUDs—hormonal and non-hormonal—are long-acting, effective contraceptives that last years.

4.11.3. Intrauterine Devices (IUDs)

Intrauterine devices, also known as IUDs, are extremely small devices that are shaped like a T and are inserted into the uterus by a medical professional (Figure 4.5).

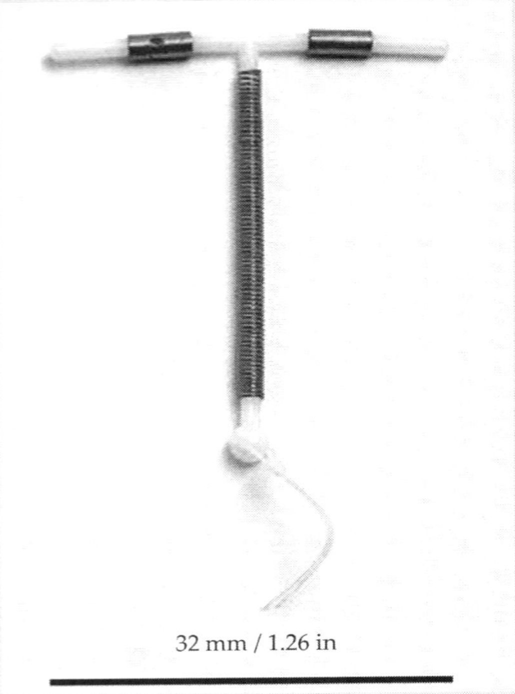

Figure 4.5. *Intrauterine devices (IUDs).*

Source: By User: Leia Wonder – File: Multiload-Gynefix-Paragard.jpg, CC BY-SA 4.0, https://commons.wikimedia.org/w/index.php?curid=62708770.

There are two primary categories of intrauterine devices (IUDs):

1. Hormonal intrauterine devices (IUDs) function by releasing progestin, a synthetic hormone that increases the viscosity of the cervical mucus and reduces the thickness of the uterine lining. This mechanism hinders the ability of sperm to reach and fertilize the egg.
2. Non-hormonal intrauterine devices (IUDs) consist of copper, which creates an unfavorable environment for sperm.

An important advantage of intrauterine devices (IUDs) is their high efficacy. Both hormonal and non-hormonal intrauterine devices (IUDs) exhibit a failure rate of less than 1%, rendering them highly dependable methods of contraception. An intrauterine device (IUD) can offer contraceptive protection for a duration of 3–10 years, depending on the specific type used. The enduring efficacy of intrauterine devices (IUDs) renders them an appealing choice for women seeking to circumvent the inconvenience of daily oral contraceptive pills or frequent visits to the pharmacy (Bailey, 2013). In addition to their effectiveness, IUDs are also highly convenient. Once inserted, an

IUD requires no maintenance or daily upkeep, unlike other forms of contraception that rely on regular use. This makes IUDs an ideal choice for women with busy lifestyles or those who may have difficulty remembering to take a pill every day. Furthermore, IUDs are reversible, meaning that fertility returns quickly after removal. This flexibility allows women to plan their pregnancies according to their own timeline.

- IUDs Have Drawbacks Despite Their Benefits:
  - Insertion may cause cramping, spotting, or menstrual bleeding in some women. Although mild and temporary, these side effects can worry some women.
  - IUD insertion may cause uterine perforation or device expulsion. These risks are rare and can be reduced by having a trained healthcare provider insert the IUD.

Women need accurate contraceptive information, including IUDs, to make reproductive health decisions. Healthcare providers should help women understand the pros and cons of various contraceptives and choose the one that best suits them. Furthermore, healthcare providers can empower women to make informed fertility decisions by openly discussing contraceptive options.

4.11.4. Condoms

There are two main types of condoms: male condoms and female condoms (Figure 4.6).

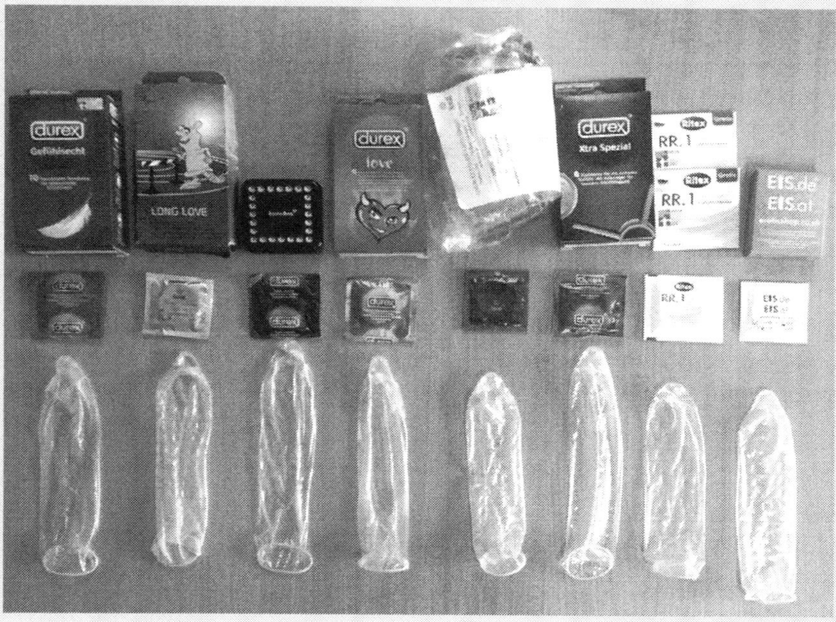

Figure 4.6. *Male condoms.*

Source: *https://hi.wikipedia.org/wiki/%E0%A4%9A%E0%A4%BF%E0%A4%A4%E0%A5%8D%E0%A4%B0:Overview_condoms_of_different_brands.jpg.*

The most common form of contraception is latex or polyurethane male condoms. They prevent sperm from entering the vagina by covering the penis during sexual activity. Pregnancy and STI prevention are excellent with male condoms. However, female condoms are less popular but have unique benefits. They are inserted into the vagina before sexual activity and are polyurethane or nitrile. Female condoms protect against pregnancy and STIs and give women more sexual health control. Since they don't need a partner, female condoms may be more comfortable for some women. Specialty condoms are available alongside traditional male and female condoms. Flavored, textured, and non-latex condoms are available for latex allergy sufferers. Specialist condoms can make sexual encounters more fun and exciting for both partners (Bailey, 2013). Choosing the right condom involves several factors.

- First, make sure the condom fits. A loose or tight condom may not prevent pregnancy or STIs.
- Checking the condom packaging's expiration date is important because expired condoms may not protect as well.
- Another factor is condom material. Latex condoms are the most popular and effective pregnancy and STI preventers. Latex-allergic people can use polyurethane or nitrile condoms. Your condom material must be safe and comfortable.

Choosing the right condom and using it correctly are both important. Condoms should be used every time you have sex, from start to finish. To properly put on and take off a condom, follow the packaging instructions. Condom misuse can reduce efficacy and increase pregnancy and STI risk.

Despite their effectiveness, condoms are not without drawbacks. For instance:

- Some people may find that condoms reduce sensitivity during sex, making it less pleasurable.
- Additionally, condoms can break or slip off during intercourse, which can lead to unintended pregnancy or STIs.

However, these risks can be minimized by using condoms correctly and consistently.

4.11.5. Diaphragms

A diaphragm is a concave, shallow cup made of silicone or latex that is inserted into the vagina prior to sexual intercourse in order to enclose the cervix and obstruct the passage of sperm towards the egg. It is a non-hormonal contraceptive method, which makes it a favored option for women who wish to evade hormonal birth control (Figure 4.7).

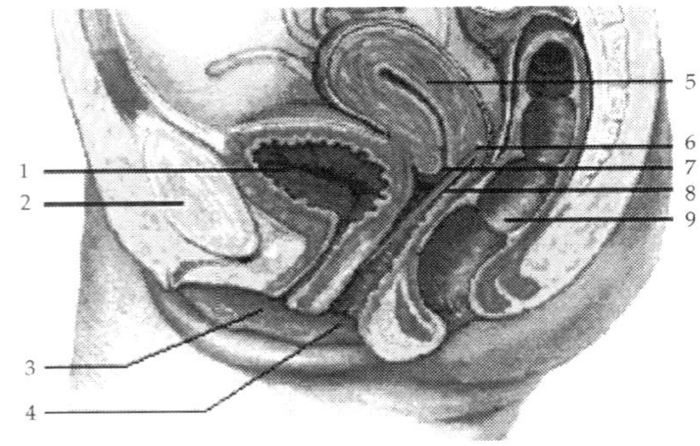

Figure 4.7. *Diaphragm birth control (8 in the figure).*

Source: *CC BY-SA 3.0, https://commons.wikimedia.org/w/index.php?curid=8759452.*

Diaphragms work well when used properly. When used with spermicide, the diaphragm fails 6% with perfect use and 12% with typical use. It is a reliable non-hormonal contraceptive option for women.

To allow sexual spontaneity, the diaphragm can be inserted hours before intercourse. The diaphragm does not need daily or monthly maintenance like the pill or patch (Bailey, 2013).

However, diaphragms have drawbacks:

- Its difficult to insert and remove
- Some women find diaphragms awkward or uncomfortable to use, and it may take practice.
- The diaphragm does not prevent STIs. Although it prevents pregnancy, it does not protect against STIs like HIV, gonorrhea, or chlamydia. To protect against STIs, women at risk should use a diaphragm and condoms.
- UTIs are another drawback of diaphragm use. Because the diaphragm covers the cervix, it can press on the bladder and urethra, allowing bacteria to enter and cause an infection. UTI-prone women may want to try alternative contraception.

Despite these drawbacks, many women prefer the diaphragm. It is safe and effective contraception without daily maintenance or hormonal manipulation. For hormone-free pregnancy prevention, the diaphragm can be effective with proper use and regular doctor visits.

4.11.6. Contraceptive Patches

The birth control patch is a diminutive, adhesive patch that is affixed to the skin and administers hormones into the bloodstream to avert pregnancy. The mechanism of action is analogous to that of birth control pills, with the key distinction being that instead of daily pill consumption, women only need to apply a fresh patch once a week for three consecutive weeks, followed by a week without any patch. This feature renders it a convenient alternative for women who may encounter challenges in recollecting to consume a pill on a daily basis (Wilson, 2002) (Figure 4.8).

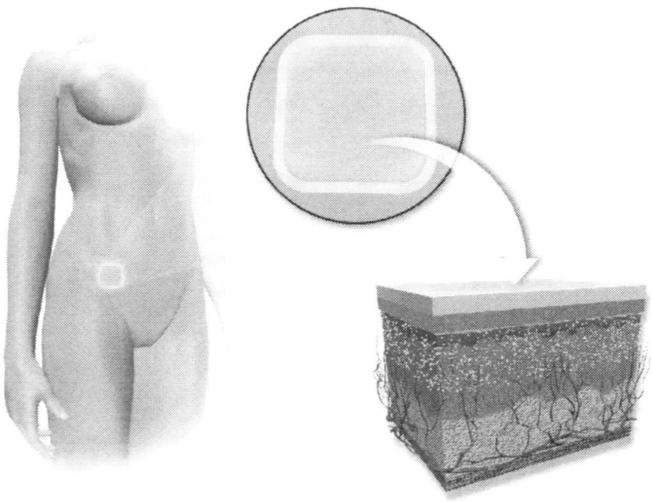

Figure 4.8. *The birth control patch.*

Source: By Bruce Blaus. When using this image in external sources it can be cited as: Blausen.com staff (2014). "Medical gallery of Blausen Medical 2014." WikiJournal of Medicine 1 (2). doi:10.15347/wjm/2014.010. ISSN 2002-4436. - Own work, CC BY 3.0, https://commons.wikimedia.org/w/index.php?curid=29600442.

There are several benefits to using the birth control patch.

- One of the main advantages is its effectiveness in preventing pregnancy when used correctly. The patch is over 99% effective at preventing pregnancy, making it one of the most reliable forms of contraception available.
- The patch can help regulate menstrual cycles, reduce menstrual cramps, and improve acne in some women.
- Another benefit of the birth control patch is its convenience. Once the patch is applied, women do not have to worry about taking a pill every day. This can be especially helpful for women with busy schedules or those who may have trouble remembering to take a pill at the same time every day.
- Additionally, the patch is discreet and can be worn under clothing, making it easy to use without drawing attention.

Despite its benefits, there are some potential drawbacks to using the birth control patch.

- Some women may experience side effects such as headaches, breast tenderness, or nausea while using the patch. These side effects are usually mild and tend to go away after a few months, but some women may find them bothersome.
- The patch does not protect against sexually transmitted infections (STIs), so women who are at risk for STIs should use condoms in addition to the patch.

It is important for women to talk to their healthcare provider before starting any form of birth control, including the patch. A healthcare provider can help determine if the patch is a suitable option based on a woman's medical history, lifestyle, and preferences. Additionally, a healthcare provider can provide information on how to use the patch correctly and what to do if a patch is accidentally removed or falls off.

4.11.7. Emergency Contraception

Emergency contraception is an essential choice for women who require immediate protection against unintended pregnancy. It is crucial for women to have knowledge about the different methods at their disposal and understand how each option functions.

1. **Morning-After Pill:** This pill contains hormones that prevent ovulation or fertilization of an egg. It is most effective when taken within 72 hours of unprotected sex, but can still be used up to five days after. The morning-after pill is available over-the-counter at most pharmacies, making it easily accessible for women in need.
2. **Emergency Contraception:** This is the copper intrauterine device (IUD). This device can be inserted by a healthcare provider up to five days after unprotected sex. The copper IUD works by creating an inhospitable environment for sperm, preventing fertilization. It is one of the most effective forms of emergency contraception, with a success rate of over 99%.
3. **Emergency Contraceptive Pills That Contain Ulipristal Acetate:** This type of pill works by delaying ovulation and is effective up

to five days after unprotected sex. Ulipristal acetate is available by prescription only, so women must visit a healthcare provider to obtain this form of emergency contraception.

It is important for women to be aware of the different options available to them and to choose the method that best fits their needs. Emergency contraception should not be used as a regular form of birth control, but rather as a backup option in case of emergency. Women should also be aware of the potential side effects of emergency contraception, which can include nausea, vomiting, and irregular bleeding (Wilson, 2002).

4.12. Family Planning Education for Women

Family planning education plays a crucial role in empowering women to make informed decisions about their reproductive health. By providing women with the necessary information and resources, family planning education can help them take control of their fertility and plan for a healthy and desired number of children.

4.12.1. Importance of Family Planning Education for Women

Family planning education plays a crucial role in empowering women to make informed decisions about their reproductive health and overall well-being. By providing women with the knowledge and resources they need to plan and space their pregnancies, family planning education can have a significant impact on their lives and the lives of their families.

- It allows women to take control of their fertility and make choices that are in line with their personal goals and aspirations. When women have access to information about contraception and family planning methods, they are better able to plan when and how many children they want to have. This can help them avoid unintended pregnancies, which can have a negative impact on their health, education, and economic opportunities.
- Family planning education can also help them space their pregnancies in a way that is beneficial for their health and the health of their children. According to research, spacing pregnancies at least two years apart can reduce the risk of maternal and infant mortality, as well as improve the overall health and well-being of both mother and child. By educating women about the importance of birth spacing, family planning education can help them make decisions that are in the best interest of their families.
- Family planning education can help women access the resources they need to plan and space their pregnancies effectively. This includes information about different contraceptive methods, as well as access to affordable and high-quality reproductive health services. By providing women with the tools they need to make informed choices about their reproductive health, family planning education can help them take control of their fertility and make decisions that are in line with their personal values and beliefs.
- Family planning education can help in promoting gender equality and women's empowerment. When women have access to information and resources that allow

them to make decisions about their reproductive health, they are better able to participate in society as equal members. By empowering women to take control of their fertility, family planning education can help them pursue their education, career, and other goals without the constraints of unintended pregnancies.

4.12.2. The Advantages of Spacing Pregnancies

When it comes to women's welfare and health, one of the most crucial aspects to consider is the spacing of pregnancies. This refers to the time interval between pregnancies, allowing a woman's body to recover fully before conceiving again. The benefits of spacing pregnancies are numerous and have a significant impact on both the mother and the child.

First and foremost, spacing pregnancies allows the mother's body to recover and replenish the nutrients that were depleted during the previous pregnancy. Pregnancy and childbirth take a toll on a woman's body, both physically and nutritionally. By spacing pregnancies, women can give their bodies the time they need to recover fully, ensuring that they are in optimal health before conceiving again. This, in turn, reduces the risk of complications during pregnancy and childbirth, leading to healthier outcomes for both the mother and the child (Wilson, 2002).

Furthermore, spacing pregnancies can help reduce the risk of maternal mortality. Women who become pregnant again too soon after giving birth are at a higher risk of complications such as pre-eclampsia, postpartum hemorrhage, and maternal mortality. By spacing pregnancies, women can reduce these risks and ensure that they are in the best possible health when they conceive again. This not only benefits the mother but also the child, as a healthy mother is more likely to have a healthy pregnancy and a healthy baby.

In addition to the physical benefits, spacing pregnancies can also have a positive impact on a woman's mental and emotional well-being. Pregnancy and childbirth are significant life events that can be both physically and emotionally draining. By spacing pregnancies, women can give themselves the time they need to recover emotionally and mentally, reducing the risk of postpartum depression and other mental health issues. This, in turn, can lead to better outcomes for both the mother and the child, as a mentally healthy mother is better able to care for her baby and herself.

Another important benefit of spacing pregnancies is the positive impact it can have on the child's health and development. Children born to mothers who have spaced their pregnancies are more likely to be born at a healthy weight and have better overall health outcomes. This is because a mother's body has had the time it needs to recover and replenish the nutrients necessary for a healthy pregnancy. Additionally, children born to mothers who have spaced their pregnancies are less likely to experience complications such as preterm birth and low birth weight, leading to better long-term health outcomes for the child.

Furthermore, spacing pregnancies can have a positive impact on a woman's socioeconomic status. Women who space their pregnancies are more likely to be able to continue their education and pursue career opportunities, leading to greater financial stability and independence. This, in turn, can benefit the entire family, as a financially stable mother is better able to provide for her children and ensure that they have access to the resources they need to thrive (Wilson, 2002).

4.12.3. Women Fertility Cycles

Given its importance in family planning and reproductive health, knowledge of fertility cycles is a critical component of women's health. The monthly process by which a woman's body gets ready for pregnancy is called the menstrual cycle, or fertility cycle. It begins with the release of an egg from the ovaries, which enters the uterus through the fallopian tubes. Pregnancy may arise from sperm fertilizing the egg. If not, during menstruation, the egg and uterine lining are shed together.

There are four main phases of the fertility cycle: menstruation, follicular phase, ovulation, and luteal phase., as shown below:

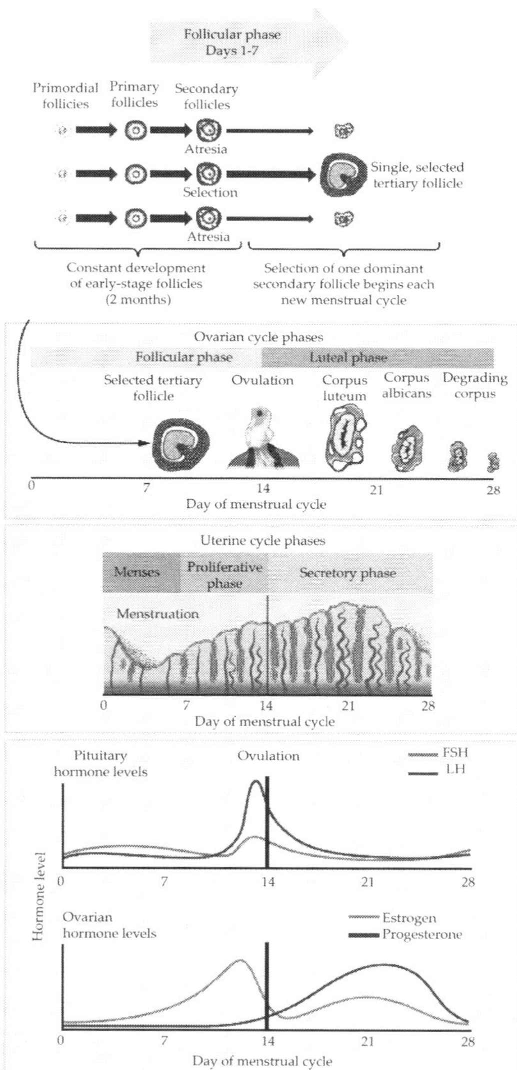

Source: By OpenStax College – Anatomy & Physiology, Connexions Web site. http://cnx.org/content/col11496/1.6/, Jun 19, 2013., CC BY 3.0, https://commons.wikimedia.org/w/index.php?curid=30148641.

Women who are trying to conceive or avoid getting pregnant should understand these stages of the fertility cycle. Women who monitor their menstrual cycles and physical changes can more accurately determine when they are most fertile and make plans accordingly.

Women can track their fertility cycles in several ways, such as by using ovulation predictor kits, tracking cervical mucus, and charting basal body temperature.

In addition to tracking fertility cycles, women should also prioritize their overall health and well-being. This includes maintaining a healthy diet, exercising regularly, getting enough sleep, and managing stress.

- Eating a balanced diet rich in fruits, vegetables, whole grains, and lean proteins can help support reproductive health. Regular exercise can help regulate hormones and improve overall well-being.
- Getting enough sleep is crucial for hormone regulation and overall health. Aim for 7–9 hours of quality sleep each night.
- Managing stress is also important for women's health. Chronic stress can disrupt hormone levels and affect fertility. Practice stress-reducing activities such as yoga, meditation, or deep breathing exercises.

4.12.4. Communicating with Partners

Effective communication about family planning options is crucial for women to make informed decisions about their reproductive health. This involves open and honest discussions about preferences, concerns, and desires, ensuring that partners understand their needs and help them make decisions that align with their values and aspirations. Couples can collaborate on designing a family plan that meets their shared goals, strengthening the relationship and promoting unity.

Good communication about family planning can prevent miscommunications and disputes, promoting harmony and understanding in the relationship. Women can assert their agency and autonomy in decision-making processes, leading to increased confidence and self-esteem. However, many women find it difficult to discuss family planning due to cultural norms, societal expectations, and personal beliefs. To overcome these obstacles, it is essential to foster an environment of support and nonjudgment in their relationships. This can involve scheduling specific times for conversations, paying attention to each other's viewpoints, and accepting each other's decisions and opinions.

Medical professionals are also essential in helping women communicate about family planning. They can provide resources, information, and advice on reproductive health and contraception, as well as counseling and other support services to help women navigate difficult conversations and make informed decisions. By creating an environment that values open communication and respect, women can overcome obstacles and make informed decisions about their reproductive health (Wilson, 2002).

4.12.5. Accessing Family Planning Resources

Access to family planning resources plays a significant role in empowering women to make informed decisions about their reproductive health.

Family planning resources encompass a range of services and information that enable women to plan and space their pregnancies, ultimately leading to healthier outcomes for both mothers and children. These resources include contraception methods, reproductive health education, counseling, and access to healthcare facilities (Bracke, 2022).

One of the key benefits of family planning is the ability to prevent unintended pregnancies. By having access to contraception methods, women can take control of their reproductive health and choose when to have children. This not only empowers women to make decisions about their future but also allows them to pursue their education and career goals without the added burden of an unplanned pregnancy.

Furthermore, family planning resources help in reducing maternal mortality rates. When women have access to quality reproductive health services, they are more likely to receive proper prenatal care and medical assistance during childbirth, leading to safer deliveries and healthier outcomes for both mothers and babies.

In addition to preventing unintended pregnancies and reducing maternal mortality rates, family planning resources also play a crucial role in promoting gender equality. When women can plan their pregnancies and access reproductive health services, they are more likely to participate in the workforce, pursue higher education, and engage in decision-making processes within their families and communities.

Despite the numerous benefits of family planning resources, many women around the world still face barriers to accessing these services. These barriers can be attributed to a lack of awareness, cultural norms, religious beliefs, financial constraints, and limited availability of healthcare facilities in rural areas.

To address these barriers and ensure that women have access to family planning resources, it is essential to implement comprehensive strategies that focus on education, advocacy, and policy change. By raising awareness about the importance of family planning and providing accurate information about contraception methods, women can make informed decisions about their reproductive health (Bracke, 2022).

Furthermore, advocacy efforts are needed to challenge harmful cultural norms and religious beliefs that may restrict women's access to family planning resources. By promoting gender equality and women's rights, societies can create an enabling environment where women are empowered to take control of their reproductive health.

Policy change is also crucial in ensuring that family planning resources are readily available and accessible to all women. Governments and international organizations must invest in healthcare infrastructure, train healthcare providers, and allocate resources to support family planning programs.

4.12.6. Addressing Cultural Beliefs Regarding Family Planning

In many societies, cultural beliefs play a significant role in shaping attitudes toward women's welfare and health, particularly when it comes to family planning. The way a society views family planning can have a direct impact on women's access to healthcare services and their overall well-being. It is important to pay specific attention to these cultural beliefs to ensure that women have the support and resources they need to make informed decisions about their reproductive health.

The cultural belief that mothers should come first can affect women's access to family planning. In some cultures, women are expected to have large families and may be stigmatized for having fewer children. Women may be afraid of judgment from their communities or families if they use contraception or other family planning services (Bracke, 2022).

Another cultural belief that can affect women's access to family planning is the idea that discussing reproductive health is taboo or inappropriate. In some cultures, talking openly about contraception or sexual health is seen as shameful, which can prevent women from seeking out the information and resources they need to make informed decisions about their bodies. This lack of education and support can have serious consequences for women's health, leading to unintended pregnancies or unsafe abortions.

We must challenge these cultural beliefs and encourage family planning acceptance. We can empower women to make healthy choices by providing accurate information about contraception and reproductive health and creating safe spaces for them to discuss these issues without judgment.

Cultural beliefs about family planning can be addressed through education and outreach. Together with community leaders, healthcare providers, and other stakeholders, we can dispel contraception and reproductive health myths. Other family planning services offered by these programs include contraception, counseling, and unintended pregnancy support.

In addition to education and outreach, it is important to involve men in conversations about family planning. In many cultures, men hold significant power and influence over women's reproductive choices, so it is crucial to engage them in discussions about contraception and family planning. By promoting gender equality and encouraging men to take an active role in supporting women's reproductive health, we can help to create a more supportive environment for women to make informed decisions about their bodies.

Additionally, women must have a variety of family planning options that meet their needs and preferences. This includes educating women about contraception and providing safe, affordable services. By providing options, we can help women find the best contraception for their needs (Bracke, 2022).

4.13. Fertility Awareness Methods

Fertility awareness is a method of natural family planning that involves tracking a woman's menstrual cycle to determine when she is most fertile. By monitoring changes in cervical mucus, basal body temperature, and other physical symptoms, women can identify their fertile window and either avoid or attempt to conceive during this time.

4.13.1. Monitoring the Process of Ovulation

Tracking ovulation is a crucial aspect of reproductive health, as it helps women understand their menstrual cycle and increases the chances of conception. By monitoring ovulation, women can also identify any irregularities in their cycle, which may indicate underlying health issues. Additionally, tracking ovulation can be a useful tool for family planning, whether a woman is trying to conceive or prevent pregnancy.

There are numerous benefits for tracking ovulation as listed below.

- It provides valuable insights into their menstrual cycle. Ovulation is the process by which an egg is released from the ovary, making it available for fertilization. By tracking ovulation, women can determine the most fertile days of their cycle, which is essential for conceiving.
- Understanding when ovulation occurs can also help women identify any irregularities in their cycle, such as irregular periods or missed periods, which may be indicative

of hormonal imbalances or other health issues.

- Tracking ovulation can also increase the chances of conception. By identifying the most fertile days of their cycle, women can time intercourse to coincide with ovulation, maximizing the likelihood of pregnancy. This is especially important for couples who are struggling to conceive, as tracking ovulation can help pinpoint the optimal time for conception.
- In some cases, tracking ovulation may even help identify potential fertility issues early on, allowing for timely intervention and treatment.
- Tracking ovulation can be a useful tool for family planning, whether a woman is trying to conceive or prevent pregnancy. For women who are trying to conceive, tracking ovulation can help them identify the best time to have intercourse and increase their chances of getting pregnant.
- For women who are looking to prevent pregnancy, tracking ovulation can help them identify their most fertile days and avoid intercourse during that time. This can be particularly helpful for women who are looking for a natural and non-hormonal method of birth control.

4.13.2. Techniques for Women to Monitor Ovulation

Various techniques are available for women to monitor ovulation, including basic tracking applications and more sophisticated fertility monitors.

4.13.2.1. Basal Body Temperature Method

By monitoring a woman's basal body temperature, one can ascertain her fertile and infertile days using the basal body temperature method, a natural family planning strategy. The term "basal body temperature" describes the body's resting temperature, which normally peaks during ovulation and falls out during sleep. Women can determine when they are most fertile and when they are most likely to ovulate by tracking changes in basal body temperature throughout the menstrual cycle (Wilson, 2002) (Figure 4.9).

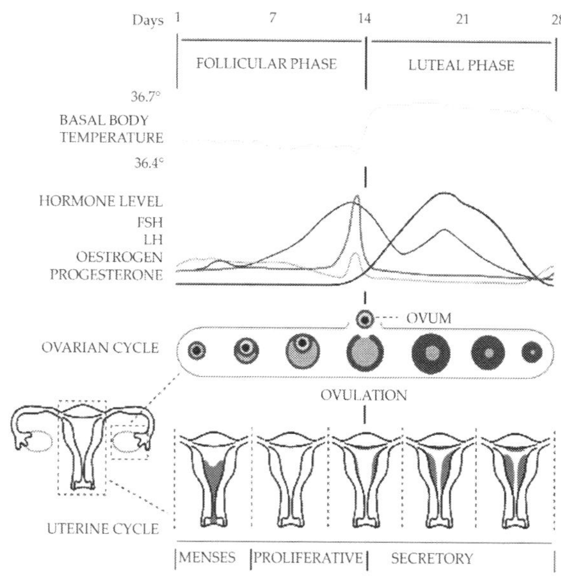

Figure 4.9. *The cycle.*

Source: By Isometrik, Kaldari; Begoon; Marnanel – Own work, CC BY-SA 3.0, https://commons.wikimedia.org/w/index.php?curid=148851325.

Women must take their temperature each morning before getting out of bed and record it on a chart to use the basal body temperature method effectively. Women can identify the days when they are most fertile by monitoring the slight rise in basal body temperature that occurs during ovulation. Depending on the woman's reproductive objectives, this information can then be utilized to either plan for or prevent pregnancy. One of the key benefits of the basal body temperature method is its non-invasiveness and lack of side effects. Unlike hormonal contraceptives or invasive procedures, the basal body temperature method relies on a woman's natural physiological signs to determine fertility. This makes it a safe and effective option for women who prefer a more natural approach to family planning (Wilson, 2002).

Additionally, the basal body temperature method can also be used to identify potential fertility issues. Consistently irregular temperature patterns or a lack of temperature rise after ovulation may indicate underlying health issues that could affect fertility. By monitoring these changes, women can gain valuable insights into their reproductive health and seek appropriate medical advice if needed.

It's crucial to remember that the basal body temperature method is not perfect and might not be appropriate for every individual. Inaccuracies in fertility prediction can result from variables that alter basal body temperature readings, including illness, stress, and irregular sleep patterns. Therefore, for extra protection, it is advised to combine the basal body temperature method with other methods of fertility awareness or barrier methods of contraception (Bailey, 2013).

To improve their understanding of their menstrual cycle, women can use fertility awareness techniques other than basal body temperature tracking. These could include using ovulation predictor kits, tracking menstrual cycles, and keeping an eye on changes in cervical mucus. By combining these methods, women can gain a more comprehensive picture of their fertility and make informed decisions about their reproductive health.

The basal body temperature method can be a useful tool for natural family planning if it is applied correctly and consistently. This approach encourages women to feel more agency and autonomy over their bodies by giving them the tools they need to take charge of their reproductive health. Because both partners can actively participate in tracking fertility and making family planning decisions, it also encourages communication and teamwork between partners (Wilson, 2002).

4.13.2.2. Cervical Mucus Method

Women's health and well-being are crucial aspects of overall family welfare. The ability to plan and space pregnancies can have a significant impact on the health and economic stability of families. Therefore, it is essential for women to have access to reliable and effective methods of family planning.

The cervical mucus method, which is categorized under fertility awareness methods, is one such technique. This technique uses variations in cervical mucus over the course of the menstrual cycle to track a woman's peak fertility. Women who are aware of these changes can determine when they are fertile and take appropriate action to either avoid or try pregnancy.

Women can naturally and non-invasively track their fertility with the cervical mucus method. Many women find it to be a safe option because it doesn't require the use of hormones or devices. Women can also feel more empowered with this method because it gives them the ability to take charge of their reproductive health and make educated decisions about family planning (Figure 4.10).

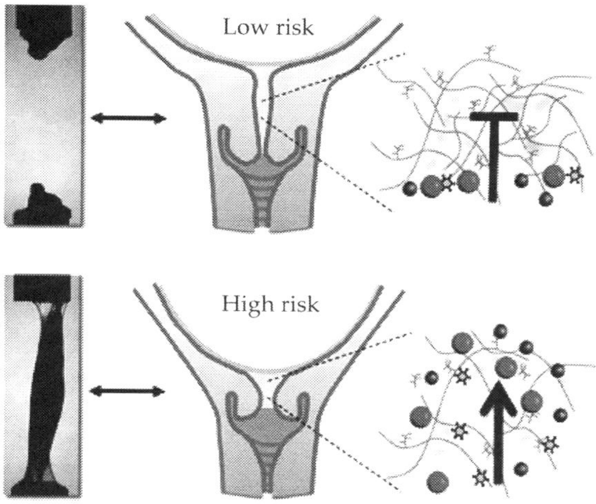

Figure 4.10. *Cervical mucus method.*

Source: By Critchfield AS, Yao G, Jaishankar A, Friedlander RS, Lieleg O, Doyle PS – Critchfield AS, Yao G, Jaishankar A, Friedlander RS, Lieleg O, Doyle PS, et al. (2013) Cervical Mucus Properties Stratify Risk for Preterm Birth. PLoS ONE 8(8): e69528, CC BY-SA 4.0, https://commons.wikimedia.org/w/index.php?curid=143483174.

To effectively use the cervical mucus method, women must first become familiar with the different types of cervical mucus and how they change throughout the menstrual cycle. Typically, cervical mucus will change from dry or sticky to creamy, watery, and then to egg -white consistency as ovulation approaches. By monitoring these changes, women can pinpoint the days when they are most likely to conceive.

It is important for women to track their cervical mucus consistently and accurately to maximize the effectiveness of this method. Keeping a daily journal or using a fertility tracking app can help women stay organized and ensure they are accurately recording their observations. Additionally, women should be aware of other factors that can affect cervical mucus, such as illness, stress, or medications, which may impact the reliability of this method (Bailey, 2013).

Although some women find the cervical mucus method to be a dependable method of family planning, it may not be appropriate for all women. The accuracy of this method can be impacted by variables like breastfeeding, irregular menstrual cycles, or specific medical conditions. Consequently, women must seek medical advice before depending exclusively on the cervical mucus method for conception or contraception.

The cervical mucus method is useful not only for family planning but also for keeping an eye on reproductive health. Variations in cervical mucus can reveal information about ovulatory problems, hormonal imbalances, and other medical conditions that may have an impact on fertility. Women who monitor these changes may be able to spot possible issues early and seek the right medical attention.

The cervical mucus method is not extensively taught or promoted in many healthcare settings, despite its many advantages. A deficiency in knowledge and instruction may hinder women's access to this beneficial method of family planning. To properly inform and assist their patients, healthcare professionals must be trained in fertility awareness techniques, such as the cervical mucus method (Wilson, 2002).

4.13.2.3. Calendar Method

The calendar method, also known as the rhythm method, is a natural family planning technique that involves tracking a woman's menstrual cycle to determine her fertile days. By understanding when ovulation occurs, couples can either avoid or plan intercourse accordingly to either prevent or achieve pregnancy (Figure 4.11).

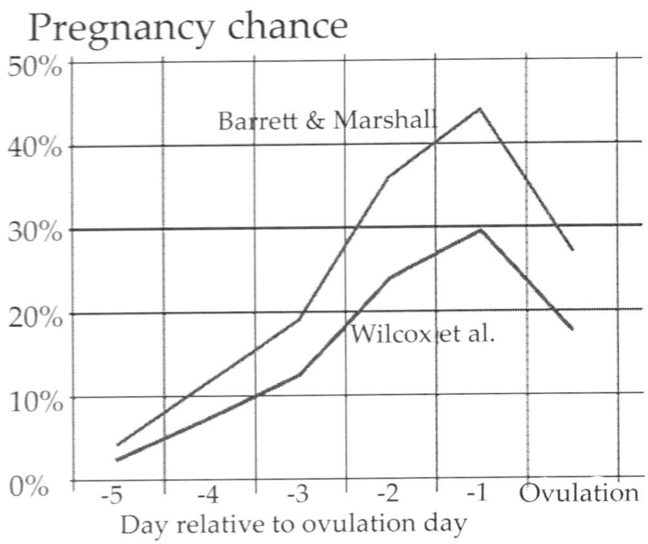

Figure 4.11. *Calendar method.*

Source: By Mikael Häggström – Own work, CC0, https://commons.wikimedia.org/w/index.php?curid=65008037.

The calendar method's accessibility and affordability are two of its main advantages. The calendar method of contraception is free of cost and side effects, in contrast to other methods like birth control pills or intrauterine devices. This makes it a desirable choice for partners seeking a safe, all-natural method of managing their fertility.

The calendar approach does, however, have certain drawbacks. It is predicated on the notion that a woman has a regular menstrual cycle, which not all women have. The duration of a woman's cycle can be influenced by a variety of factors, including stress, illness, and lifestyle modifications, making it challenging to precisely predict ovulation. Couples who are not in a mutually monogamous relationship may also need to think about other forms of protection, as the calendar method does not offer protection against STIs.

Even with these drawbacks, when applied properly, the calendar method can be a reliable method of birth control. According to studies, the calendar method can prevent pregnancy up to 95% of the time when used correctly. If the method is not consistently followed, there is a higher risk of an unintended pregnancy, as the typical use effectiveness rate is approximately 76% (Bailey, 2013).

In addition to its use as a contraceptive method, the calendar method can also be used to help couples achieve pregnancy. By tracking a woman's menstrual cycle, couples can identify the most fertile days and time for intercourse accordingly. This can be particularly helpful for couples who are struggling with infertility or who want to maximize their chances of conceiving.

When it comes to women's and family welfare, the calendar method can play a significant role in empowering women to take control of their reproductive health. By understanding their menstrual cycle and fertility patterns, women can make informed decisions about when to have children and when to avoid pregnancy. This can help to reduce the risk of unintended pregnancies and improve maternal and child health outcomes (Bailey, 2013).

Due to limited access to family planning services and contraception in many parts of the world, natural methods such as the calendar method are a valuable option for women. Healthcare providers can empower women to make decisions consistent with their reproductive goals by educating and supporting FAM techniques. Women's general health and well-being as well as the health of their families may benefit from this.

It is crucial to remember that there are numerous fertility awareness methods accessible to women, the calendar method being just one of them. In addition to providing more information about a woman's fertility, other techniques like basal body temperature tracking and cervical mucus monitoring can also improve the efficacy of natural family planning.

4.13.2.4. Symptothermal Method

The Symptothermal method is a natural family planning method that involves tracking a woman's fertility signs to determine her fertile and infertile days. This method relies on monitoring changes in basal body temperature, cervical mucus, and other symptoms to identify the most fertile time in a woman's menstrual cycle. By understanding these signs, women can effectively prevent or achieve pregnancy without the use of hormonal contraceptives.

The Symptothermal method is a valuable tool for promoting women's health and family welfare. By enabling women to comprehend and manage their fertility, this approach fosters body literacy and self-awareness. Women who use the Symptothermal method have a greater sense of awareness of their bodies and can recognize abnormalities or possible health problems earlier. This may result in the early identification and management of diseases like polycystic ovarian syndrome, thyroid issues, and hormone imbalances (Bailey, 2013).

Moreover, the symptothermal method encourages partners to communicate and work together. When using this method, couples have to collaborate to track fertility indicators and decide how to plan their family. This shared accountability can enhance mutual understanding, support, and relationship strength. Gender equality and shared decision-making in family planning are encouraged by the symptothermal method, which involves men in the process of fertility awareness.

Additionally, compared to hormonal contraceptives, the symptothermal method is more affordable and ecologically friendly. By using this method, women can avoid getting pregnant without the need for costly contraceptives or other devices. This can help women in underdeveloped nations or low-income communities have easier access to family planning. Additionally, women can lessen their exposure to synthetic hormones and any possible side effects by not using hormonal contraceptives.

Despite these benefits, the symptothermal method is not without its challenges. One of the main barriers to the widespread adoption of this method is the lack of awareness and education. Many women are not familiar with the symptothermal method or do not have access to accurate information about how to practice it effectively. This highlights the need for comprehensive education and training programs to promote fertility awareness and empower women to make informed choices about their reproductive health.

Another challenge is the stigma and misconceptions surrounding natural family planning methods. Some people mistakenly believe that the symptothermal method is unreliable or ineffective compared to hormonal contraceptives. However, research has shown that when practiced correctly, the symptothermal method can be just as effective as other forms of contraception. By dispelling myths and providing accurate information, we can help more women feel confident in using this method to manage their fertility (Wilson, 2002).

To overcome these challenges and promote the symptothermal method as a Fertility Awareness Method, we must take a multi-faceted approach. This includes funding courses and training programs for teachers, community leaders, and healthcare professionals. By providing these stakeholders with the necessary knowledge and abilities to raise awareness about fertility, we can accurately inform more women and families about the symptothermal method.

Furthermore, in order to prove the efficacy and security of the symptothermal method, we need to give research and evidence-based practices a top priority. We can make a compelling case for this method's inclusion in family planning programs and policies by carrying out research and gathering data on the results of utilizing it. It will be necessary for advocates, legislators, and researchers to work together to make sure that the symptothermal method is accepted as a good choice for working mothers and their families.

4.13.2.5. Standard Days Method

The Standard Days Method is a type of natural family planning that can be used by women to track their menstrual cycles and determine their fertile days. This method is based on the fact that most women have a menstrual cycle that lasts between 26 and 32 days, with ovulation typically occurring around day 14. By tracking their cycles and avoiding unprotected sex during their fertile window, women can effectively prevent unwanted pregnancies.

To ascertain the duration of their cycles and determine their fertile days, women using the Standard Days Method must monitor their menstrual cycles for a few months. Day 1 of the menstrual cycle is the first day of the menstrual period, and days 8 through 19 are thought to comprise the fertile window. Women are advised to either avoid having sex during this time or use barrier contraception, like condoms, to avoid getting pregnant.

The Standard Days Method's non-invasive, hormone-free method of contraception is one of its main advantages. This makes it a desirable choice for women who would rather use a more natural method of family planning or who are worried about the negative effects of hormonal contraceptives. Women who are attempting to conceive can also use the Standard Days Method, as it can help them determine the most fertile days of their cycle and improve their odds of getting pregnant.

It's crucial to remember that the Standard Days Method is not infallible and might not be appropriate for every woman. Women who can accurately track their cycles and have regular menstrual cycles are the ones who benefit from it the most. This method may not be suitable for women who have irregular cycles or medical conditions that impact their fertility (Bailey, 2013).

Like all forms of natural family planning, the success of the Standard Days Method relies heavily on the commitment and cooperation of both partners. It is important for couples to communicate openly and honestly about their intentions and to work together to ensure that they are following the method correctly. Additionally, women who are using the Standard

Days Method should be prepared for the possibility of an unplanned pregnancy and have a plan in place in case their method fails.

4.13.2.6. Two-Day Method

The Two-Day Method is a simple and effective Fertility Awareness Method (FAM) that can be used by women to monitor their fertility status based on cervical secretions.

With this approach, a daily check is made to determine whether cervical secretions are present or absent. After wiping, women are advised to check for secretions by feeling the opening in their vagina or by looking at the toilet paper. On any given day, if secretions are seen, the woman is deemed fertile. The woman is deemed infertile if there are no secretions for two days in a row. This approach is predicated on the knowledge that cervical secretions undergo volume and consistency changes during the menstrual cycle, with the most fertile secretions being transparent, elastic, and slick.

Research has demonstrated that, when applied appropriately, the Two-Day Method can be a dependable method of natural family planning. Its efficacy as a FAM has been examined in a variety of contexts. The Two-Day Method has a perfect use effectiveness rate of 96.3% and a typical use effectiveness rate of 89.4%, according to a study done in the Philippines. These rates are in line with other FAMs, including the Symptothermal Method and the Standard Days Method (Bailey, 2013).

The Two-Day Method is not only very effective but also inexpensive and non-invasive, with women being able to learn it with ease in a range of contexts. This makes it an important tool for advancing the welfare of women and their families, particularly in areas with limited resources where access to contemporary contraceptive methods may be restricted. The Two-Day Method gives women the tools to track and understand their fertility cycles, enabling them to plan pregnancies following their preferences and make educated decisions about their reproductive health. Women who are attempting to conceive can also use the Two-Day Method. Women can determine when they are most fertile and schedule sexual activity to maximize their chances of becoming pregnant by keeping an eye on their cervical secretions. The ability to track ovulation naturally and non-invasively can be especially useful for women who have irregular cycles or other fertility problems, as it increases the likelihood of conception.

However, it is important to note that the Two-Day Method, like all FAMs, requires a certain level of commitment and consistency to be effective. Women must be diligent in tracking their cervical secretions every day and following the guidelines for determining fertility status. Additionally, the Two-Day Method may not be suitable for women with certain health conditions or irregular menstrual cycles, as it relies on the presence or absence of cervical secretions to determine fertility status (Wilson, 2002).

4.14. Safe Abortion Services

Abortion is a sensitive and complex issue that requires careful consideration of legal, medical, and ethical factors. When it comes to women's health and well-being, safe abortion services are essential to ensure that women have access to the care they need in a supportive and non-judgmental environment (Bracke, 2022).

4.14.1. Legal Considerations for Abortion

In many countries, abortion is legal under certain circumstances, such as when the woman's life is at risk, in cases of rape or incest, or when the fetus has severe abnormalities. It is important for women to be aware of their rights and the legal framework surrounding abortion in their country to ensure they can access safe and legal services (Bracke, 2022).

4.14.2. Types of Abortion Procedures

There are two main types of abortion procedures: medical abortion and surgical abortion. Medical abortion involves taking medication to induce a miscarriage, while surgical abortion involves a procedure to remove the fetus from the uterus.

Both medical and surgical abortion are safe and effective methods of terminating a pregnancy. The choice between the two methods will depend on factors such as how far along the pregnancy is, the woman's medical history, and her personal preferences. Medical abortion may be preferred by some women because it can be done at home and does not require a surgical procedure, while surgical abortion may be recommended in certain situations, such as if the pregnancy is further along or if there are medical complications.

4.14.3. Post-Abortion Care

After an abortion, it is important for women to receive appropriate post-abortion care to ensure their physical and emotional well-being. This may include follow-up appointments with a healthcare provider, counseling, and access to support services. Women should be informed about what to expect after an abortion and how to care for themselves during the recovery process.

4.14.4. Counselling and Support for Women Seeking Abortion

Women who are considering an abortion may benefit from counseling and support to help them make an informed decision and cope with any emotional challenges they may face. Counselling can provide women with a safe space to express their feelings, ask questions, and explore their options. Support services can also help women access practical assistance, such as transportation to and from appointments or financial assistance.

4.14.5. Addressing Stigma Around Abortion

One of the biggest barriers to accessing safe abortion services is the stigma and shame that is often associated with abortion. It is important to challenge these negative attitudes and create a supportive and non-judgmental environment for women who are seeking abortion care. This may involve educating the public about the realities of abortion, promoting open and honest discussions about reproductive health, and providing resources for women who are facing stigma.

4.14.6. Accessing Abortion Services

Access to safe abortion services is essential for women's health and well-being. Women should be able to access abortion care in a timely and affordable manner, without facing unnecessary barriers or restrictions. This may involve ensuring that healthcare providers are trained and equipped to provide abortion services, that facilities are safe and hygienic, and that women are treated with respect and dignity throughout the process.

4.15. Promoting Optimal Pregnancies

A woman's pregnancy is a unique period in her life that calls for extra consideration and care. Pregnancy health is crucial for the mother's and the unborn child's welfare. There are various aspects of women and family welfare during pregnancy, including prenatal care, nutrition, exercise, managing discomforts, screening tests, preparing for labor and delivery, and postpartum support for new mothers.

Throughout pregnancy, prenatal care is essential for keeping an eye on the mother's and the unborn child's health. Frequent prenatal visits with a medical professional can help identify any possible problems early on and guarantee the health of the mother and unborn child. To track the baby's growth and development, physical examinations, ultrasounds, and blood tests may be part of these check-ups.

A healthy pregnancy is largely supported by nutrition. Consuming a diet rich in whole grains, lean meats, fruits, and vegetables will help guarantee that mother and child are getting all the nutrients they require. Prenatal vitamins are also essential as they can supplement the diet and promote the growth of the unborn child.

Maintaining a healthy pregnancy also requires exercise during pregnancy. The majority of women can safely participate in low-impact activities like walking, swimming, and prenatal yoga, though it's still important to speak with a healthcare professional before beginning any exercise program. Maintaining an active lifestyle during pregnancy can enhance circulation, lower stress levels, and lower the risk of gestational diabetes.

Managing pregnancy discomforts is another important aspect of women and family welfare during pregnancy. Common pregnancy discomforts like nausea, exhaustion, and back pain affect a lot of women. It's crucial to discuss management options for these discomforts with a healthcare professional. These options may include medication, lifestyle modifications, or other therapies.

Pregnancy screening tests are essential for identifying any possible problems that could compromise the mother's or the unborn child's health. Blood tests, ultrasounds, and other diagnostic procedures to check for genetic disorders, preeclampsia, gestational diabetes, and other conditions may be part of this testing regimen. Making sure that mother and child receive the care they require can be facilitated by early detection of these issues.

Pregnancy-related preparation for labor and delivery is crucial for the wellbeing of pregnant women and their families. It's critical to create a birth plan that details preferences for pain management, labor positions, and other labor and delivery-related topics after discussing birth preferences with a healthcare professional. Attending childbirth education classes is also essential if you want to learn about the labor process and how to handle pain and discomfort.

For new mothers to transition to motherhood smoothly, postpartum support is crucial. After giving birth, a lot of new mothers go through a range of emotions, such as happiness, sadness, and anxiety. It's critical to ask for help during this period from medical professionals, relatives, and friends. Assistance with caring for the newborn, mental health counseling, and lactation support are examples of postpartum support.

4.16. Care after Childbirth

Postpartum care is an essential component of women's health and the well-being of their families. Postnatal care is the term used to describe the care and support given to a woman following childbirth. The postnatal period, also referred to as the puerperium, is a phase characterized by notable physiological and psychological transformations in women. Ensuring adequate postpartum care is crucial for the overall welfare of both the mother and the newborn.

There are several components of postpartum care. These include postpartum contraception options, physical recovery after childbirth, emotional well-being postpartum, breastfeeding and contraception, family planning after childbirth, postpartum check-ups, and contraception options for women with medical conditions (Seifer, Minkoff, & Merhi, 2015).

Postpartum contraception options are important for women who have recently given birth. It is crucial to discuss with your healthcare provider the best method of contraception for you, taking into consideration factors such as breastfeeding, medical history, and personal preferences. Some common options include birth control pills, intrauterine devices (IUDs), contraceptive injections, and barrier methods like condoms.

Physical recovery after childbirth is a gradual process that can take several weeks. It is important to rest, eat well, and stay hydrated to aid in your recovery. Gentle exercises, such as walking or pelvic floor exercises, can also help strengthen your muscles and speed up the healing process. It is normal to experience discomfort and bleeding in the days and weeks following childbirth, but if you have severe pain or excessive bleeding, be sure to contact your healthcare provider.

Emotional well-being postpartum is just as important as physical recovery. Many women experience a range of emotions after giving birth, including joy, sadness, anxiety, and overwhelm. It is normal to feel a mix of emotions during this time, but if you are feeling overwhelmed or unable to cope, it is important to seek help from a healthcare provider or mental health professional.

Breastfeeding and contraception are closely linked, as some contraceptive methods can affect milk supply. It is important to discuss with your healthcare provider which contraception options are safe to use while breastfeeding. Barrier methods like condoms are often recommended for breastfeeding mothers, as they do not interfere with milk production.

Family planning after childbirth is an important consideration for many women. It is important to discuss with your partner and healthcare provider your plans for future pregnancies and the spacing of children. Family planning can help you achieve your reproductive goals and ensure that you have the support and resources you need for your family (Seifer, Minkoff, & Merhi, 2015).

Postpartum check-ups are essential for monitoring your health and well-being after childbirth. Your healthcare provider will likely schedule a follow-up appointment to check on your physical recovery, discuss any emotional concerns, and guide contraception and family planning. It is important to attend these check-ups to ensure that you are on track for a healthy postpartum recovery.

Contraception options for women with medical conditions may vary depending on the condition and individual circumstances. It is important to discuss with your healthcare provider the best contraceptive method for you, taking into consideration any medical conditions or medications you may be taking. Some contraceptive methods may not be suitable for women with certain medical conditions, so it is important to explore all options and find the best fit for your health and well-being.

By discussing postpartum contraception options, physical recovery, emotional well-being, breastfeeding, family planning, postpartum check-ups, and contraception for women with medical conditions, we can better support women during this important time in their lives. It is important to seek guidance from healthcare providers and mental health professionals to ensure a healthy and successful postpartum recovery (Seifer, Minkoff, & Merhi, 2015).

4.17. Birth Control Myths and Facts

There are numerous myths about birth control. One prevalent myth is that birth control pills make you gain weight. While some individuals may experience slight weight fluctuations, studies have shown that most women do not gain weight because of taking birth control pills. Another myth is that birth control is only for preventing pregnancy. While birth control is indeed an effective method of preventing pregnancy, it also offers numerous other benefits, such as regulating menstrual cycles, reducing acne, and managing symptoms of conditions like endometriosis (Wilson, 2002).

One common misconception about contraception is that using birth control will make it harder to get pregnant in the future. In fact, most forms of birth control do not have a long-term impact on fertility, and individuals can typically conceive shortly after discontinuing the use of contraception. Another misconception is that birth control is only for women. While many forms of birth control are designed for women, there are also options available for men, such as condoms and vasectomies.

It's important to understand that no form of birth control is 100% effective, but when used correctly, most methods are highly reliable. For example, birth control pills have a failure rate of less than 1% when taken consistently and correctly. Additionally, long-acting reversible contraceptives (LARCs) like IUDs and implants are over 99% effective at preventing pregnancy, making them some of the most reliable forms of contraception available.

It's essential to recognize that different individuals may experience varying side effects when using contraception. Common side effects of birth control pills can include nausea, headaches, and mood changes, but these symptoms typically subside after a few months as the body adjusts to the hormones. It's important to speak with a healthcare provider if you experience severe or persistent side effects while using birth control, as they may be able to recommend a different method that better suits your needs.

Beyond preventing pregnancy, birth control offers a range of additional benefits. For example, hormonal birth control can help regulate menstrual cycles, reduce the severity of menstrual cramps, and improve acne. In some cases, birth control may also be prescribed to manage symptoms of conditions like polycystic ovary syndrome (PCOS) or endometriosis. By discussing your individual health needs and concerns with a healthcare provider, you can determine which form of birth control may offer the most benefits for you (Wilson, 2002).

When it comes to choosing the right birth control method, there are several factors to consider. These may include your lifestyle, medical history, and preferences regarding convenience and effectiveness. Some individuals may prefer a low-maintenance option like an IUD or implant, while others may opt for a method that allows for more flexibility, such as birth control pills or condoms. By discussing your options with a healthcare provider, you can make an informed decision about which form of contraception is best suited to your needs.

Some individuals worry that using birth control for an extended period may have negative effects on their health. While all forms of contraception come with potential risks and side effects, most individuals can safely use birth control for many years without experiencing any adverse consequences. Regular check-ups with a healthcare provider can help monitor your health while using birth control and ensure that any potential issues are addressed promptly (Wilson, 2002).

4.18. Reproductive Rights and Access

Access to reproductive healthcare is a fundamental human right. One of these rights is the freedom to make decisions regarding one's own body, such as whether or not to have children and if so, when and how many. Even with the legal safeguards in place, many women still encounter obstacles when attempting to obtain reproductive healthcare services (Bracke, 2022).

The scarcity and high cost of reproductive healthcare services constitute major obstacles to accessing it. Reproductive healthcare services are not widely available in many parts of the world, particularly in low-income areas. This might be the result of a shortage of medical facilities, qualified personnel, or funding. Many women consequently lack access to crucial reproductive healthcare services, including safe abortion procedures, family planning, and prenatal care.

The stigma and discrimination that many women experience when seeking reproductive healthcare services is another obstacle to accessing these services. Women who seek reproductive healthcare services—particularly those about abortion—frequently encounter criticism and disapproval from their peers, medical professionals, and even relatives. This stigma may keep women from getting the care they require, which could have detrimental effects on their health and general wellbeing.

To remove these obstacles and guarantee that all women have access to the healthcare services they require, advocacy for reproductive rights is essential. Promoting access to reproductive healthcare services for all women, fighting discriminatory laws and policies, and increasing public awareness of reproductive rights are the goals of advocates. We can guarantee that women have the freedom to make decisions about their own bodies and have access to the care they require to live healthy lives by fighting for reproductive rights (Bracke, 2022).

Beyond individual rights, reproductive justice is a framework that prioritizes the group welfare of marginalized communities. The goal of reproductive justice is to defend everyone's right to procreate, refrain from procreating, and raise their children in secure and healthful environments. This framework seeks to address the intersecting oppressions of race, class, and gender while acknowledging the connections between reproductive rights and other social justice issues.

A crucial aspect of reproductive rights is ensuring access to contraception, which is necessary for giving women the agency to make decisions about their own bodies. Women can plan their pregnancies, space out their kids, and avoid unplanned pregnancies by using contraception. For marginalized communities, who might encounter additional obstacles in accessing reproductive healthcare services, access to contraception is especially crucial.

Reproductive rights have a substantial effect on public health. Women who have access to reproductive healthcare services are more likely to plan their families in a way that best suits them, as well as to have healthy pregnancies and deliveries. This may result in decreased rates of unwanted pregnancies, better outcomes for the health of mothers and their children, and lower rates of maternal mortality.

Diverse national and international viewpoints exist regarding reproductive rights. While some nations offer comprehensive reproductive healthcare services and protections, others have laws and policies that restrict women's access to care. Mother mortality rates are lower, women have greater access to healthcare services, and contraceptive use is more common in nations where reproductive rights are upheld and supported. However, women may encounter major obstacles to receiving care and may be more vulnerable to unfavorable health outcomes in nations where reproductive rights are restricted (Bracke, 2022).

4.19. Advocating for Comprehensive Family Planning Services

Comprehensive family planning services play a crucial role in promoting women's health and well-being, as well as ensuring the overall welfare of families. By providing access to a range of contraceptive methods and reproductive health services, comprehensive family planning programs empower individuals to make informed decisions about their reproductive futures. This not only helps to prevent unintended pregnancies but also allows individuals to space and time their pregnancies according to their own preferences and circumstances.

Funding for family planning programs is essential to ensure that individuals have access to the services they need. Adequate funding can help to expand the availability of contraceptive methods, improve the quality of care provided, and reach underserved populations. By investing in family planning programs, policymakers can help to reduce healthcare costs associated with unintended pregnancies and improve the overall health and well-being of women and families (Shartzer & Johnston, 2016).

Integrating family planning into healthcare services is another important step in ensuring that individuals have access to comprehensive family planning services. By incorporating family planning into routine healthcare visits, healthcare providers can help individuals to make informed decisions about their reproductive health and access the services they need. This can help to reduce unintended pregnancies, improve maternal and child health outcomes, and promote overall well-being.

Addressing disparities in family planning access is crucial to ensuring that all individuals have access to the services they need. Disparities in access to family planning services can be influenced by factors such as income, education, geography, and race. By targeting resources to underserved populations and addressing barriers to access, policymakers can help to ensure that all individuals have access to comprehensive family planning services.

Educating policymakers on the benefits of family planning is essential to garnering support for comprehensive family planning programs. By highlighting the positive impact of family planning on women's health, economic empowerment, and overall well-being, advocates can help to build a strong case for investing in family planning programs. Educating policymakers on the cost-effectiveness of family planning services can also help to demonstrate the long-term benefits of investing in these programs (Shartzer & Johnston, 2016).

Advocacy strategies for promoting family planning services can include engaging with policymakers, building coalitions with like-minded organizations, and mobilizing grassroots support. By working together to raise awareness about the importance of family planning, advocates can help to build support for policies that expand access to these services. By leveraging the power of storytelling and personal experiences, advocates can help to humanize the issue of family planning and demonstrate its impact on individuals and families.

Collaborating with community organizations is another key strategy for improving access to family planning services. By partnering with local organizations that serve underserved populations, advocates can help to reach individuals who may not have access to traditional healthcare services. Community organizations can also provide valuable insights into the unique needs and challenges faced by their communities, helping to inform the development of targeted family planning programs.

By investing in family planning programs, integrating family planning into healthcare services, addressing disparities in access, educating policymakers, and collaborating with community organizations, advocates can help to expand access to these critical services. By working together to promote the importance of family planning, advocates can help empower individuals to make informed decisions about their reproductive health and improve the health and well-being of women and families (Shartzer & Johnston, 2016).

A Closer Look

Family Planning

Family planning plays a crucial role in ensuring the well-being of families and communities by enabling individuals to make informed decisions about the timing and number of children they have. It encompasses a range of methods and strategies designed to help people manage their reproductive health, including contraceptive options, fertility awareness, and access to reproductive health education. By providing individuals with the tools and knowledge needed to plan their pregnancies, family planning helps to promote healthier pregnancies, reduce unintended pregnancies, and improve maternal and child health outcomes.

Access to family planning services can also have profound socio-economic benefits. For instance, when women and couples can plan their families, they are better able to invest in their children's education and well-being, which can contribute to breaking the cycle of poverty. Furthermore, family planning supports gender equality by empowering women to make decisions about their reproductive health, allowing them to pursue education and career opportunities on their terms.

Despite its benefits, access to family planning services can be uneven, with disparities often linked to geographic, economic, and social factors. Addressing these disparities requires a multifaceted approach that includes improving access to affordable and effective contraceptive methods, enhancing educational outreach, and ensuring that family planning services are culturally sensitive and accessible to all.

Summary

This chapter covers the unique health challenges faced by women, emphasizing the importance of understanding their bodies and advocating for their well-being.

It explores the biological, social, and cultural factors that influence women's health across the lifespan, from adolescence to menopause and beyond. It discusses common issues such as reproductive health, mental health, and chronic diseases, highlighting the need for personalized care and proactive health management.

The chapter also addresses the significance of education, access to healthcare, and supportive environments in empowering women to make informed decisions about their health.

Recognizing the diverse needs of women and promoting a holistic approach to healthcare, this chapter aims to inspire women to take charge of their health and lead healthier, more fulfilling lives.

References

1. World Health Organization. Health in 2015: from MDGs to SDGs. 2015. http://apps.who.int/iris/bitstream/10665/200009/1/9789241565110_eng.pdf?ua=1 (accessed 22 July 2024).
2. World Health Organization. Global Health Estimates 2014 Summary Tables. 2014. http://www.who.int/healthinfo/global_burden_disease/estimates/en/index1.html (accessed 22 July 2024).
3. Norton R, Peters S, Jha V et al.. Women's health: a new global agenda. Oxford: Oxford Martin School, 2016.
4. Secretary-General UN. Global strategy for women's and children's health. New York: The Partnership for Maternal, Newborn and Child Health, 2010.
5. Every Women Every Child. Saving lives protecting futures. Progress report on the global strategy for women's and children's health 2010–2015. New York: Every women Every Child, 2015.
6. Desalegn H, Solberg E, Kim JY. The Global Financing Facility: country investments for every woman, adolescent, and child. Lancet 2015;386:105–6. 10.1016/S0140-6736(15)61224-7
7. Every Women Every Child. The global strategy for women's, children's and adolescents' health (2016–2030). New York: Every Women Every Child, 2015.
8. United Nations. Sustainable Development Goals: 17 goals to transform our world. http://www.un.org/sustainabledevelopment/sustainable-development-goals/ (accessed 22 July 2024).
9. World Health Organization. Special theme: women's health beyond reproduction—a new agenda. Bull World Health Organ 2015;91:621–715.
10. Langer A, Meleis A, Knaul FM et al.. Women and health: the key for sustainable development. Lancet 2015;386:1165–210. 10.1016/S0140-6736(15)60497-4
11. Melloni C, Berger JS, Wang TY et al.. Representation of women in randomized clinical trials of cardiovascular disease prevention. Circ Cardiovasc Qual Outcomes 2010;3:135–42. 10.1161/CIRCOUTCOMES.110.868307
12. US Government Accountability Office. Drug Safety: Most Drugs Withdrawn in Recent Years Had Greater Health Risks for Women. 2001. http://www.gao.gov/new.items/d01286r.pdf

13. Gupta A, Lampropulos JF, Bikdeli B et al.. Most important outcomes research papers on cardiovascular disease in women. Circ Cardiovasc Qual Outcomes 2013;6:e1–7. 10.1161/CIRCOUTCOMES.112.970202
14. Mosca L, Barrett-Connor E, Wenger NK. Sex/gender differences in cardiovascular disease prevention: what a difference a decade makes. Circulation 2011;124:2145–54. 10.1161/CIRCULATIONAHA.110.968792
15. Mosca L, Benjamin EJ, Berra K et al.. Effectiveness-based guidelines for the prevention of cardiovascular disease in women—2011 update: a guideline from the American Heart Association. J Am Coll Cardiol 2011;57:1404–23. 10.1016/j.jacc.2011.02.005
16. Leening MJ, Ferket BS, Steyerberg EW et al.. Sex differences in lifetime risk and first manifestation of cardiovascular disease: prospective population based cohort study. BMJ 2014;349:g5992.
17. George J, Rapsomaniki E, Pujades-Rodriguez M et al.. How does cardiovascular disease first present in women and men? Incidence of 12 cardiovascular diseases in a contemporary cohort of 1,937,360 People. Circulation 2015;132:1320–8. 10.1161/CIRCULATIONAHA.114.013797
18. Anderson RD, Pepine CJ. Gender differences in the treatment for acute myocardial infarction: bias or biology? Circulation 2007;115:823–6. 10.1161/CIRCULATIONAHA.106.685859
19. Cabana MD, Kim C. Physician adherence to preventive cardiology guidelines for women. Womens Health Issues 2003;13:142–9.
20. Humphries KH, Pu A, Gao M et al.. Angina with "normal" coronary arteries: sex differences in outcomes. Am Heart J 2008;155:375–81. 10.1016/j.ahj.2007.10.019
21. Huxley RR, Woodward M. Cigarette smoking as a risk factor for coronary heart disease in women compared with men: a systematic review and meta-analysis of prospective cohort studies. Lancet 2011;378:1297–305. 10.1016/S0140-6736(11)60781-2
22. Peters SA, Huxley RR, Woodward M. Diabetes as risk factor for incident coronary heart disease in women compared with men: a systematic review and meta-analysis of 64 cohorts including 858,507 individuals and 28,203 coronary events. Diabetologia 2014;57:1542–51. 10.1007/s00125-014-3260-6
23. Peters SA, Huxley RR, Woodward M. Diabetes as a risk factor for stroke in women compared with men: a systematic review and meta-analysis of 64 cohorts, including 775,385 individuals and 12,539 strokes. Lancet 2014;383:1973–80. 10.1016/S0140-6736(14)60040-4

Chapter 5

IMPROVING MATERNAL AND CHILD HEALTH THROUGH INTEGRATED HEALTHCARE SERVICES

Contents

Introduction

Women and family welfare are vital components of public health, with an emphasis on advancing the health and happiness of women and children. Maternal and Child Health (MCH) is a significant focus within this field, to enhance the well-being of mothers and children through diverse interventions and programs. MCH services encompass a broad array of activities, which include prenatal care.

Postnatal care refers to the medical attention and support provided to a woman and her newborn baby after childbirth. Immunizations and nutrition programs, among other services, are provided.

These services are crucial in reducing maternal and child mortality rates, as well as fostering optimal growth and development.

Maternal and child health (MCH) programs mitigate the occurrence of complications during pregnancy and childbirth, enhance the growth and development of children, and enhance the overall health of women and their families by delivering high-quality healthcare services.

Orientation and Directional Terms

Term	Definition	Illustration
Fetal Development	The process of growth and maturation of the fetus during pregnancy, from conception to birth.	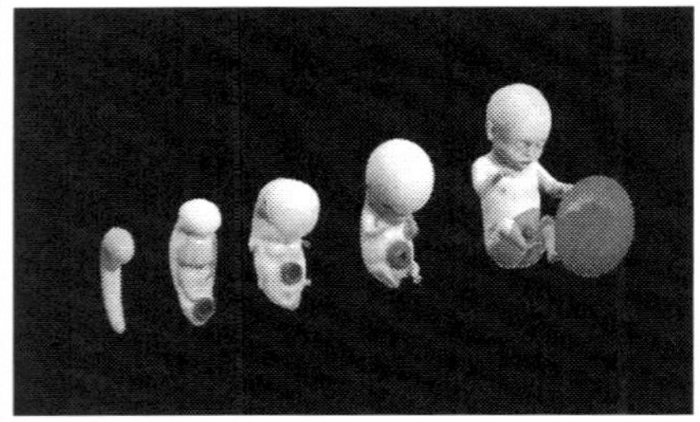
Genetic Testing	A medical test that analyzes DNA to identify changes or mutations in genes that could indicate a genetic disorder or risk.	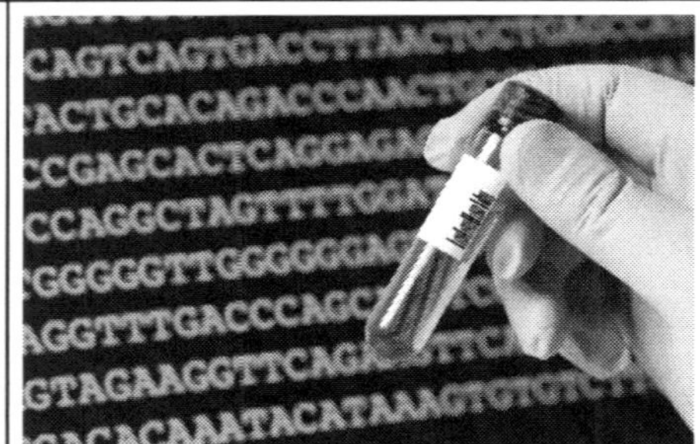
Childbirth Education	The process of teaching expectant parents about labor, delivery, and newborn care to prepare them for childbirth and parenting.	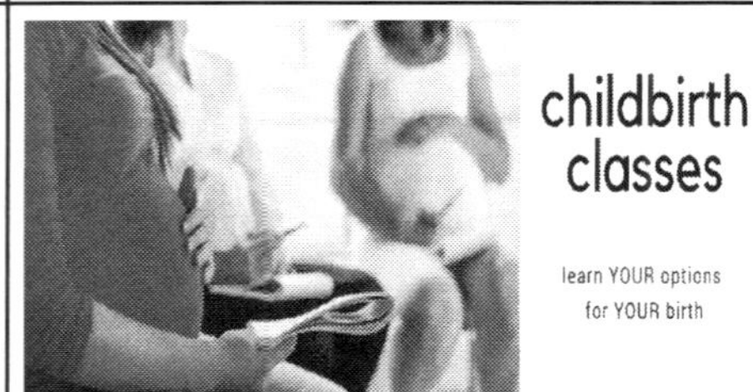
Postpartum Care	The medical and emotional care provided to a mother following the birth of her baby, including recovery, support, and counseling.	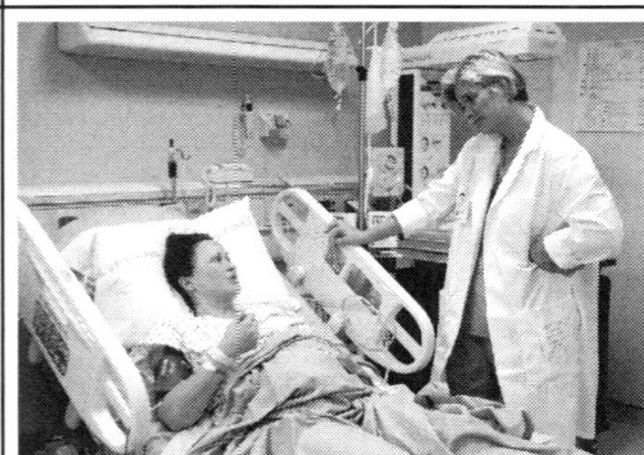
Breastfeeding	The practice of feeding an infant with breast milk directly from the mother's breast, providing essential nutrients and bonding opportunities.	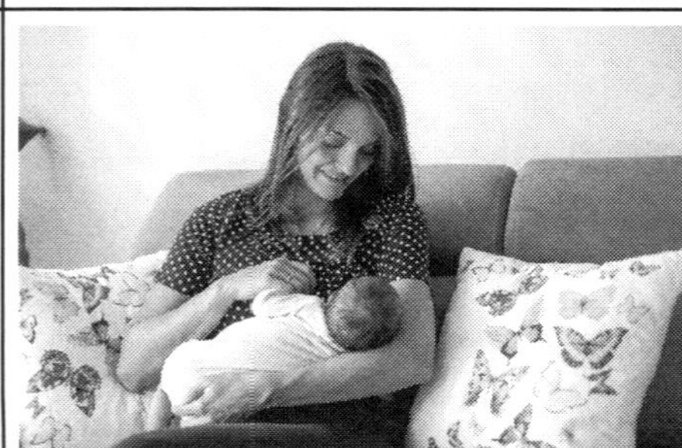

5.1. Prenatal Care and Screening

Ensuring proper prenatal care is crucial for the well-being of both the mother and the fetus. It entails periodic medical examinations and screenings to monitor the progress of the pregnancy and detect any potential problems. Consistent prenatal care assists pregnant women in preventing complications during pregnancy and childbirth.

5.1.1. Nutrition During Pregnancy

Optimal nutrition during pregnancy is essential for the physical and mental well-being of both the mother and the developing fetus. Women must prioritize their diet and ensure they receive all the essential nutrients required to maintain a healthy pregnancy.

- Pregnant women should prioritize consuming a diverse range of fruits, in addition to the aforementioned essential nutrients, as part of a well-balanced diet.
- Edible plants
- Whole grains.
- Nutritious lipids.
- Pregnant women should prioritize maintaining hydration by consuming ample amounts of water throughout the day.
- Pregnant women should refrain from consuming or restrict their intake of specific foods during pregnancy. These include: – Uncooked or partially cooked meat
- Consuming fish, eggs, and unpasteurized dairy products.
- Pregnant women should refrain from consuming deli meats, soft cheeses, and fish that contain high levels of mercury.
- Pregnant women should consult their doctor regarding their dietary intake and supplementation. Healthcare providers can customize advice based on the specific needs of both the mother and the baby. In addition to maintaining a balanced diet, it is important for pregnant women to adopt a health-conscious way of living. Included are regular exercise, adequate rest, and effective stress management.
- Engaging in smoking, alcohol consumption, and the use of recreational drugs is detrimental to the health of pregnant women.
- Ensuring proper prenatal care is crucial for the well-being of both the mother and the child.
- Pregnant women should schedule regular appointments with their healthcare provider to closely monitor the progress of their pregnancy and promptly address any issues or worries. Physicians will assess the mother's weight, blood pressure, and overall well-being during prenatal appointments. In addition, routine tests will be conducted to screen for gestational diabetes and preeclampsia.
- Pregnant women should also be mindful of potential complications such as intense abdominal pain, vaginal bleeding, and abrupt swelling of the hands and face. Pregnant women should promptly seek medical attention if they experience these symptoms.

5.1.2. Monitoring Fetal Development

It is crucial to monitor the progress of fetal development during pregnancy to detect any possible problems at an early stage and take appropriate measures to deal with them.

Monitoring fetal development offers a multitude of advantages:

In order to ensure optimal growth and development of the fetus. By monitoring the growth and development of the fetus, healthcare professionals can detect any abnormalities or delays that may necessitate additional investigation or intervention.

Assists in guaranteeing that the fetus is obtaining a sufficient provision of nutrients and oxygen from the mother, which is crucial for appropriate growth.

Genetic screening tests such as NIPT or amniocentesis are used to identify any genetic or chromosomal abnormalities that may be present. These tests can detect conditions such as Down syndrome, cystic fibrosis, or sickle cell anemia. Timely diagnosis enables parents to make well-informed decisions regarding their pregnancy and adequately prepare for medical interventions.

Prenatal care additionally entails the surveillance of the mother's physical condition and overall welfare. Fetal development can be impacted by gestational diabetes, preeclampsia, and infections, necessitating vigilant monitoring and treatment. Routine prenatal screenings can identify and address these problems before they escalate into more severe conditions.

Various techniques are employed to observe the progress of fetal growth during prenatal care and screening. Ultrasound imaging, a frequently used technique, employs high-frequency sound waves to generate images of the fetus inside the uterus. Ultrasound imaging can yield significant data regarding the dimensions, orientation, and general progress of the fetus, while also detecting any possible anomalies or complications (Limwattananon, Tangcharoensathien, & Prakongsai, 2010) (Figure 5.1).

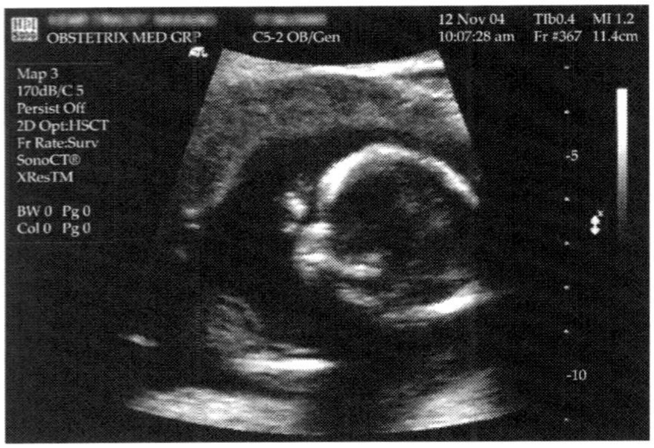

Figure 5.1. *Cross-section ultrasound image of a fetus.*

Source: https://en.wikipedia.org/wiki/File:Obsteric_ultrasonograph.jpg.

Fetal monitoring is a crucial method for monitoring the development of the fetus. It entails the tracking of the fetal heart rate and movements. Fetal monitoring aids in evaluating the fetal condition and identifying any indications of distress or abnormality. This data can be utilized to ascertain the necessity for additional examination or intervention, such as a cesarean section or induction of labor.

Genetic screening tests, such as Non-Invasive Prenatal Testing (NIPT) or amniocentesis, are crucial tools for monitoring the progress of fetal development. These tests can detect genetic or chromosomal abnormalities in the fetus, enabling parents to make informed decisions about their pregnancy and prepare for any required medical interventions or treatments. Genetic screening tests are commonly provided to women who are older in terms of their reproductive age or those who have a familial background of genetic disorders (Limwattananon, Tangcharoensathien, & Prakongsai, 2010).

5.1.3. Genetic Testing

Genetic testing conducted as part of prenatal care and screening is an essential element in safeguarding the health and welfare of both the mother and the developing fetus. Prenatal genetic testing offers significant insights into the baby's genetic composition, enabling healthcare professionals to promptly detect and assess any potential hazards or irregularities during the early stages of pregnancy. By identifying these problems at an early stage, parents and healthcare professionals can make well-informed choices regarding the most appropriate steps to guarantee the well-being and safety of both the mother and the infant.

Several genetic tests are conducted as part of prenatal care, including:

Early pregnancy screening: This test utilizes a combination of blood analysis and ultrasound imaging to identify chromosomal abnormalities, such as Down syndrome. The mother's blood test assesses the levels of proteins and hormones, while the ultrasound evaluates the nuchal translucency, which refers to the thickness of the baby's neck. These tests can assist physicians in forecasting chromosomal abnormalities in infants.

Cell-free fetal DNA testing involves the analysis of small fragments of fetal DNA present in the mother's blood. Healthcare providers can precisely diagnose trisomy 21 (Down syndrome), trisomy 18 (Edwards syndrome), and trisomy 13 (Patau syndrome) by examining these fragments with accuracy. Cell-free fetal DNA testing is typically provided to women who are 35 years of age or older, or who have a familial background of genetic disorders.

Diagnostic genetic testing may be recommended if a possible problem is detected during prenatal care. Diagnostic procedures such as chorionic villus sampling (CVS) and amniocentesis examine genetic material from samples of the placenta or amniotic fluid to detect any abnormalities. These tests can definitively diagnose genetic conditions and assist healthcare professionals and parents in making informed decisions regarding pregnancy.

Prenatal genetic testing is crucial for both detecting genetic disorders and reassuring expectant parents. Acquiring the outcomes of these examinations can assist parents in making emotional and financial arrangements in anticipation of the birth of a child with exceptional requirements. Additionally, it enables healthcare providers to formulate a strategy for monitoring and addressing any potential health concerns that may arise throughout the pregnancy or postpartum period.

Although prenatal genetic testing can offer valuable insights, it is crucial for parents to comprehend the constraints associated with these tests. There is no test that is completely accurate, and it is possible to have results that are either false-positive or false-negative. Parents must engage in a discussion with their healthcare provider regarding the outcomes of genetic testing and, if needed, pursue genetic counseling. Genetic counselors assist parents in comprehending the outcomes of genetic tests, examining the various choices available to them, and making well-informed decisions regarding their pregnancy.

5.1.4. Pregnancy Complications Management

Proper prenatal care and screening are essential for expectant mothers to safeguard the health and well-being of both the mother and the baby during pregnancy. Nevertheless, certain pregnancies may be hindered by diverse factors that necessitate supplementary administration and surveillance to avert potential hazards and complexities.

Common Pregnancy Complications		
Condition	**Characteristics**	**Management**
Gestational Diabetes	Pregnancy-induced high blood sugar. Macrosomia, preterm birth, and preeclampsia can result from this condition.	Expectant mothers with gestational diabetes may need to monitor their blood sugar, follow a diet, and take insulin.
Preeclampsia	Hypertension and protein in the urine occur after 20 weeks of pregnancy. Seizures and eclampsia can result from preeclampsia.	Preeclampsia can be managed by lowering blood pressure with medication, monitoring blood pressure and urine protein levels, and delivering the baby early if severe.
Preterm Labor	Contraction-induced cervix opening before 37 weeks. Preterm labor and birth can cause respiratory distress syndrome and developmental delays.	Preterm labor may require bed rest, contraction-stopping medications, and medical monitoring to prevent early delivery.
Multiple Gestations	Multiple pregnancies can cause preterm birth, low birth weight, and preeclampsia.	Multiple gestation mothers may need more prenatal visits, ultrasounds, and monitoring to ensure baby health and growth.
Miscarriages or Stillbirths	Pregnancy monitoring and care may be needed after miscarriages or stillbirths.	These women may need more prenatal visits, ultrasounds, and testing to detect complications early and avoid complications.

Healthcare providers must conduct a thorough screening of expectant mothers for pregnancy complications during prenatal care to detect any potential risk factors and administer suitable management and monitoring. Screening tests, including blood tests, ultrasounds, and urine tests, can identify conditions like gestational diabetes, preeclampsia, and preterm labor at an early stage. This early detection helps prevent complications and enhances outcomes for both the mother and the baby (Limwattananon, Tangcharoensathien, & Prakongsai, 2010).

5.1.5. Getting Ready for Labor and Delivery

Pregnancy is an extraordinary process that necessitates meticulous preparation for childbirth. Prenatal care and screening are essential for promoting a healthy pregnancy and ensuring a safe delivery for both the mother and the baby. Expectant mothers can enhance their physical, emotional, and mental readiness for labor and delivery by adhering to the instructions given by healthcare professionals.

Regular attendance at prenatal care appointments is an initial and crucial step in preparing for labor and delivery. These appointments enable healthcare providers to monitor the progression of the pregnancy, evaluate the well-being of both the mother and the baby, and deal with any concerns or complications that may emerge. Prenatal care offers expectant mothers the chance to inquire, obtain advice on nutrition and physical activity, and get ready for labor and delivery (Nakamura, 2010).

ealthcare providers may suggest specific screenings and tests during prenatal care appointments to monitor the well-being of both the mother and the baby. These screenings can detect any potential complications that could impact the pregnancy or delivery, enabling healthcare providers to implement necessary measures to ensure a safe and healthy outcome. Common diagnostic procedures include blood tests, ultrasounds, and genetic screenings.

Expectant mothers can enhance their physical preparedness for labor and delivery by attending prenatal care appointments, undergoing screenings and tests, and taking additional measures. Engaging in physical activity and adhering to a healthy lifestyle during pregnancy can enhance one's strength, endurance, and flexibility, thereby facilitating the management of the physical challenges associated with childbirth. Engaging in prenatal exercise classes, practicing yoga, and participating in swimming are all effective methods to maintain physical activity and condition the body in anticipation of childbirth. Expectant mothers should prioritize consuming a nutritious and well-balanced diet throughout their pregnancy. Optimal nutrition is crucial for the well-being of both the mother and the baby, and can aid in the prevention of complications during childbirth. Healthcare providers may advise individuals to follow specific dietary recommendations, including consuming more fruits, vegetables, whole grains, and lean proteins, while avoiding foods that are high in sugar, salt, and unhealthy fats (Nakamura, 2010).

Aside from physical readiness, it is crucial for pregnant women to also mentally and emotionally prepare themselves for the process of giving birth. The process of giving birth can be a demanding and daunting ordeal, and it is common for pregnant women to experience feelings of anxiety, fear, or uncertainty regarding what lies ahead. Engaging in conversations with a partner, family member, or friend regarding fears and concerns, participating in childbirth education classes, and regularly practicing relaxation techniques can effectively diminish anxiety and enhance self-assurance in managing the process of labor and delivery.

Before the impending deadline, pregnant women should create a birth plan that clearly states their desired choices for the process of giving birth. A birth plan serves to communicate the mother's preferences to healthcare providers and facilitate decision-making during labor. A birth plan encompasses the mother's preferences for pain management, labor positions, interventions, and postpartum care, as well as any specific considerations or concerns she may have.

Expectant mothers should not only prepare themselves physically, emotionally, and mentally for labor and delivery, but they should also assemble a hospital bag containing necessary items for their stay at the hospital. Essential items to pack in a hospital bag are comfortable attire, personal care products, food, a camera, and any required documents like insurance details and a birth plan. Preparing a hospital bag in advance can alleviate anxiety and ensure that the mother is equipped for unforeseen circumstances (Nakamura, 2010).

5.2. Childbirth Education

Childbirth education is an essential element in equipping prospective parents with the necessary knowledge and skills to prepare for the birth of their upcoming child. It offers valuable information and resources to assist parents in making well-informed decisions regarding their childbirth experience. Childbirth education provides parents with the necessary knowledge and skills to confidently navigate the birthing process, including understanding the stages of labor and learning about pain management techniques (Figure 5.2).

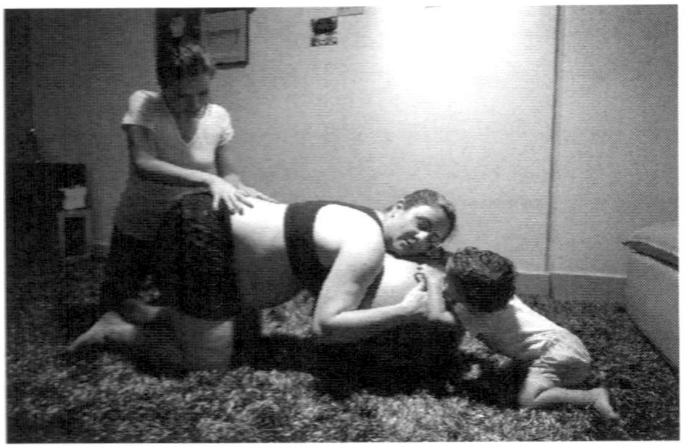

Figure 5.2. *Childbirth preparation.*

Source: By Jefferson Rudy/Senado Federal - Fotos produzidas pelo Senado, CC BY 2.0, https://commons.wikimedia.org/w/index.php?curid=47836939.

The primary objective of childbirth education is to equip parents with the knowledge and skills necessary to assert their rights and make informed decisions for themselves and their infants throughout the process of labor and delivery. Parents can align their choices with their values by comprehending the available options. Childbirth education equips and enables parents to make informed decisions regarding the use of medication, the location of birth (home or hospital), and whether to have a medicated or unmedicated birth.

Childbirth education encompasses not only the dissemination of knowledge about the process of giving birth, but also includes instruction on subjects such as the care of newborns, the act of breastfeeding, and the recovery period following childbirth. This comprehensive strategy guarantees that parents are adequately prepared to provide care for their newborn and themselves during the days and weeks after childbirth. Childbirth education fosters a supportive and informative atmosphere, enabling parents to enhance their confidence and preparedness for the trials of early parenthood.

Childbirth education should also equip parents with the knowledge and skills to handle unforeseen labor and delivery complications. Acquire knowledge about typical interventions and procedures designed to enhance parents' assurance in making prompt decisions. Gaining insight into the potential hazards and advantages of various interventions can provide parents with a sense of authority and mastery, even in challenging circumstances. Childbirth education facilitates effective communication and collaboration between parents and doctors. Childbirth education facilitates transparent and sincere communication, enabling parents to establish confidence in their care team and experience enhanced support during the birthing process. The adoption of this cooperative method fosters the practice of making decisions together and showing regard for one another, resulting in advantages for both parents and infants (Nakamura, 2010).

Childbirth education additionally diminishes anxiety related to labor and delivery. Childbirth education enhances parents' confidence and preparedness for the birthing experience by offering precise information and debunking prevalent myths and misconceptions. Parents can enhance their ability to regulate their emotions and adjust their expectations, thereby fostering a more positive and empowering birth experience. Parents who prefer to learn at home can access online and virtual childbirth education classes. These platforms offer convenient and flexible access to valuable information and resources, without the need to attend class. Parents who have demanding schedules or limited opportunities to attend in-person classes may find this beneficial.

5.2.1. Process of Labor and Delivery

Gaining a comprehensive comprehension of the labor and delivery process is essential for expectant mothers as it enables them to adequately prepare themselves mentally and physically for the significant event. Childbirth education is crucial in equipping women with the necessary knowledge and resources to effectively navigate the process of labor and delivery.

The process of labor can be divided into three distinct stages:

- **The Initial Phase:** This stage is characterized by the initiation of labor and continues until the cervix is completely dilated to 10 centimeters. This stage is subdivided into three distinct phases: early labor, active labor, and transition.
- Early labor is characterized by sporadic contractions that gradually increase in intensity.
- During active labor, the contractions become more intense and occur at shorter intervals as the cervix expands from 4 to 7 centimeters.
- Transition is the most critical phase of labor, characterized by the cervix expanding 8–10 centimeters and contractions reaching their maximum intensity.
- The second stage of childbirth typically begins when the cervix is completely dilated and concludes with the delivery of the baby.
- During the expulsion stage, the mother is required to exert force during each contraction to propel the baby through the birth canal.
- The duration of this stage can vary from a few minutes to several hours, depending on the baby's position and the intensity of the mother's pushing.
- The third stage of childbirth involves the expulsion of the placenta, typically occurring within 15–30 minutes after the baby's birth.
- During this phase, individuals typically experience mild contractions and bleeding.
- Following the delivery of the placenta, the mother's uterus undergoes contractions to regulate bleeding and revert to its original size before pregnancy.

A significant number of women experience apprehension regarding the discomfort associated with childbirth. Both natural techniques such as breathing exercises and relaxation, as well as medical interventions like epidurals and analgesics, can alleviate pain. It is imperative for women to engage in a conversation with their doctor regarding pain management and formulate a birth plan. Childbirth education classes offer expectant mothers valuable knowledge about pain management techniques, such as breathing exercises, massage, and visualization. These classes provide a comprehensive analysis of the advantages and disadvantages of epidurals and analgesics, assisting women in making informed decisions regarding pain management.

Childbirth education classes not only address pain management but also emphasize the emotional and psychological aspects of labor and delivery. Women commonly undergo a variety of emotions during childbirth, such as fear, anxiety, and excitement. Childbirth education classes assist women in comprehending these emotions and offer effective coping strategies to manage them (Nakamura, 2010).

Childbirth education highlights the importance of receiving assistance and encouragement throughout the process of giving birth. During the process of giving birth, emotional support, encouragement, and reassurance can be provided by a partner, family member, or doula. Childbirth education classes prioritize the importance of a support person and offer guidance on how they can effectively assist the mother during labor. Pregnant women should be aware of the indicators of labor to determine the appropriate time to proceed to the hospital or birthing facility. Common contractions, lumbar discomfort, and rupture of the amniotic sac are indicative of labor. Women acquire the ability to identify these indicators and determine the appropriate time to seek medical assistance through childbirth education classes. Childbirth education should also equip women with the knowledge and skills to handle unforeseen labor and delivery outcomes. The majority of births are uneventful, however, unforeseen complications may necessitate medical intervention. Childbirth education classes provide women with information about typical complications during childbirth, such as fetal distress, umbilical cord prolapse, and placental abruption, as well as the methods used to handle these complications.

Postpartum care is a crucial subject that is addressed in childbirth education classes. The postpartum period, also referred to as the fourth trimester, is a period during which women undergo physical and emotional adaptation. Childbirth education classes offer women comprehensive knowledge regarding postpartum recuperation, breastfeeding, infant care, and self-care techniques aimed at facilitating healing and enhancing overall health (Nakamura, 2010).

5.2.2. Pain Management Options

Childbirth is a remarkable and transformative event, yet it is also accompanied by excruciating agony. It is imperative for pregnant women to have a comprehensive understanding of the different pain relief choices that are accessible to them during childbirth. Through comprehending their options, women can make well-informed choices that are in line with their personal preferences and values.

Multiple pain management techniques are available for use during the process of childbirth. Below, a few of them are discussed.

Epidurals: An epidural is a form of regional anesthesia that effectively inhibits pain in a targeted area of the body. During the process of childbirth, an anesthesiologist administers medication through injection into the lower back, specifically near the spinal cord, to block the sensation of pain by numbing the nerves. Epidurals are widely favored due to their efficacy in alleviating pain and facilitating a childbirth experience devoid of pain (Figure 5.3).

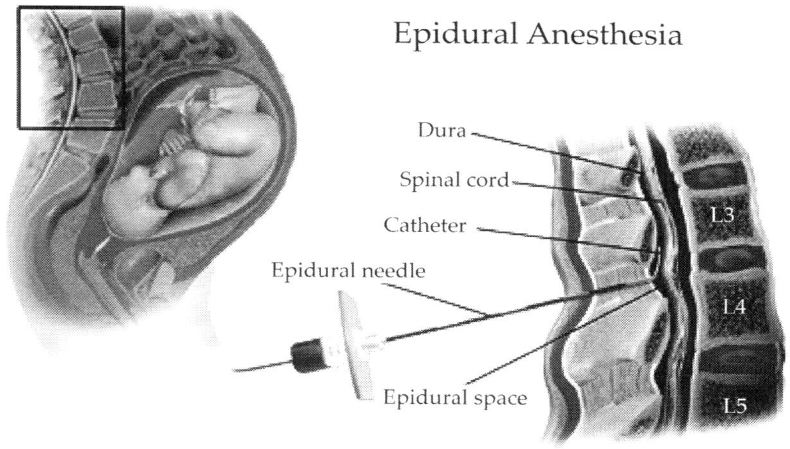

Figure 5.3. *Epidural anesthesia.*

Source: https://en.m.wikipedia.org/wiki/File:Epidural_Anesthesia.png.

The utilization of nitrous oxide, commonly referred to as laughing gas: Mask-inhaled nitrous oxide is both colorless and odorless. It aids women in managing contractions by diminishing anxiety and inducing relaxation. Nitrous oxide is safe for both the mother and the baby, and it does not have any long-term consequences. Nitrous oxide is often preferred by women during labor due to its efficacy in pain relief and the absence of side effects commonly associated with other pain medications. Non-pharmacological methods for managing pain: These techniques prioritize natural methods for alleviating pain and inducing relaxation. Several widely used non-pharmacological methods for managing pain include:

- Respiration techniques
- Massage and visualization techniques.
- Hydrotherapy

These techniques can assist women independently or in conjunction with other analgesics, in effectively managing labor contractions. A significant number of women experience a sense of empowerment and control over their childbirth process through the use of non-pharmacological pain management techniques.

Acupuncture and acupressure: Thin needles are inserted into specific body points to stimulate energy flow and relieve pain in acupuncture. Acupressure relieves pain and relaxes by applying pressure to specific body points. Both acupuncture and acupressure can reduce labor pain and be useful in a woman's pain management plan.

Expectant mothers need to discuss their pain management options with their healthcare provider and create a birth plan that outlines their preferences for pain relief during labor. A birth plan is a written document that communicates a woman's preferences for her childbirth experience, including her desired pain management options, labor positions, and interventions.

By creating a birth plan, women can advocate for their needs and preferences during labor and ensure that their healthcare providers are aware of their wishes (Wang & Pies, 2004).

Childbirth education classes are a valuable resource for expectant mothers to learn about their pain management options and prepare for labor and delivery. These classes provide information on the different types of pain relief available, as well as techniques for coping with labor pain. Childbirth education classes also teach women about the stages of labor, the role of the birth partner, and strategies for managing stress and anxiety during childbirth. By attending childbirth education classes, women can gain the knowledge and skills they need to make informed decisions about their pain management options and feel confident and empowered during labor and delivery.

5.2.3. Formulating a Birth Plan

Developing a birth plan as part of childbirth education is a crucial measure in getting ready for the birth of your child. A birth plan is a written document that specifies your preferences and desires for the process of giving birth, including labor, delivery, and postpartum care. It functions as a directive for your healthcare providers and support team to guarantee that your desires are honored and adhered to the utmost extent of their capabilities.

wHEN creating a birth plan, it is essential to prioritize adaptability and a receptive mindset. Anticipating unforeseen changes or complications is essential, as childbirth is an unpredictable and intricate procedure. Aside from expressing your preferences and desires in your birth plan, it is crucial to maintain adaptability and contemplate alternative options and interventions when necessary (Althabe et al., 2008). Participating in childbirth education classes can enhance your preparedness for the process of labor and delivery, as well as assist you in formulating a birth plan. Childbirth education classes provide valuable knowledge and tools to acquire information on pain management techniques, comprehend the process of giving birth, and develop effective coping mechanisms for when labor begins. Additionally, they provide an opportunity to engage with other prospective parents, inquire about any concerns, and establish a network of support for the upcoming journey. Enrolling in birth education classes can also aid you in formulating a birth plan that accurately represents your principles and preferences. To create a birth plan that reflects your wishes and goals for labor and delivery, discuss your preferences for pain management, labor positions, interventions, and postpartum care with your childbirth educator (Wang & Pies, 2004).

5.2.4. Postpartum Care

Postpartum care is an essential component of childbirth education, providing the necessary physical, emotional, and social assistance required by a new mother following childbirth. The "fourth trimester" refers to a period of adaptation and recovery for both the mother and the baby. Gaining a comprehensive understanding of postpartum care is essential for ensuring the health and well-being of both the mother and the baby. Postpartum physical care entails closely observing the mother's recuperation from childbirth, encompassing her healing progress and overall physical health. These items include (Figure 5.4):

- Evaluating for indications of infection
- Observing hemorrhaging
- Ensuring the mother receives sufficient rest and adequate nutrition.

New mothers should prioritize paying attention to their bodies and promptly seek medical assistance if they encounter any atypical symptoms or complications.

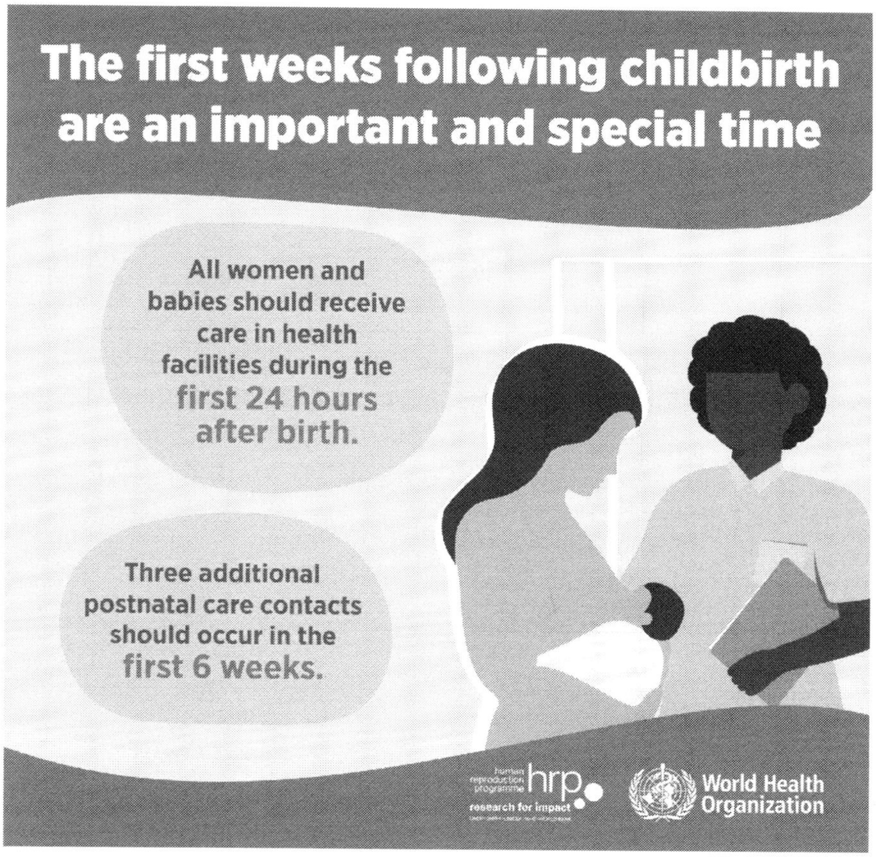

Figure 5.4. *Postpartum care.*

Source: *Postpartum Care – Los Angeles, CA, n. d. https://cdn.who.int/media/images/default-source/infographics/maternal-health/postnatal-1.tmb-549v.jpg?sfvrsn=110f453d_32.*

During the postpartum period, new mothers may undergo a variety of emotional states, including happiness, enthusiasm, as well as sadness or anxiety. Therefore, it is crucial to provide adequate emotional support during this period. New mothers often experience feelings of being overwhelmed or exhausted, and it is essential for them to seek assistance from their partners, family members, or healthcare providers. Healthcare professionals should conduct screenings for postpartum depression and provide appropriate support and treatment, as it is a significant condition that can impact new mothers. During the postpartum period, social support plays a crucial role as new mothers may experience feelings of isolation or overwhelming pressure due to the demands of caring for a newborn. New mothers must establish connections with fellow mothers and seek community assistance, be it through online forums, support groups, or alternative methods. Having a partner during this period is crucial as they can provide emotional assistance, assist with household tasks, and help with the care of the newborn. Maternal education is crucial for providing new mothers with the necessary knowledge and skills to effectively care for themselves and their newborns, thereby preparing them for the postpartum period. Childbirth education classes commonly address subjects such as breastfeeding, emotional well-being, postpartum recovery, and newborn care. Attending these classes can provide new mothers with the knowledge and skills to effectively handle the emotional and physical changes that they may experience during the postpartum period. Empowering new mothers with the information and skills to make informed choices regarding their postpartum care is a key benefit of childbirth education. By providing information on the various postpartum care options, new mothers can choose the approach that aligns most effectively with their needs and preferences. For example, certain new mothers may opt to depend on their friends or family for assistance during the postpartum period, whereas others may choose to employ a doula or postpartum nurse (Wang & Pies, 2004).

Education regarding childbirth facilitates the acquisition of essential abilities required by new mothers to attend to their newborns in the postpartum period. This involves acquiring knowledge of efficient breastfeeding techniques, mastering the art of soothing a crying infant, and developing the ability to identify signs of illness or discomfort in the infant. Acquiring knowledge and skills can help new mothers feel more prepared and confident in caring for their newborns during the initial days and weeks after giving birth. Childbirth education not only imparts knowledge and skills but also helps new mothers establish a support network consisting of other mothers and medical professionals. Enrolling in childbirth education classes allows new mothers to connect with other mothers who are going through similar experiences, providing an opportunity to exchange questions, concerns, and advice. Healthcare professionals who teach childbirth education classes can provide ongoing support and guidance to new mothers during the postpartum phase (Althabe et al., 2008).

5.2.5. Assistance for Breastfeeding

- Breastfeeding is an essential component of infant care that offers a multitude of advantages for both the infant and the mother. Hence, it is imperative for healthcare providers to provide sufficient assistance and instruction on breastfeeding during childbirth classes.
- Primarily, providing breastfeeding support during childbirth education enhances the self-assurance and readiness of new mothers to breastfeed their infants. When initiating breastfeeding for the first time, numerous women experience feelings of anxiety or uncertainty. Childbirth educators can diminish these anxieties and enable mothers to breastfeed by instructing them on breastfeeding techniques, proper positioning, and addressing common problems.
- Moreover, providing breastfeeding support during childbirth education can enhance the results of breastfeeding. Research indicates that mothers who receive sufficient breastfeeding education are more inclined to initiate breastfeeding, engage in exclusive breastfeeding, and achieve overall success in their breastfeeding journey. Childbirth educators can facilitate successful breastfeeding by instructing mothers on the necessary techniques and methods. Childbirth educators not only provide information on breastfeeding techniques but also offer emotional support to new mothers. A significant number of women experience challenges and strong emotional responses when it comes to breastfeeding, particularly during the initial weeks after giving birth. Childbirth educators can assist mothers in managing breastfeeding difficulties by offering a secure environment for mothers to engage in open discussions. Another

crucial element of childbirth education is the provision of assistance and guidance in dealing with typical obstacles encountered during breastfeeding. New mothers may face a range of challenges when breastfeeding, including latch difficulties and insufficient milk production. By engaging in open discussions about these challenges and offering practical solutions and resources, childbirth educators can assist mothers in resolving issues and maintaining successful breastfeeding (Wang & Pies, 2004).

- Additionally, providing breastfeeding assistance during childbirth education can promote a feeling of camaraderie and bonding among new mothers. Certain women experience feelings of solitude and seclusion during the act of breastfeeding, particularly in the absence of a robust network of assistance. Childbirth educators can foster a supportive and inclusive environment by bringing together breastfeeding expectant mothers to exchange experiences, offer advice, and form enduring friendships.
- Childbirth educators must also emphasize the significance of partner support in breastfeeding. Mothers require emotional, practical, and uplifting support from their partners. Childbirth educators can assist the new family in establishing a robust support system by providing education to partners regarding the advantages of breastfeeding, their responsibilities in supporting it, and how they can contribute to the mother's success (Wang & Pies, 2004).

5.3. Nutrition for Infants and Children

- Optimal nutrition is essential for the robust growth and maturation of infants and children. Children undergo rapid physical and cognitive transformations from infancy to adolescence, necessitating sufficient nutrients for their well-being. Parents and caregivers should recognize the significance of providing their children with a well-rounded diet.
- Advantages of Breastfeeding: Infant nutrition is most effectively provided through breastfeeding, a widely acknowledged method. Human breast milk contains a comprehensive array of essential nutrients that are necessary for the growth and development of a baby. Additionally, it provides infants with immunity against infections and diseases through the presence of antibodies. Breastfeeding diminishes the likelihood of developing obesity, diabetes, and other long-lasting ailments in the future. The optimal recommendation is to exclusively breastfeed for the initial six months, and subsequently introduce solid foods until at least one year of age.
- Introduction to Complementary Feeding: At approximately six months of age, infants are generally prepared to commence consuming solid foods alongside breast milk or formula.

- Expose infants to a diverse range of foods to acquaint them with various flavors and textures.
- Commence by combining pureed fruits and vegetables, gradually progressing to more intricate puree mixtures.
- Avoidance of honey, cow's milk, and foods that pose a choking hazard is recommended.
- Be vigilant for any food allergies or sensitivities, such as the occurrence of a rash, vomiting, or diarrhea. If any of these symptoms arise, it is advisable to seek medical advice from a doctor (Figure 5.5).

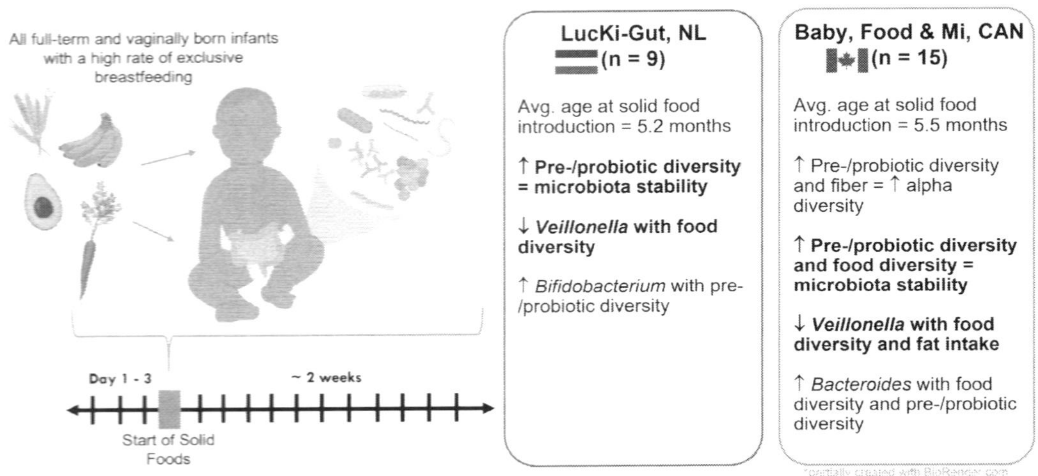

Figure 5.5. *Starting solids and baby's first foods.*

Source: *Homann C-M, Rossel CAJ, Dizzell S, Bervoets L, Simioni J, Li J, Gunn E, Surette MG, de Souza RJ, Mommers M, et al. Infants' First Solid Foods: Impact on Gut Microbiota Development in Two Intercontinental Cohorts. Nutrients. 2021; 13(8):2639. https://doi.org/10.3390/nu13082639.*

Allergies and Food Sensitivities: Infants and children often have food allergies. Common allergens include cow's milk, eggs, peanuts, tree nuts, soy, wheat, fish, and shellfish. These foods should be introduced slowly and monitored for side effects. If a food allergy is suspected, seek medical advice and possibly allergy testing. However, food sensitivities can cause digestive, skin, or behavioral issues. A food diary can help identify triggers and make eliminating problem foods easier:

- **Healthy Eating:** Healthy eating habits must start early for long-term health.
  - Kids should eat a variety of fruits, vegetables, whole grains, lean proteins, and dairy.
  - Cut back on sugar, salt, and fat.
  - Eat healthy and involve kids in meal prep to set an example.
  - Limit processed foods and sugary drinks and offer fruits, vegetables, nuts, and yogurt.
  - Avoid using food as a reward or punishment and teach kids to recognize hunger and fullness.

- Meal Planning for Children:
  - Meal planning helps kids get the nutrients they need to grow.
  - At each meal, try different foods from all food groups.
  - Plan meals and snacks in advance to avoid unhealthy last-minute choices.
  - Get kids involved in meal planning and preparation to foster a love of cooking and healthy eating.
  - Sit down as a family and avoid screens to enjoy meals.
  - Encourage children to try new foods and be patient if they hesitate.

5.4. Vaccination and Immunization

Vaccination and Immunization play a critical role in maintaining public health by shielding people from dangerous illnesses and halting the spread of infectious diseases. Vaccinations have reduced measles, polio, and influenza rates, making them crucial. By stimulating the immune system to produce antibodies against pathogens, vaccines boost immunity and prevent infections (Althabe et al., 2008).

The recommended vaccination schedule delineates the appropriate timing and dosage of vaccinations that individuals should receive over the course of their lifetime, as advised by medical professionals.

This regimen is designed to protect against many diseases from childhood to adulthood. Following the vaccination schedule can protect people from infectious diseases and prevent community outbreaks. Despite overwhelming research showing vaccinations' efficacy and safety, many myths persist. Numerous scientific studies have disproven the widespread myth that vaccines cause autism. Another common misconception is that vaccines contain trace amounts of harmful substances like formaldehyde or mercury and have regulatory approval. A crucial idea in public health, herd immunity—also referred to as community immunity—highlights the significance of high vaccination rates within a population. A protective barrier that stops the disease from spreading to people who are not vaccinated, such as young children, the elderly, and people with weakened immune systems, is created when a significant portion of the population is immune against it. Communities can successfully manage the spread of infectious diseases and stop outbreaks by developing herd immunity.

Regulatory organizations and healthcare providers place a high premium on vaccine safety. Before being used, a vaccine is extensively tested for safety and efficacy. This process includes animal preclinical research and human clinical trials to evaluate the vaccine's side effects and immune response. Post-marketing surveillance detects rare or unexpected adverse events in vaccines (Althabe et al., 2008).

5.5. Early Childhood Development

Early Childhood Development refers to the physical, cognitive, social, and emotional growth that occurs in children from birth through around age eight. This period is crucial for shaping a child's future health, happiness, success, and overall well-being (Figure 5.6).

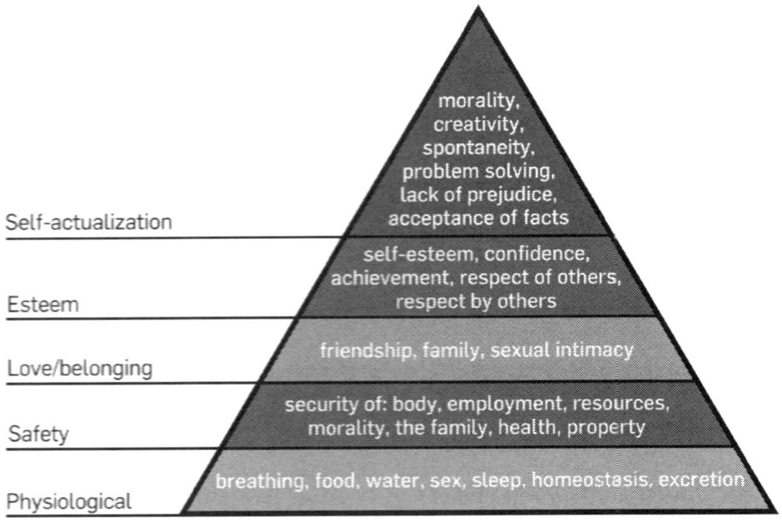

Figure 5.6. *Early childhood development.*

Source: By Saul McLeod – http://www.simplypsychology.org/maslow.html, CC BY-SA 4.0, https://commons.wikimedia.org/w/index.php?curid=47784797.

During early childhood, children experience rapid growth and development in all areas.

- Physical changes manifest in height, weight, and motor skills.
- Cognitive development includes language, memory, problem-solving, and abstract thinking.
- Children develop social skills, including forming relationships, interacting with peers, and exhibiting empathy and compassion.
- They learn to control their emotions and recognize and respond to others.

Early childhood experiences have a lasting impact on a child's development. Positive experiences, such as nurturing relationships, a safe environment, and opportunities for play and exploration, can lead to healthy development and positive outcomes later in life. On the other hand, adverse experiences, such as neglect, abuse, or exposure to violence, can have detrimental effects on a child's development and well-being.

Parents, caregivers, teachers, and other adults are crucial to early childhood development. Adults can help children reach their potential by providing a loving and stimulating environment, responsive interactions, and learning and growth opportunities.

5.5.1. Key Events in Child Development

During the period of early childhood development, children experience a series of significant milestones that indicate their progress and maturation. These milestones are pivotal benchmarks that serve as reliable indicators of a child's development and can provide parents and caregivers with valuable insights into what to anticipate during various phases of their child's life.

There are several significant stages in early childhood development, which will be discussed below.

- Physical Growth:
  - Children undergo rapid physical changes from birth to age five, including height, weight gain, and muscle strength.
  - Children typically walk, run, and climb stairs with help by age two.
  - By five, they can bike and play sports.
- Cognitive Development:
  - Children learn to think, problem-solve, and decide during this stage.
  - Most three-year-olds can follow simple instructions, recognize shapes and colors, and play imaginatively.
  - They can count to ten, recognize letters and numbers, and understand cause and effect by age five.
- Social and Emotional Development:
  - This milestone is crucial to early childhood development.
  - Children learn to communicate, express emotions, and form relationships during this stage.
  - Most children can play cooperatively, show empathy, and express their feelings by age three.
  - By five, they can share toys, make friends, and understand fairness.
- Language Development:
  - This is another crucial early childhood milestone.
  - Children learn to speak, listen, and understand during this stage.
  - Most children can speak sentences, ask questions, and have conversations by age three.
  - Children can tell stories, use complex vocabulary, and understand basic grammar by age five.
- Motor Skills Development:
  - This marks an important early childhood development milestone.
  - This stage helps children develop fine and gross motor skills needed for daily tasks.
  - Most three-year-olds can use scissors, draw simple shapes, and dress themselves.
  - They can write their name, tie their shoes, and do coordinated, balanced activities by five.
- Self-Help Skills Development:
  - Children become more independent and self-sufficient during this stage.
  - Most three-year-olds can feed, potty, and clean themselves.
  - By age five, they can dress, brush, and follow a routine without prompts.

5.5.2. Cognitive Development

Cognitive development is an essential component of early childhood development. It involves the development and advancement of a child's cognitive skills, including their capacity to think, analyze, solve problems, and comprehend their surroundings. The period from ages 2 to 6 is marked by substantial cognitive development and acquisition of skills in children.

An important achievement in cognitive development during early childhood is the acquisition of symbolic thinking. Cognitive representation involves the utilization of language, visual depictions, and physical movements to mentally depict objects and concepts. Children employ symbolic cognition to engage in play, comprehend the concept of time, and facilitate communication. Abstract thinking and problem-solving skills are also developed through it.

Memory and attention experience significant growth during early childhood, contributing to cognitive development. As children grow older, their memory and attention span develop, resulting in enhanced ability to remember and retrieve information. This advancement facilitates children's ability to concentrate, adhere to instructions, and retain significant information, which is essential for achieving academic excellence.

In addition, the cognitive development that occurs during early childhood encompasses the growth of executive functions. These cognitive abilities assist children in regulating their thoughts, emotions, and behaviors. Executive functions encompass impulse control, planning, organization, and self-regulation. These skills enable children to effectively navigate social situations, regulate their emotions, and make informed decisions.

Early childhood cognitive development encompasses not only symbolic thinking, memory, attention, and executive functions, but also the acquisition and refinement of language skills. Language is a crucial tool for children to acquire communication skills, express their thoughts and emotions, and gain knowledge about the world. Language proficiency develops with age, enabling children to engage in intricate discussions, narrate anecdotes, and acquire novel ideas.

Furthermore, the cognitive development that occurs in early childhood is shaped by a multitude of factors, such as genetics, environment, and experiences. Specific genes influence a child's intelligence, memory, and other cognitive abilities. Children acquire knowledge and skills by observing and interacting with their caregivers, peers, and surroundings. Consequently, the environment also plays a significant role in shaping cognitive development. Engaging in activities such as stimulating tasks, reading, and educational games can enhance cognitive development during early childhood.

Parents, caregivers, and educators should prioritize providing assistance and fostering cognitive growth in young children. Adults can facilitate the development of crucial cognitive skills and abilities in children by offering them opportunities to participate in activities that foster cognitive growth, such as reading, playing games, and solving puzzles. In addition, adults can establish a stimulating and supportive atmosphere that motivates children to engage in exploration, learning, and critical thinking (Thomsen et al., 2011).

5.5.3. Development of Interpersonal and Intrapersonal Skills

The social and emotional development that occurs in early childhood is a crucial component of a child's overall growth and well-being. During this developmental stage, typically occurring between the ages of 2 and 6, children acquire the skills to engage with their peers, manage their emotions, and establish social connections.

To guarantee future success, it is imperative for parents and caregivers to comprehend and endorse early social and emotional development. An essential component of social development in early childhood is the capacity to participate in constructive interactions with peers. During this stage of development, children acquire the skills of sharing, taking turns, and cooperating. These skills are crucial for social development as they facilitate the establishment of relationships and friendships. Parents and caregivers can assist by providing children with opportunities for play, instructing them in conflict resolution, and exemplifying positive conduct.

Emotional development during early childhood is also significant, as children learn to identify and express their emotions in healthy ways. Children rapidly develop emotional regulation and stress management during this time. Children's emotions can be validated, coping strategies taught, and a safe space for expression provided by parents and caregivers.

Another critical aspect of social and emotional development during early childhood is the formation of secure attachments. This age helps children trust and feel secure in their caregivers, which is crucial for healthy emotional development. Being responsive to their child's needs, providing consistent care and affection, and creating a nurturing, safe, and secure environment can help. As children progress through early childhood, they begin to develop a sense of self-awareness and empathy towards others. This milestone in social and emotional development provides the foundation for understanding and respecting others' feelings. Parents can help by teaching children about emotions, encouraging them to consider others' perspectives, and modeling empathy (Thomsen et al., 2011).

During early childhood, children also begin to develop a sense of independence and autonomy. As children gain independence while still needing their caregivers, this can be difficult for parents and children. Parents and caregivers can help by giving children choices and responsibilities while setting clear and consistent boundaries for their safety and well-being. As children approach school age, their social and emotional development becomes increasingly important for academic success. Strong social and emotional skills help kids focus, regulate their behavior, and get along with teachers and peers. Encourage social and emotional learning, problem-solving, and conflict resolution, and create a supportive home environment (Figure 5.7).

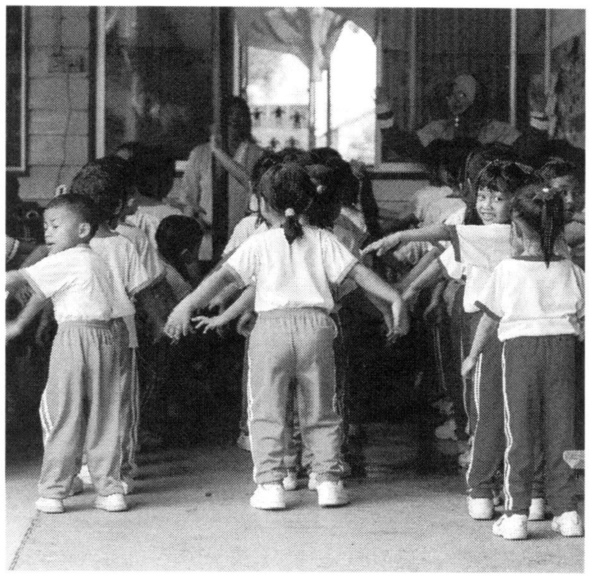

Figure 5.7. *Social development during early childhood.*

Source: By Photo by CEphoto, Uwe Aranas or alternatively © CEphoto, Uwe Aranas, CC BY-SA 3.0, https://commons.wikimedia.org/w/index.php?curid=33475265.

5.5.4. Language Development

Language acquisition in early childhood is a crucial component of a child's holistic development. Their capacity to communicate, articulate, and engage with others is contingent upon it. Language skills progress rapidly as children acquire the ability to communicate, comprehend, and utilize language in increasingly intricate manners.

Speech emergence is a significant milestone in the development of language.

The majority of 2-year-olds possess the ability to articulate a limited number of words and phrases.

By the age of three, children are capable of constructing more intricate sentences and possess a broader range of words in their vocabulary.

This phenomenon of rapid language development is commonly referred to as the "language explosion," as children acquire new vocabulary and linguistic abilities at a swift pace.

An additional crucial element of language acquisition in early childhood is the progression of grammar and syntax. Children acquire knowledge of subject-verb agreement and word order. In addition, they employ more intricate sentence structures and possess comprehension of past, present, and future tenses.

During early childhood, children not only acquire speech and grammar but also enhance their listening and comprehension abilities. They acquire the ability to adhere to instructions, respond to inquiries, and engage in conversation. Listening and comprehension are essential for effective communication and social interaction.

The process of language development in early childhood is shaped by multiple factors, such as genetics, environment, and social interactions. Children acquire language by emulating the speech patterns of others, honing their linguistic abilities through play and social engagement, and receiving guidance and encouragement from caregivers and peers.

Parents and caregivers have a vital role in facilitating and encouraging language development in young children. They can facilitate children's acquisition of language and vocabulary through verbal communication, reading, and engaging in play activities with them. Parents should additionally furnish books, music, and other language-acquisition materials within their household.

Early childhood educators have a crucial role in facilitating language development in young children. By establishing an environment in the classroom that is abundant in language, offering activities that promote language development, and offering assistance and guidance to children as they acquire and practice new language abilities, educators can facilitate the growth of language skills in children and equip them for success in academics (Thomsen et al., 2011).

5.5.5. Engagement in Play Facilitates the Process of Acquiring Knowledge and Skills

Play is an essential component of early childhood development, functioning as a crucial mechanism for learning and advancement. Children utilize play as a means to investigate their surroundings, cultivate fundamental abilities, and comprehend their encounters (Figure 5.8).

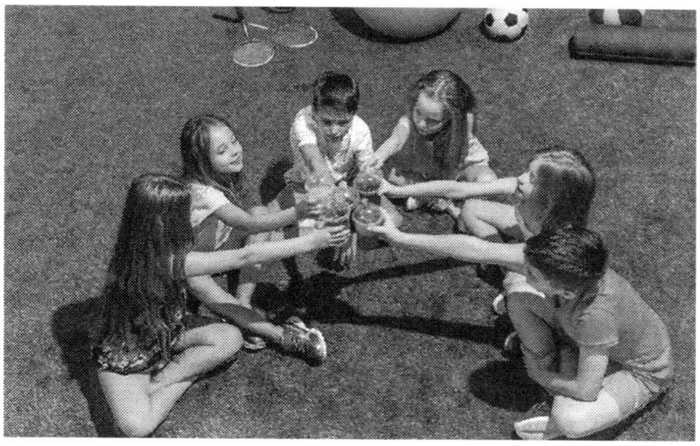

Figure 5.8. *Play during early childhood development.*

Source: https://personalitydevelopmentskills.wordpress.com/wp-content/uploads/2021/06/why-social-development-in-early-childhood.jpg?w=800&h=510&crop=1.

There are numerous benefits of playing

- Play provides children with the opportunity to engage in hands-on, experiential learning. Children explore, manipulate, and interact through play. This hands-on learning method helps children connect what they know to what they're experiencing, solidifying their worldview.
- Play promotes the development of essential skills that are crucial for academic success. For instance, pretend play helps kids develop empathy, cooperation, and problem-solving. Success in school, social interactions, and beyond requires these skills. Play helps kids develop these skills in a safe, supportive environment, preparing them for success.
- Play also fosters creativity and imagination in children. Children can create new worlds, explore different perspectives, and think creatively through imaginative play. This type of creative thinking is necessary for 21st-century success in problem-solving, innovation, and adaptability. Parents and educators can foster creativity and innovation in young learners by encouraging imaginative play.
- Play provides children with the opportunity to practice and reinforce academic concepts in a fun and engaging way. Educational games help kids practice counting, sorting, and letter recognition. These hands-on learning experiences help kids understand academic concepts and make learning fun. Using play in the classroom can help kids love learning for life.

It is important to note that play is not just a frivolous activity but a vital component of early childhood development. Research shows that play helps children develop their brains, bodies, and social-emotional skills. Play helps children develop neural connections, fine and gross motor skills, and emotional regulation. These skills are essential for academic success and well-being. Early childhood educators can improve children's learning and development by emphasizing play (Thomsen et al., 2011).

5.6. Ensuring the Safety of Children and Preventing Injuries

Ensuring the safety of children is of utmost importance to parents and caregivers. It is imperative to implement precautions to mitigate injuries and accidents that pose a risk to children. By acknowledging potential hazards and implementing measures to mitigate risks, we can establish a secure setting for children to develop and flourish.

5.6.1. Securing Your Home for Child Safety

Childproofing your home is a crucial measure for ensuring the safety of children. This entails ensuring that all hazardous objects are inaccessible to children, fastening furniture and appliances that have the potential to topple, and affixing safety gates on staircases. It is crucial to ensure that small objects that may pose a choking risk are kept out of reach of young children. Additionally, it is necessary to properly secure cabinets and drawers that store cleaning products or other hazardous items. By implementing these measures, you can establish a secure setting for your child to investigate and engage in recreational activities.

5.6.2. Ensuring the Safety of Car Seats

Another vital element of child safety is guaranteeing that your child is appropriately secured in a car seat whenever you are operating a vehicle. It is crucial to select a car seat that is suitable for your child's age and dimensions, and to ensure its proper installation in your vehicle. It is imperative to ensure that your child is consistently and securely fastened into the car seat, with the harness straps tightly fitted against their body. By adhering to these instructions, you can aid in safeguarding your child in the occurrence of a vehicular collision.

5.6.3. Ensuring Accident Prevention

Although accidents can occur in any location, there are measures you can implement to minimize the likelihood of harm to your child. An essential measure to avert accidents is to closely monitor your child, particularly when they are engaged in outdoor activities or in proximity to bodies of water. It is crucial to educate your child on safety protocols, such as practicing proper road crossing by checking both directions and wearing a protective helmet while cycling. By exemplifying proper behavior and instructing your child on safety measures, you can proactively mitigate the occurrence of accidents.

5.6.4. Aquatic Safety

Water-related fatalities are a prominent cause of mortality among young children, thus it is crucial to implement measures to ensure your child's safety in aquatic environments. It is imperative to never leave your child unsupervised in the vicinity of a pool or any other water source. Additionally, it is crucial to ensure that they consistently wear a life jacket while engaging in boating or swimming activities. It is crucial to instruct your child in swimming at a young age to ensure their ease in water and their ability to maintain safety. By adhering to these instructions, you can effectively mitigate water-related incidents and ensure the safety of your child.

5.6.5. Child First Aid

Despite taking the utmost precautions, accidents can still occur. Therefore, it is crucial to possess the knowledge and skills required to provide immediate medical assistance to your child during a critical situation. Proficiency in life-saving techniques such as CPR and the Heimlich maneuver, as well as the ability to provide first aid for minor injuries like cuts and burns, are essential. It is crucial to possess a readily accessible first aid kit at all times to promptly address any injuries that may arise. By being proactive and possessing the knowledge to react effectively during a crisis, you can contribute to expediting the necessary medical attention for your child.

5.7. Pediatric Healthcare Accessibility

Children require access to pediatric healthcare to uphold their physical and mental health and overall welfare. Accessing pediatric healthcare involves multiple sequential steps. These encompass:

- Searching for a pediatrician for check-ups
- Overseeing long-term health conditions
- Specialists in the field of pediatrics Pediatric telemedicine

Securing the services of a pediatrician is an essential measure to guarantee that children obtain the requisite medical attention. Parents can initiate the process by seeking referrals from acquaintances, relatives, or their primary healthcare provider. Opting for a pediatrician who is board-certified and possesses extensive experience in treating children is crucial. In addition, parents should take into account the geographical proximity of the pediatrician's office and their accessibility for scheduling appointments. Developing a strong rapport with a pediatrician is crucial for parents to feel at ease when discussing their child's health issues and receiving expert advice on how to provide optimal care for their child.

Well-child visits are a crucial component of pediatric healthcare, as they enable pediatricians to closely observe a child's growth and development. During these visits, pediatricians will conduct a comprehensive physical examination, evaluate the child's growth and development, and administer essential immunizations. Well-child visits provide parents with the opportunity to address any concerns they may have regarding their child's health or development. Regular well-child visits are essential for parents to ensure their child receives the requisite medical care and attention to promote their overall health and well-being (Minkovitz et al., 2002).

Continuously providing care and support from healthcare providers is necessary for managing chronic conditions in children. Children who have chronic conditions, such as asthma, diabetes, or ADHD, may need consistent monitoring and treatment in order to effectively manage their condition. Pediatricians have a vital role in organizing care for children with chronic conditions, collaborating closely with other healthcare providers to guarantee that the child receives comprehensive care. Parents of children with chronic conditions should collaborate closely with their pediatrician to establish a comprehensive care plan that caters to their child's distinct requirements and guarantees they receive the essential assistance to effectively handle their condition.

Pediatric specialists are essential in delivering specialized medical care to children with intricate medical requirements. Children afflicted with ailments such as cancer, cardiac conditions, or developmental disorders may necessitate the proficiency of pediatric specialists to receive optimal care. Pediatric specialists, such as pediatric oncologists, cardiologists, or developmental pediatricians, possess specialized expertise and training in addressing the medical needs of children with specific conditions. Collaborating closely with pediatric specialists enables children with intricate medical requirements to access the specialized care and assistance necessary for effectively managing their condition and enhancing their quality of life (Minkovitz et al., 2002).

Telemedicine has gained popularity among children as it offers convenient access to healthcare services from the comfort of their own homes. Telemedicine enables children to access medical care and guidance from healthcare professionals through virtual appointments, phone consultations, or secure messaging. Telemedicine offers significant advantages for children residing in remote regions or facing challenges in accessing conventional healthcare services. Telemedicine enables children to access prompt medical care and assistance without the necessity of physically going to a healthcare facility. Parents should collaborate closely with their pediatrician to ascertain the appropriateness of telemedicine for their child's healthcare requirements.

5.8. Encouraging the Well-Being of Families

Families often struggle to prioritize their health in the modern, fast-paced world. Families often neglect their physical and emotional well-being as a result of busy schedules, work demands, and excessive reliance on technology. Promoting a wholesome lifestyle within the family is essential for the overall welfare of all individuals. By implementing modifications and incorporating wholesome practices into their daily routines, families can improve their physical health, strengthen their relationships, and cultivate a nurturing environment for individual development (Minkovitz et al., 2002).

5.8.1. Family Bonding Activities

Family time is crucial for bonding and creating memories. Family activities like game nights, outdoor adventures, and cooking can strengthen bonds. These activities can strengthen family bonds through open communication, laughter, and shared experiences. Spending time together doing fun things can strengthen family bonds.

5.8.2. Communication Skills

Healthy family relationships require good communication. Family members can improve communication and bond by actively listening, sharing thoughts and feelings, and being empathetic. Open and honest family communication can help resolve conflicts, prevent misunderstandings, and build trust and understanding. Families can foster a supportive, nurturing environment where everyone feels heard and valued by prioritizing communication and listening.

5.8.3. Conflict Resolution

Family conflicts are normal, but how they are resolved can affect the family's well-being. Family members should learn conflict resolution through active listening, compromise, and problem-solving. Avoiding conflicts from escalating can protect relationships. Respectful and constructive conflict resolution can help families resolve issues. To strengthen relationships and foster family unity, family members should talk openly, share their concerns, and work together to find solutions.

5.8.4. Building Resilience

Being resilient can help families overcome challenges and obstacles. Supporting family members in stress management, change adaptation, and recovery can boost their resilience and ability to overcome obstacles. Family members should be encouraged to develop healthy coping skills, self-care, and seek support when needed. This can keep them positive during tough times. Resilience helps families overcome life's challenges and grow stronger.

5.8.5. Creating a Supportive Environment

Fostering emotional health and family bonds requires a supportive environment. By supporting, encouraging, and validating each other, families can create a safe, nurturing environment where everyone feels valued. Empathy, listening, and encouraging words can help family members feel understood and supported. By fostering understanding and support, families can foster the sense of connection and belonging needed for a happy and healthy life.

A Closer Look

Multiple Gestations

Multiple gestations, involving the simultaneous development of two or more embryos or fetuses in the uterus, present unique medical, ethical, and social challenges. The prevalence of multiple pregnancies has risen significantly due to advancements in assisted reproductive technologies (ART) and the increased maternal age at conception. Twins, the most common form of multiple gestations, can be either monozygotic (identical), resulting from a single fertilized egg splitting, or dizygotic (fraternal), originating from the fertilization of two separate eggs.

The medical implications of multiple gestations are profound. Mothers carrying multiples face a higher risk of complications, including preeclampsia, gestational diabetes, and preterm labor. The fetuses are at an increased risk for preterm birth, low birth weight, and intrauterine growth restriction (IUGR). Monozygotic twins, sharing a single placenta, can experience twin-to-twin transfusion syndrome (TTTS), a condition where blood flow between the twins is unbalanced, leading to complications for both fetuses. Regular and intensive prenatal monitoring is essential to manage these risks effectively.

Ethical considerations also arise in the context of ART, where the implantation of multiple embryos can lead to high-order multiple pregnancies (triplets or more). Selective reduction, the practice of reducing the number of fetuses to improve the chances of survival and health for the remaining ones, poses ethical dilemmas and emotional distress for prospective parents.

Socially, families with multiples often require additional support and resources. The financial burden of raising multiple infants simultaneously can be substantial, encompassing the costs of medical care, childcare, and education. Psychological support is also crucial for parents, as the stress of managing multiple births can be overwhelming.

Summary

- Maternal and child health is a crucial aspect of public health, encompassing the well-being of mothers and children from preconception to adolescence.
- It is essential for reducing child mortality and improving overall health outcomes.
- Key components include access to prenatal care, skilled attendance at birth, postnatal care for mother and baby, and childhood immunizations.
- Maternal health focuses on the health of women during pregnancy, childbirth, and the postnatal period, addressing issues such as maternal mortality and morbidity, prenatal care, and family planning.
- Child health, on the other hand, focuses on the physical, mental, and social well-being of children, including nutrition, immunizations, and early childhood development. Improving maternal and child health requires a comprehensive approach, including access to healthcare services, education, and social support.

References

1. Bacon, S. L., Bouchard, A., Loucks, E. B., & Lavoie, K. L. (2009). Individual-level socioeconomic status is associated with worse asthma morbidity in patients with asthma. *Respiratory Research, 10*, 125. https://doi.org/10.1186/1465-9921-10-125.
2. Beard, J. R., Cerda, M., Blaney, S., Ahern, J., Vlahov, D., & Galea, S. (2009). Neighborhood characteristics and change in depressive symptoms among older residents of New York City. *American Journal of Public Health, 99*(7), 1308–1314. https://doi.org/10.2105/AJPH.2008.149823.
3. Burra, T. A., Moineddin, R., Agha, M. M., & Glazier, R. H. (2009). Social disadvantage, air pollution, and asthma physician visits in Toronto, Canada. *Environmental Research, 109*(5), 567–574. https://doi.org/10.1016/j.envres.2009.03.009.
4. Curry, A., Latkin, C., & Davey-Rothwell, M. (2008). Pathways to depression: The impact of neighborhood violent crime on inner-city residents in Baltimore, Maryland, USA. *Social Science & Medicine, 67*, 23–30. https://doi.org/10.1016/j.socscimed.2008.03.006.
5. Cutrona, C. E., Wallace, G., & Wesner, K. A. (2006). Neighborhood characteristics and depression: An examination of stress processes. *Current Directions in Psychological Science, 15*(4), 188–192. https://doi.org/10.1111/j.1467-8721.2006.00438.x.
6. Dear, M. (2002). Los Angeles and the Chicago school: Invitation to a debate. *City & Community, 1*(1), 5. https://doi.org/10.1111/1540-6040.00002.
7. Farfel, A., Tirosh, A., Derazne, E., Garty, B. Z., & Afek, A. (2010). Association between socioeconomic status and the prevalence of asthma. *Annals of Allergy, Asthma & Immunology, 104*(6), 490–495. https://doi.org/10.1016/j.anai.2010.03.002.
8. Finkelstein, M. M., Jerrett, M., DeLuca, P., Finkelstein, N., Verma, D. K., Chapman, K., & Sears, M. R. (2003). Relation between income, air pollution and mortality: A cohort study. *Canadian Medical Association Journal, 169*(4), 397–402. https://doi.org/10.1503/cmaj.1038518.
9. Foster, H., & Brooks-Gunn, J. (2009). Toward a stress process model of children's exposure to

physical family and community violence. *Clinical Child and Family Psychology Review, 12*(1), 71–94. https://doi.org/10.1007/s10567-008-0043-3.

10. Franzini, L., Caughy, M., Spears, W., & Eugenia Fernandez Esquer, M. (2005). Neighborhood economic conditions, social processes, and self-rated health in low-income neighborhoods in Texas: A multilevel latent variables model. *Social Science & Medicine, 61*(6), 1135–1150. https://doi.org/10.1016/j.socscimed.2004.12.024.
11. Garner, R., & Kohen, D. (2008). Changes in the prevalence of asthma among Canadian children. *Health Reports, 19*(2), 45–50.
12. Gee, G. C., & Payne-Sturges, D. (2004). Environmental health disparities: A framework integrating psychosocial and environmental concepts. *Environmental Health Perspectives, 112*(17), 1645–1653. https://doi.org/10.1289/ehp.7074.
13. Gupta, R. S., Zhang, X., Sharp, L. K., Shannon, J. J., & Weiss, K. B. (2008). Geographic variability in childhood asthma prevalence in Chicago. *Journal of Allergy and Clinical Immunology, 121*(3), 639–645. https://doi.org/10.1016/j.jaci.2007.11.011.
14. Gupta, R. S., Zhang, X., Springston, E. E., Sharp, L. K., Curtis, L. M., Shalowitz, M., Shannon, J. J., & Weiss, K. B. (2010). The association between community crime and childhood asthma prevalence in Chicago. *Annals of Allergy, Asthma & Immunology, 104*(4), 299–306. https://doi.org/10.1016/j.anai.2010.01.021.
15. Haczku, A., & Panettieri Jr, R. A. (2010). Social stress and asthma: The role of corticosteroid insensitivity. *Journal of Allergy and Clinical Immunology, 125*(3), 550–558. https://doi.org/10.1016/j.jaci.2009.11.041.
16. Henderson, C., Roux, A. V., David, R. J., Kiefe, C. I., West, D., & Williams, D. R. (2005). Neighborhood characteristics, individual level socioeconomic factors, and depressive symptoms in young adults: The CARDIA study. *Journal of Epidemiology and Community Health, 59*(4), 322–328. https://doi.org/10.1136/jech.2004.025478.
17. Hwang, B. F., Lee, Y. L., Lin, Y. C., Jaakkola, J. J. K., & Guo, Y. L. (2005). Traffic related air pollution as a determinant of asthma among Taiwanese school children. *Thorax, 60*(6), 467–473. https://doi.org/10.1136/thx.2004.031823.
18. Kozyrskyj, A. L., & Becker, A. B. (2004). Rural-urban differences in asthma prevalence: Possible explanations. *Journal of Allergy and Clinical Immunology, 113*(2), S306. https://doi.org/10.1016/j.jaci.2003.12.1484.
19. Kozyrskyj, A. L., Hayglass, K. T., Sandford, A. J., Paré, P. D., Chan-Yeung, M., & Becker, A. B. (2009). A novel study design to investigate the early-life origins of asthma in children (SAGE study). *Allergy, 64*(8), 1185–1193. https://doi.org/10.1111/j.1398-9995.2009.01999.x.
20. Kozyrskyj, A. L., Kendall, G. E., Jacoby, P., Sly, P. D., & Zubrick, S. R. (2010). Association between socioeconomic status and the development of asthma: Analyses of income trajectories. *American Journal of Public Health, 100*(3), 540–546. https://doi.org/10.2105/AJPH.2008.151886.
21. Kozyrskyj, A. L., Mai, X. M., McGrath, P., HayGlass, K. T., Becker, A. B., & MacNeil, B. (2008). Continued exposure to maternal distress in early life is associated with an increased risk of childhood asthma. *American Journal of Respiratory and Critical Care Medicine, 177*(2), 142–147. https://doi.org/10.1164/rccm.200705-735OC.

22. Laraia, B., Messer, L., Kaufman, J., Dole, N., Caughy, M., O'Campo, P., & Savitz, D. (2006). Direct observation of neighborhood attributes in an urban area of the US south: Characterizing the social context of pregnancy. *International Journal of Health Geographics, 5*, 11. https://doi.org/10.1186/1476-072X-5-11.

23. Lee, J. T., Son, J. Y., Kim, H., & Kim, S. Y. (2006). Effect of air pollution on asthma-related hospital admissions for children by socioeconomic status associated with area of residence. *Archives of Environmental & Occupational Health, 61*(3), 123–130. https://doi.org/10.3200/AEOH.61.3.123-130.

24. Lightbody, J. (1978). The reform of a metropolitan government: The case of Winnipeg, 1971. *Canadian Public Policy/Analyze de Politiques, 4*(4), 489–504.

25. MacLeod, K. E., Gee, G. C., Crawford, P., & Wang, M. C. (2008). Neighborhood environment as a predictor of television watching among girls. *Journal of Epidemiology and Community Health, 62*(4), 288–292. https://doi.org/10.1136/jech.2006.059972.

26. Mair, C., Diez Roux, A. V., & Morenoff, J. D. (2010). Neighborhood stressors and social support as predictors of depressive symptoms in the Chicago community adult health study. *Health & Place, 16*(5), 811–819. https://doi.org/10.1016/j.healthplace.2010.04.002.

27. Matheson, F. I., Moineddin, R., Dunn, J. R., Creatore, M. I., Gozdyra, P., & Glazier, R. H. (2006). Urban neighborhoods, chronic stress, gender and depression. *Social Science & Medicine, 63*(10), 2604–2616. https://doi.org/10.1016/j.socscimed.2006.06.025.

28. Morello-Frosch, R., & Shenassa, E. D. (2006). The environmental riskscape and social inequality: Implications for explaining maternal and child health disparities. *Environmental Health Perspectives, 114*(8), 1150–1153. https://doi.org/10.1289/ehp.8811.

29. Mulvaney, C., & Kendrick, D. (2005). Depressive symptoms in mothers of pre-school children. *Social Psychiatry and Psychiatric Epidemiology, 40*(3), 202–208. https://doi.org/10.1007/s00127-005-0867-8.

30. Myers, T., & Tomasio, L. (2011). Asthma: 2015 and beyond. *Respiratory Care, 56*(10), 1389–1410.

31. O'Campo, P., Salmon, C., & Burke, J. (2009). Neighborhoods and mental well-being: What are the pathways? *Health & Place, 15*, 56–68. https://doi.org/10.1016/j.healthplace.2008.02.004.

32. Persky, V. W., Slezak, J., Contreras, A., Becker, L., Hernandez, E., Ramakrishnan, V., & Piorkowski, J. (1998). Relationships of race and socioeconomic status with prevalence, severity, and symptoms of asthma in Chicago school children. *Annals of Allergy, Asthma & Immunology, 81*(3), 266–271. https://doi.org/10.1016/S1081-1206(10)62820-6.

33. Pittman, T. (2011). The association between neighborhood stressors and asthma prevalence of school children in Winnipeg. *Allergy, Asthma & Clinical Immunology, 6*(1), 1. https://doi.org/10.1186/1710-1492-6-1.

34. Sampson, R. J. (2009). Disparity and diversity in the contemporary city: Social (dis) order revisited. *British Journal of Sociology, 60*(1), 1–31. https://doi.org/10.1111/j.1468-4446.2009.01217.x.

35. Sampson, R. J., Morenoff, J. D., & Felton, E. (1999). Beyond social capital: Spatial dynamics of collective efficacy for children. *American Sociological Review, 64*(5), 633–660. https://doi.org/10.2307/2657367.

36. Shankardass, K., McConnell, R. S., Milam, J., Berhane, K., Tatalovich, Z., Wilson, J. P., & Jerrett, M. (2007). The association between contextual socioeconomic factors and prevalent asthma in a cohort of Southern California school children. *Social Science & Medicine, 65*(8), 1792–1806. https://doi.org/10.1016/j.socscimed.2007.05.032.

37. Smargiassi, A., Kosatsky, T., Hicks, J., Plante, C., Armstrong, B., Villeneuve, P. J., & Goudreau, S. (2009). Risk of asthmatic episodes in children exposed to sulfur dioxide stack emissions from a refinery point source in Montreal, Canada. *Environmental Health Perspectives, 117*(5), 653–659. https://doi.org/10.1289/ehp.0800151.

38. Statistics Canada. (2009). *1996 Census of Population: All Tables, Winnipeg (157 areas) (table), 1996 Census of Population (43 Large Urban Centres, Census Tracts (neighbourhoods)) (database), Using E-STAT (distributor)*. Ottawa, Canada.

39. Steptoe, A., & Feldman, P. J. (2001). Neighborhood problems as sources of chronic stress: Development of a measure of neighborhood problems, and associations with socioeconomic status and health. *Annals of Behavioral Medicine, 23*(3), 177–185. https://doi.org/10.1207/S15324796ABM2303_3.

40. Sternthal, M. J., Coull, B. A., Chiu, Y. H. M., Cohen, S., & Wright, R. J. (2011). Associations among maternal childhood socioeconomic status, cord blood IgE levels, and repeated wheeze in urban children. *Journal of Allergy and Clinical Immunology, 128*(2), 337–345. https://doi.org/10.1016/j.jaci.2011.04.033.

41. Sternthal, M. J., Jun, H. J., Earls, F., & Wright, R. J. (2010). Community violence and urban childhood asthma: A multilevel analysis. *European Respiratory Journal, 36*(6), 1400–1409. https://doi.org/10.1183/09031936.00012310.

42. Subbarao, P., Becker, A., Brook, J. R., Daley, D., Mandhane, P. J., Miller, G. E., Turvey, S. W., & Sears, M. R. (2009). Epidemiology of asthma: Risk factors for development. *Expert Review of Clinical Immunology, 5*(6), 777–795. https://doi.org/10.1586/eci.09.63.

43. Szreter, S., & Woolcock, M. (2004). Health by association? Social capital, social theory, and the political economy of public health. *International Journal of Epidemiology, 33*(4), 650–667. https://doi.org/10.1093/ije/dyh013.

44. To, T., Gershon, A., Wang, C., Dell, S., & Cicutto, L. (2007). Persistence and remission in childhood asthma: A population-based asthma birth cohort study. *Archives of Pediatrics & Adolescent Medicine, 161*(12), 1197–1204. https://doi.org/10.1001/archpedi.161.12.1197.

45. Wilkins, R. (2009). *PCCF+ Version 5D User's Guide. Automated Geographic Coding Based on the Statistics Canada Postal Code Conversion Files, Including Postal Codes Through September 2008 (Statistics Canada, Catalogue 82F0086-XDB)*. Ottawa, Canada.

46. Wright, R. J. (2006). Health effects of socially toxic neighborhoods: The violence and urban asthma paradigm. *Clinics in Chest Medicine, 27*(3), 413–421. https://doi.org/10.1016/j.ccm.2006.04.007.

47. Wright, R. J., & Cohen, S. (2002). Parental stress as a predictor of wheezing in infancy: A prospective birth-cohort study. *American Journal of Respiratory and Critical Care Medicine, 165*(3), 358–365. https://doi.org/10.1164/ajrccm.165.3.2101124.

48. Wright, R. J., & Fisher, E. B. (2003). Putting asthma into context: Community influences on risk, behavior, and intervention. In I. Kawachi & L. F. Berkman (Eds.), *Neighborhoods and Health* (pp. 182–210). Oxford University Press.

49. Wright, R. J., & Steinbach, S. F. (2001). Violence: An unrecognized environmental exposure that may contribute to greater asthma morbidity in high-risk inner-city populations. *Environmental Health Perspectives, 109*(11), 1085–1089. https://doi.org/10.2307/3454692.

Chapter

PROMOTING HEALTH FOR OLDER ADULTS

6

Contents

Introduction

With the increasing lifespan and growing population of older individuals in both industrialized and developing nations, a crucial concern arises: will this aging population experience long-term or enhanced health, an improved quality of life, and adequate social and economic support? The solution to this question depends on the capacity of families and communities, as well as contemporary social, political, economic, and health service delivery systems, to offer the best possible assistance to older individuals. Nevertheless, although all contemporary societies are dedicated to offering healthcare and social services to their population, these systems are constantly changing, influenced by various and developing national and regional policy frameworks. There is significant variation in the health, social, and economic policies for older individuals across developed countries. Conducting cross-national research to analyze these variations can greatly aid in developing effective policies to improve the health, social, and economic well-being of elderly populations. One of the key policy concerns related to health and lifespan is the future financial sustainability of pension, health, and social insurance systems, whether they are run by the government or private entities. Additionally, it is important to consider how these systems affect the rates of savings and investment. The duration of one's employment, tax contributions, and savings will play a significant role in the outcomes of population aging. A significant number of individuals already have a work span that is less than half of their lifetime due to prolonged periods of education and training during their early years, earlier retirement, and increased life expectancy. This presents a challenge to the long-term viability of systems that are intended to provide support for the elderly. If the current trend of longer lifespans continues without a corresponding increase in the duration of working years, the strain on these systems could become even more significant.

The involvement of individuals in the workforce, their investment and saving habits, and the availability of health services are intricate phenomena that are interconnected at both the individual and societal levels (Quinn & Burkhauser, 1994; Smith, 1999). Government and employer incentives significantly influence labor force participation. Potential strategies to promote longer working lives include minimizing the financial disincentives for individuals to work beyond the typical retirement age and reducing the expenses associated with employing and potentially retraining older individuals. However, when creating these incentives, policymakers must have a clear understanding of the duration for which individuals can be expected to continue working. What is the extent of physical and mental abilities in older individuals? What is the course of health and function as individuals progress in age? Is it possible to sustain and improve productivity in older individuals, and if so, what are the associated expenses? Does productivity and engagement vary with age? How can healthcare services be delivered in a way that ensures the highest level of health and functionality? At its core, policymakers are faced with the challenging task of determining how to distribute scarce resources to protect and enhance public health. What are the strategies to attain optimal health without incurring excessive expenses? Should additional resources be allocated towards behavioral modification and other initiatives aimed at promoting health and preventing diseases, including improving health during the early stages of life? Alternatively, should more resources be focused on treating patients with advanced-stage diseases? What is the optimal investment amount for the development of new healthcare technologies, service delivery enhancements, and professional training?

An emphasis on the health status of a nation at the national level and how it changes over time is crucial for multiple reasons. The state of one's health is a crucial measure of overall welfare, and it significantly influences the amount of money spent on healthcare and social services for older individuals. Social and political policies and programs have a reciprocal impact on health status. Moreover, the health status can be modified through the implementation of top-notch health promotion and disease prevention initiatives, alongside efficient medical services. Many national programs and policies that focus on the health and healthcare services for older individuals have significant consequences and intricate connections with other sectors of the economy. Table 6.1 presents illustrations.

Table 6.1. Relationship of Public-Sector Programs and Policies to Health Services for Older Persons

Sector	Relation to the Provision of Health Services for Older Persons
Housing	Provision of suitable-quality housing, both in the community and within institutions, to sustain health. Reconstruction of housing to accommodate disabled older persons.
Public Health	Creation of prevention and health promotion programs that affect older persons.
Education	Training of all levels of health professionals and ancillary workers in special skills related to the problems of older persons.
Manufacturing	Provision of increasingly complex mechanical and electronic devices for the treatment and rehabilitation of older persons.
Urban Design	Location of housing for older persons so as to optimize access to health, nutritional, recreational, and social services. Opportunities for generativity and engagement by older persons.
Transportation	Provision of public transportation and facilitation of personal transport to enhance mobility and its social outcomes.

Source: May, J. F. (2016). The Politics of Family Planning Policies and Programs in sub-Saharan Africa. Population and Development Review, 43(S1), 308–329.

This chapter focuses on the importance of health status and change in shaping health, social, and economic policy development. Initially, we delineate the fundamental concerns that need to be investigated regarding the health condition of older individuals. Next, we introduce a theoretical model that outlines the factors that influence an individual's health condition. This model will serve as a basis for the subsequent discussion. Next, we will examine the fundamental indicators of health status, providing specific instances of basic global patterns and trends. Subsequently, a concise examination of the attributes of national health systems ensues. The chapter also examines the data sources used for conducting cross-national research on the health status of the elderly, along with the advantages and disadvantages of this type of research.

Orientation and Directional Terms

Term	Definition	Illustration
Geriatrics	The branch of medicine focused on the health care of elderly people, aiming to promote health and prevent and treat diseases in older adults.	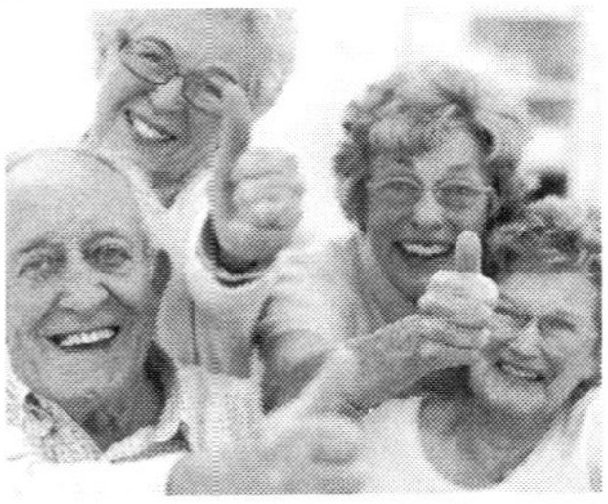
Frailty	A clinical syndrome in older adults characterized by decreased strength, endurance, and physiologic function, which increases vulnerability to adverse health outcomes.	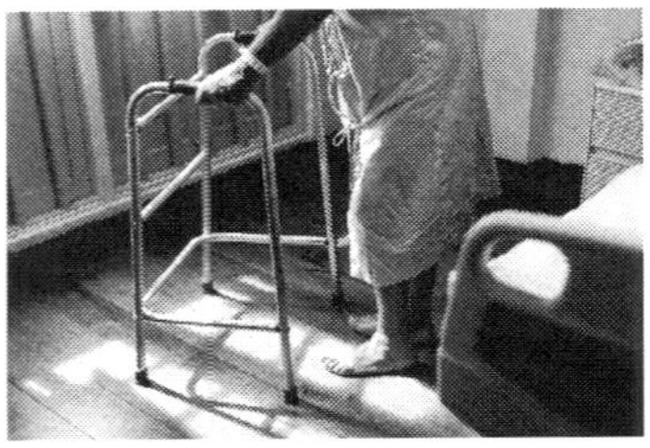
Cognitive Decline	The gradual loss of cognitive abilities, including memory, attention, and problem-solving skills, often associated with aging and conditions like dementia.	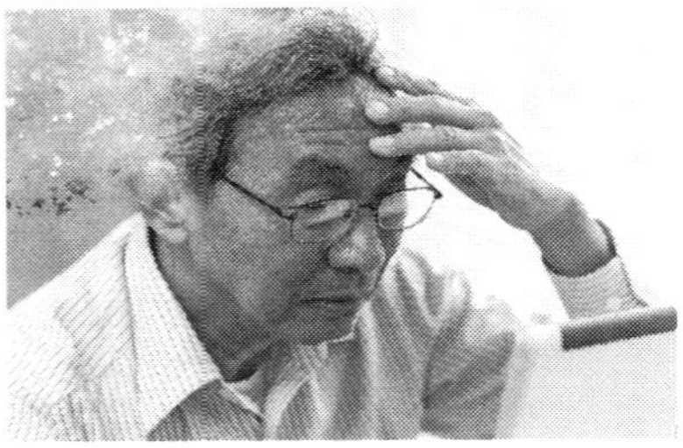
Polypharmacy	The use of multiple medications by a single patient, often seen in older adults, which can increase the risk of adverse drug interactions and side effects.	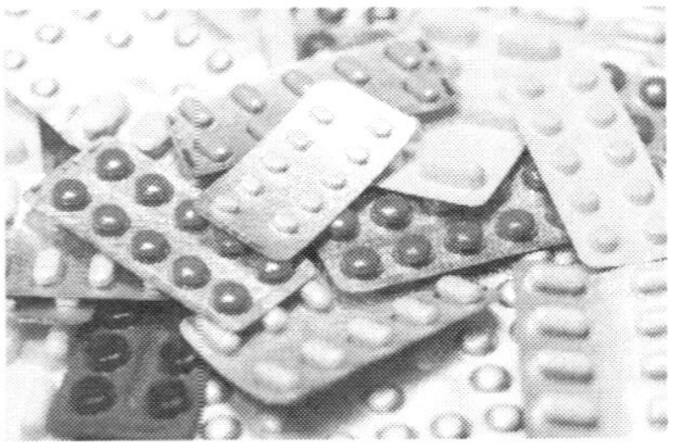
Osteoarthritis	Osteoarthritis is a degenerative disease that worsens over time, often resulting in chronic pain.	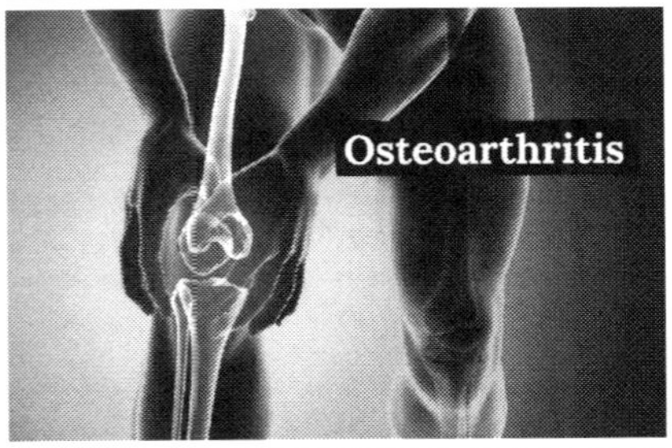

6.1. Key Issues

The complexity of national health policy decisions regarding older individuals is growing due to various factors. The populations of elderly individuals and those in the oldest age group have experienced a significant surge in most developed countries. Nations with a significant elderly population will experience a growing proportion of elderly individuals in the future, along with the associated social and economic requirements. Furthermore, countries need to make arrangements for the increasing population of younger individuals with disabilities who are living longer due to advancements in healthcare. Policy decisions regarding the provision of health services for the elderly have become intricate due to technological, fiscal, and ethical considerations. Furthermore, it is important to highlight that health services are closely interconnected with the delivery of social services and economic assistance, such as housing, nutrition, institutional care, and other related endeavors. The inclusion of preventive and rehabilitative services has increased both the expenses of healthcare and the possibility of enhancing function, mobility, and social interaction. Healthcare for older individuals differs from that provided to other age groups in various ways. These include greater resource requirements, the integration of professional health services with social services, the frequent occurrence of ethical dilemmas, a higher prevalence of physical and mental disabilities, and a relatively limited scientific evidence base for determining effective preventive and medical interventions. Within this particular framework, it is important to highlight the following matters of significance.

- What is the significance of one's health condition on their retirement preferences and patterns? What is the correlation between health status and retirement age? Have the recent trends in declining age-specific rates of disability resulted in higher and more prolonged engagement in the labor force?
- What is the influence of health on families? How has the evolving health condition of elderly individuals impacted the productivity and economic standing of families and households? What strategies do families employ to financially support ailing parents, and how does this impact their participation in the workforce? How does the declining health of elderly individuals, specifically the development of physical weakness, impact their ability to provide care for a sick or disabled spouse or relative? What economic arrangements do families establish to ensure the long-term care of older individuals, whether they are living in the community or in chronic care facilities? How do these provisions align or coordinate with public and voluntary assistance and care programs?
- What is the significance of health in relation to wealth and economic status? What empirical evidence supports the direct impact of health status on an individual's wealth, assets, and economic productivity? The healthcare system plays a crucial role in preventing, treating, and rehabilitating illnesses. It works to uphold individuals' economic status by ensuring their health and well-being. What is the impact of health shocks on future economic status and personal and family wealth, taking into account the underlying socioeconomic status?

- What is the impact of economic status and educational levels on the health of individuals throughout their lives? Through which mechanisms and to what extent does economic status contribute to improved health status? During which age groups does economic status exert the most significant influence on health status? How does the allocation of wealth, income, and economic productivity within a country impact the maintenance, improvement, or deterioration of health status, regardless of individual and family socioeconomic characteristics? What is the impact of providing health services on long-term health outcomes? Developing policies and systems for delivering health services to older individuals necessitates a constant stream of information, including quantitative data on population health status, trends, and the resources allocated to the healthcare system. Specifically, the utilization of global experiences in the field of health and healthcare has the potential to significantly enhance the effectiveness of these policies and systems. In addition, conducting research across different countries can facilitate the development of assessment methods that would typically be impractical within a single country due to the uniformity of medical practices and administrative cultures. This research can also assist in resolving the issues by offering a variety of observations regarding changes that occur over time and, potentially, early indications of emerging health patterns. Comparative research can enhance our comprehension of how specific diseases and conditions manifest as disability in different work, social, policy, and living settings. This, in turn, offers valuable insights into which modifications in these environments would yield the greatest cost-effectiveness.

6.2. Conceptual Model of the Determinants of Health Status

As noted above, the determinants of health are complex and comprise multiple policy domains. One basic but important conceptual model that can be used to illustrate the breadth of these determinants is shown in Figure 6.1. This construct represents the health of all demographic groups in a society, although the emphasis here is on the health of older persons. The determinants are presented in a set of concentric circles, with the community population at the center. Outermost, and often difficult to quantify, are the general social, economic, cultural, and environmental (physical-chemical) conditions that have important long-term health effects. The next circle contains society's basic social, health, and economic institutions, which sustain or impair a healthy existence. The next circle emphasizes the critical role of social and community interactions and exchanges, whereby individuals make their collective decisions. The circle next to the core highlights the importance of individual behavioral choices (e.g., cigarette smoking, risk-taking behaviors) in the determination of health status.

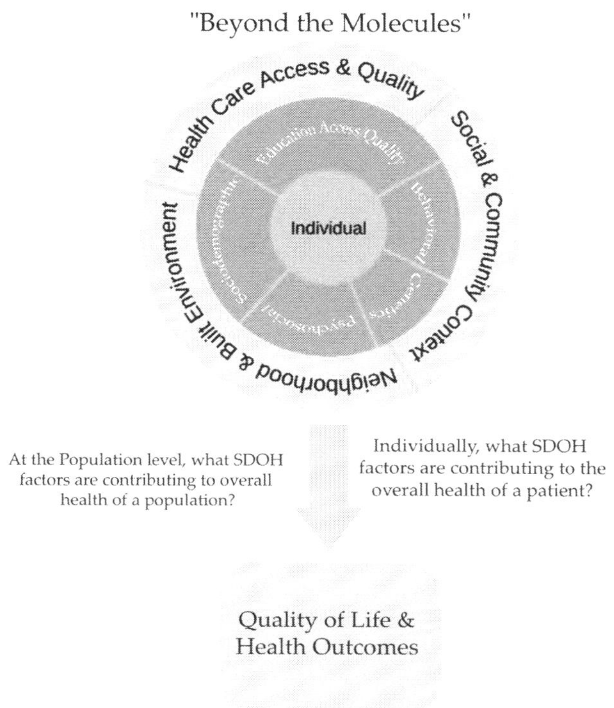

Figure 6.1. *Social determinants of health status.*

Source: *Davidson J, Vashisht R, Butte AJ. (2022). From genes to geography, from cells to community, from biomolecules to behaviors: the Importance of social determinants of health. Biomolecules, 12(10), 1449. https://doi.org/10.3390/biom12101449.*

A limitation of a two-dimensional representation is the lack of temporal dimension. Other models provide a more comprehensive analysis of the impact of infancy, childhood, and the environment on health outcomes in later life. However, the model depicted in Figure 6.1 is advantageous in various aspects. As an illustration, it emphasizes the close connection between economic and employment conditions and health. As a consequence, the model assigns professional health services a significant but not overriding role among the institutional forces that influence health status. The model appropriately highlights the importance of fundamental public health factors, such as the physiochemical environment and the provision of safe and sufficient food and sanitary services. Furthermore, the model demonstrates an acknowledgment of the personal accountability for one's health condition, both in the choice of actions and in the joint determinations made by individuals. Ultimately, the model demonstrates that policy interventions in a single institution or domain can either succeed or fail to achieve the intended outcome due to the involvement of various sectors. Therefore, policy outcomes can only be improved by implementing interventions at multiple points. Conversely, interventions in one sector may result in unforeseen consequences in other sectors.

6.3. Measuring Health Status

In the 20th century, significant shifts occurred in population health and survival rates in both developed and developing nations. During the early part of the century, there was a significant reduction in mortality rates for infants, children, and pregnant women in industrialized nations. These enhancements persist up to the current moment. Subsequently, during the later part of the century, significant decreases in death rates among elderly individuals were observed in almost all advanced nations. These reductions were primarily due to declines in fatalities caused by heart disease, as well as other major causes of death. Furthermore, there has been a transition among elderly individuals towards not only surviving but also flourishing despite the presence of common chronic ailments like different heart conditions and arthritis. Surveys of the population have also shown that the occurrence of physical disability at different ages has decreased in certain countries (Jacobzone et al., 1998). Developing nations have experienced slower progress compared to more developed nations in terms of reducing mortality rates and transitioning from a higher prevalence of infectious and parasitic diseases to a higher prevalence of chronic and degenerative diseases. Nevertheless, the disparity between highly developed nations and less developed nations has significantly diminished.

In the latter part of the 20th century, there was a notable increase in how the health status of a population could be described. This was achieved by adding additional measures to mortality data, such as personal clinical signs and symptoms, diseases and conditions, and functional disabilities. The increased potential availability of more precise health data has significantly expanded the range of quantitative tools for health policy and planning, especially for older individuals, who have higher rates of disease and disability compared to other demographic groups.

Forecasting healthcare needs and formulating policies for older individuals rely heavily on accurately determining the trends of significant health indicators. However, the task of defining "health" and determining the health status of individuals is a complex and challenging endeavor. Even in ideal conditions and without limitations on resources, it is difficult to thoroughly evaluate the physical condition of individuals, comprehend the characteristics and factors influencing personal or social behavior, and anticipate the extent and severity of the consequences of environmental challenges (such as those encountered in the workplace or elsewhere in the community). Furthermore, it is challenging to anticipate the specific impacts that different medical services or interventions will have on individuals. With the advent of advanced and accurate health status assessments, significant progress can be made.

The assessment of health status can be approached from different angles, depending on the objectives and applications of the data. Personal health can be evaluated through subjective self-report, objective physiological and biochemical measurements, or standardized indicators of diseases and disabilities. Indeed, each of these viewpoints holds significance and serves to enhance one another. In addition, the health status can be classified based on key areas such as physical health (e.g., the performance of the heart and lungs), mental health (e.g., the existence of a depressed mood), and physical and social functional health (e.g., the capability to climb stairs or engage in a specific occupation). Health can also be conceptualized in terms of its temporal and longitudinal aspects. For instance, what are the changes in the individual's health status, or did the individual survive or perish? Changes in health status can also be observed through variations in the extent of healthcare resource utilization, including the use of pharmaceuticals, institutional care, or rehabilitative services. The temporal viewpoint is crucial and results in a focus on longitudinal, cohort data sources.

Although there is no universally accepted method for characterizing health status, there are multiple significant ways to evaluate and describe an individual's health. Access to this data may be limited in computerized or easily accessible formats, but it can typically be obtained by extracting information from clinical records or conducting surveys of patients, healthcare professionals, administrators, or populations within a specific geographic region. Section 6.9 provides a comprehensive description of the health status measures that are frequently employed for survey and administrative data collection. These measures encompass clinical signs, symptoms, and syndromes; specific medical conditions; self-assessed health; functional abilities and disabilities; physiological and pathological indicators; mortality data and related measures; as well as aging and mental illness.

6.4. Characteristics of Healthcare Systems

There are many public health measures as well as personal behaviors that have an impact on health status. There is a possibility that health promotion activities aimed at older people will not involve direct contact with the formal healthcare system. Some examples of the latter activities include education programs and the provision of good preventive nutrition, safe transportation to enhance mobility, and the guarantee of adequate housing. In light of this, the only way to evaluate the effectiveness and overall impact of numerous fundamental public health programs, along with the costs that are already incurred, is to make use of information obtained from population surveys in addition to the data obtained from clinical sources. When it comes to older adults, a decrease in the use of toxic substances, an increase in the amount of exercise and structured leisure activities, and even paid and unpaid work are all associated with improved function, a reduction in the occurrence of physical and emotional illness, and an improvement in quality of life. Therefore, to have effective national and regional policies for the promotion of health among older people, it is necessary to identify significant deficiencies in these areas. It is possible that population surveys are the only method that can bring about accurate information regarding issues such as the consumption of cigarettes and alcohol, the perception of elder abuse, the availability and utilization of exercise and other leisure and recreational programs, as well as the levels of mobility and social interaction for the elderly.

The ability to provide community-based preventive services, which are typically provided within the context of primary care, is another essential component of the national health policy of the United States for older people. According to Bloom et al. (2000), the presence of such services has been utilized as a benchmark for determining the overall quality of care in nations such as the United States and other countries. The provision of appropriate immunizations and screening for early and treatable conditions, such as colon and breast cancer, high blood cholesterol, high blood pressure, and depression, are among the activities that are included in this category. There is a recommendation for the implementation of explicit geriatric screening and management programs for the prevention and treatment of falls, early cognitive impairment, physical disability, and inappropriate medication use. By providing these services, the elderly can maintain or improve their function, which in turn leads to an improvement in their quality of life. Despite the presence of obvious illness, a methodical approach to the complicated functional and medical issues that older people face, which is commonly known as geriatric assessment, can be of assistance in preserving useful function. Health professionals may recommend certain preventive activities, but other people will actually carry them out. Providing ramps rather than stairs and handrails in the appropriate locations is an example of environmental screening that can be beneficial in preventing falls and improving mobility. This is an important example.

It is essential for the various sectors involved to coordinate public and clinical policies that are relevant to health promotion and disease prevention in order for these policies to have the desired positive effects on the health status of older people. There are many different sectors involved. International comparisons of preventive service delivery programs may assist in determining which programs have the most desirable outcomes and which individual programs have the potential to be usefully implemented in several different countries. For instance, standardized specific blood cholesterol levels can predict very different rates of heart disease in various countries (Kromhout, 1999). This could potentially result in different priorities for prevention programs when it comes to cholesterol levels. One more time, representative household surveys of older people are the most efficient method for gathering the information that is required for such international research.

As far as structure, function, and administration are concerned, every single national health system is extremely complicated. The complexity and diversity of these health systems make it difficult to classify them, a challenge that is made even more difficult by the fact that all health systems are continuously evolving in accordance with ongoing political and economic forces. Regardless of how broadly one interprets the term, the complexity of the situation makes it extremely difficult to initiate and evaluate policy. In the same vein, however, the majority of contemporary healthcare systems, particularly those found in developed nations, are confronted with the following collective forces and challenges: rapid and costly technological innovation; the increasing infusion of business practices to contain the costs of delivering care; growing consumer demands for care that is uniformly distributed geographically and socioeconomically; the provision of effective quality assurance programs; the need to identify funding for the breadth of health services demanded by communities, to balance the needs of primary and specialty care programs, and to respond to complementary and alternative medical practices; and, in many cases, the decentralization of authority in previously monolithic systems.

Within the context of the comparative study of health systems, several different classification systems have been proposed and utilized; however, there has not been the development of a taxonomy that is generally accepted. Mechanic and Rochefort (1996) provide a comprehensive analysis of a wide variety of health system typologies. These typologies place varying degrees of emphasis on various aspects, including political organization and control, economics and fiscal management, population demands and utilization, the role of market forces, universality of coverage, cultural influences on professional practice, the degree of professional dominance, and adherence to a variety of social movements and principles.

People who are older tend to make significant use of formal health services. This is primarily because as people get older, they experience higher rates of morbidity and disability. These kinds of services require a significant amount of resources, and one of the most important policy questions that all nations must attempt to answer is how to allocate the resources that are available in a manner that will produce the best possible health outcomes through the most effective means. Once more, cross-national comparative research is an important avenue for addressing this issue. This research investigates international variations in the organization, financing, delivery, and evaluation of elder health services. Specifically, Figure 6.2 illustrates the international variation in the utilization of nursing homes on a per capita basis across 20 countries, while Figure 6.3 illustrates the variation in spending for health services among the seven nations that make up the G7. The relationship between the organization, administration, and financing of the health system and the health status and outcomes is something that is considered to be one of the most important macro-analytical policy questions. In spite of the fact that there has been relatively little research conducted in this field, cross-national analyzes provide the most effective method for comprehending the ways in which major factors, such as the amount of money invested in new technology, influence health outcomes.

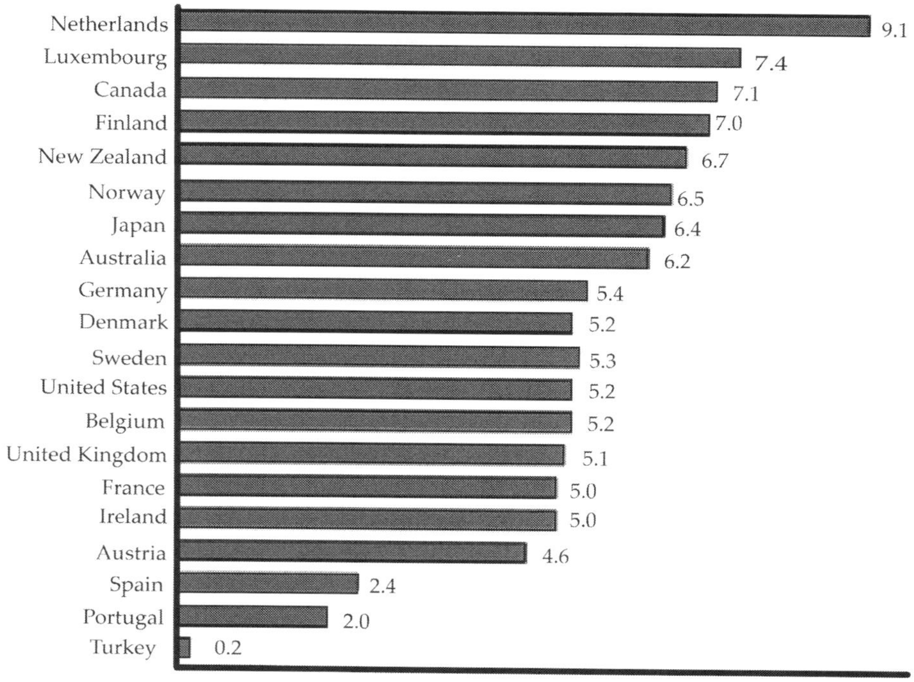

Figure 6.2. *Percent of elderly population in residential care: Circa 1991.*

Source: Organization for Economic Co-Operation and Development (1996).

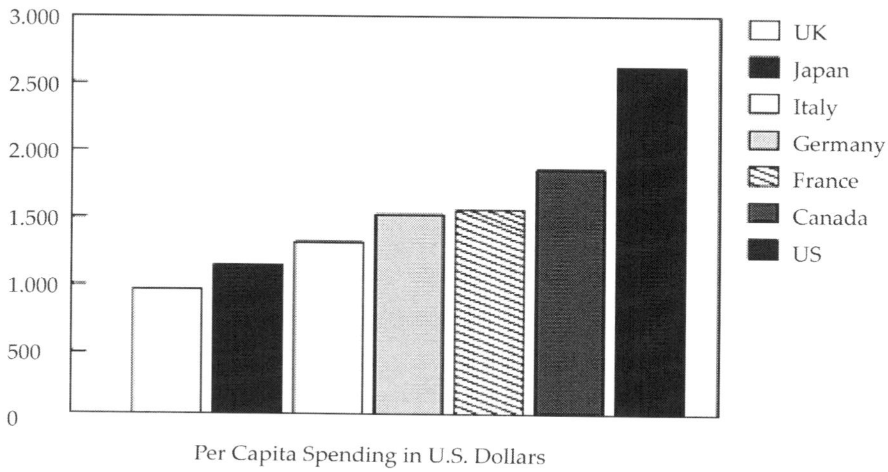

Figure 6.3. *Healthcare expenditure in the G7 nations: 1990.*

Source: Cutler (1999).

Depending on the problems that are being addressed, there are a variety of different units of analysis that can be used to characterize health systems. A selection of examples of analytical variables that are frequently utilized to describe health systems at either the national or regional level is provided in Table 6.2. It is important to keep in mind several concerns when utilizing these variables because they involve a significant amount of conceptual complexity. As was mentioned earlier, the units of health service that are provided merely play a role in determining the health status of an individual. For reasons that are difficult to quantify, health systems provide a wide variety of preventive care and public health services. In every age group, but especially among older people, there is a significant amount of self-care, as well as varying levels of alternative and complementary healthcare practices. These practices include self-medication with herbs and the utilization of alternative practitioners, both of which have the potential to influence the outcomes of health care. Furthermore, it is possible that both preventive and clinical care will not have an effect on health outcomes and quality of life until the following decades, and it may be challenging to effectively evaluate this latency in analytical studies. In point of fact, many of the fundamental professional activities of health systems may be of critical importance to patients and their families, but it is not reasonable to anticipate that these activities will result in objective, quantitative health outcomes. Some examples of these activities include ensuring that illness is not present, providing prognostic information, assisting with care administration issues, and providing family-friendly hospice care. Nevertheless, in spite of these conceptual challenges, cross-national studies provide the best opportunity to determine how different health system structures, funding mechanisms, and management mechanisms affect health outcomes.

Table 6.2. Chosen Units of Analysis for Describing Health Systems

Category	Variables
Type of Formal Care: Location/ Institutional Nature	Acute general hospital Intermediate care facilities Long-term institutional care (e.g., mental health, mental retardation, rehabilitation, infectious disease) Community-based, primary care facility Home-based care Pharmaceutical/dental/mental health services Emergency care facilities

Basic Funding Mechanisms	Fee-for-service Personal insurance, with or without copayments Employer insurance, with or without copayments Government-provided insurance, with or without copayments, including taxation systems Mixed payment systems and other contractual systems
Community-Based Care Typologies	Clinical public health services Health education programs Workplace health programs and services Health-oriented recreational and leisure programs Informal care, including family and self-care Complementary and alternative care modalities
Healthcare Utilization Measures	Episodes of attendance at various units of health care Access to care based on distance to provider(s) Access to care based on consumer satisfaction, including culturally acceptable care
Patient-Centered Measures	Continuity of care over time and different medical services Cultural appropriateness of care Presence of patient education programs

Source: *(Public Health Reports, 1995)*

Irrespective of the level of sophistication, modernity, and comprehensiveness of health services in a country, the utilization of these services is frequently uneven and can differ based on socioeconomic status, ethnicity, geographic location, and various other factors. Furthermore, it is crucial to consider that there could be specific factors associated with the characteristics of an illness and an individual's personality that influence their behavior within the healthcare system. These factors can complicate the study of health outcomes. Furthermore, it is important to note that all healthcare systems can have negative consequences that may reduce the overall positive impact on health outcomes. Typical instances include infections acquired in hospitals, incorrect use of treatments, and unintended negative effects of medications and devices. It is crucial to recognize these negative effects, as many of them can be corrected. There is ultimately diversity among national health systems in terms of the level of care and the programs implemented to ensure and maintain quality. Many modern health systems have shown significant variation in the utilization rates of medical/surgical procedures and health outcomes within small areas. Furthermore, certain services may exhibit a lower level of sophistication in rural or frontier areas, as well as in other geographical locations. This variation emphasizes the necessity of having extensive, wide-ranging, or countrywide data to carry out appropriate research.

6.5. Health Data Pertaining to Older Individuals: Categorization, Accessibility, and Reliability

The data necessary for conducting cross-national research on the health status of the elderly can be obtained from various sources, and it is not always possible to predict in advance which variables will be required. Furthermore, the elderly population possesses distinct characteristics that differentiate their health data requirements from those of other demographic groups:

The frequency of health events is generally higher among the elderly compared to other age groups, which highlights the importance of collecting longitudinal (panel) data on cohorts of older individuals.

Elderly individuals exhibit numerous clinical manifestations, symptoms, and functional limitations that require particular consideration, as they are not encompassed by conventional administrative data systems that prioritize disease prevalence.

Due to the prevalence of multiple medical conditions and functional impairments among older individuals, it is necessary to create concise measures of comorbidity and health status to effectively manage the existing health and administrative data. Examining the circumstances and limitations faced by older individuals in isolation may, at times, hinder the progress of worldwide policy formulation.

Having access to data on the physical and social environments of older individuals is crucial for the effective delivery of health services. Understanding the social context is crucial for the significant population of older adults who experience mobility or self-care limitations. It is also vital for ensuring the accurate administration of prescribed medical treatments in both home and community environments. Accurate information about the physical environment is crucial for reducing falls, injuries, and the advancement of disability. In certain situations, it can also help prevent deaths caused by climate-related factors.

The elderly population, especially those in the oldest age group, frequently experience cognitive and mental impairments. These impairments can result in a deficiency of social support and interaction, failure to adhere to medical treatment plans, inability to carry out self-care tasks, and an elevated requirement for structured supervision and institutionalization. Therefore, it is crucial to gather data on the prevalence and factors associated with mental impairments in the elderly population to inform health and healthcare policies. Since certain impairments make it impossible to directly interview the individuals involved, it is necessary to use techniques for obtaining proxy data. When comparing older individuals to other age groups, it is evident that they have significantly higher rates of living in institutions and utilizing long-term care services in their homes and communities. To gain a thorough understanding of this significant and expanding group, it is necessary to have data on the health condition of these individuals as well as the type of long-term and institutional care they are receiving.

This section will discuss the different sources of health data on the elderly and explore potential methods to enhance the usefulness of this data for cross-national research and policy development.

6.5.1. Sources of National Health Data

Extensive data on health and health status is readily accessible in most developed countries and is increasingly becoming available in developing countries as well. It is important to handle this data with caution and acknowledge its limitations. Table 6.3 (adapted from Andrews, 1999) summarizes health data sources and their potential limitations.

Table 6.3. Sources of Health Data and Their Possible Constraints

Source	Potential Limitations
Census Data	Infrequent collection; generally little health content
National Household Surveys	Target population, sample size, periodicity, comprehensiveness, survey design
Mortality Vital Records	Age accuracy among elders, analytical access
Morbidity Information	Accuracy, access, geographic coverage, variation in format and vocabulary/coding
Health Administrative Data	Timeliness, lack of analysis, format variation
Special Research Studies	Relevance, quality, presentation, national coverage, availability for analysis
Healthcare Evaluations	Availability, timeliness, accuracy
Outcomes Research	Varying conceptual frameworks, availability, utility, legal implications
Longitudinal Cohorts/Panels	Design, costs, timeliness, relevance
Qualitative Studies	Design, coverage, relevance
Market Research	Target population, relevance, accuracy
Institutional Sources	National coverage, costs, data access, identification of all relevant populations, type of data

Source: Andrews (1999).

Table 6.3 demonstrates that several obstacles could hinder the effective utilization of these data sources, which have the potential to be highly informative. Firstly, in numerous cases, there might be a lack of adequate or suitable data gathered or accessible, and the collected data may have limited precision. Furthermore, there is a lack of uniformity in how administrative data is collected and presented among different countries, which may also apply to computer software and file formats. Timely access to information is often hindered by significant delays, sometimes spanning several years. Policy and decision-makers may have a limited understanding of how information is relevant for research applications, and researchers may have a limited understanding of the policy process. However, when political perspectives are imposed on research, it can be harmful to everyone involved. Political, fiscal, and ethical constraints may hinder the smooth dissemination of the data to suitable analysts. There might be a lack of appropriate analytical methodology to effectively summarize and interpret complex and extensive datasets. Therefore, a coordinated administrative and political endeavor is necessary to gather the data essential for capitalizing on the possibilities of international research.

6.5.1.1. International Repositories of Health Data

The health data sources listed in Table 6.3 are often limited by issues of availability and access. Although certain datasets may have restricted distribution, it would be beneficial to make others available in repositories or cataloged for administrative and research analysts. Currently, there is no single centralized database that contains health information specifically gathered from population surveys or health system administrative data pertaining to older individuals. Significant compilations of catalogs are being undertaken by esteemed organizations such as the United Nations (Agree & Myers, 1998), the Organization for Economic Cooperation and Development (OECD) (Gudex & Lafortune, 2000), the European Union (Hupkens, 1997), and the U.S. National Institute on Aging (2000). Furthermore, the University of Michigan's Interuniversity Consortium for Political and Social Research manages a National Archive of Computerized Data on Aging (accessible at http://www.icpsr.umich.edu/NACDA/index.html) which has been expanding its global reach. The endeavors of these organizations will persist in their significance in discerning the requisite data for international comparative research.

6.5.1.2. The Concept of the Graduated Minimum Dataset

The varied operational requirements of healthcare organizations and agencies that tackle aging concerns, both domestically and internationally, present a difficulty in attaining the necessary data consistency to address numerous overarching inquiries that go beyond specific local populations. Each unit constructs administrative data systems and gathers data following its specific requirements and understanding of usefulness. An issue that often arises is the inability to enhance analytical capabilities through the comparison of local experiences with those of other populations or regions.

One-way national governments can address this problem is by creating minimum and/or core datasets that include clear definitions for each data element. By doing this, it allows for the use of standard methods to report data on important health statistics and to analyze information across different population groups, service system components, and the utilization and costs of healthcare. The National Center for Health Statistics in the United States collaborates with other agencies in the Department of Health and Human Services, and with guidance from the National Committee on Vital and Health Statistics, sets standardized minimum datasets, data elements, and data definitions that are uniformly used across the Department of Health and Human Services. Although these activities play a significant role in establishing shared naming conventions and data standards, it is necessary to have dedicated data repositories for the information collected in developed countries and, whenever feasible, in developing countries as well. The World Health Organization has actively and persistently pursued this objective.

Many nations are still in the process of standardizing the terminology used in the administration of health services. As an illustration, the United States is progressing towards establishing a uniform dataset for long-term care that includes the following categories: demographic information, health status information, service information, and procedural information. Demographic variables encompass biological sex, date of birth, racial background, ethnic origin, marital status, typical living arrangements (including type and location), and any legal restrictions imposed by a court. A comprehensive list could be significantly expanded to include additional categories such as educational attainment, income from diverse sources, received entitlements, and religion and religious involvement. The list can be modified following political, social, or economic influences, as well as internationally accepted terminology whenever feasible.

The differences in data collection methods between countries significantly exacerbate the challenges of obtaining comparable information. Slight deviations in the definition, formulation of questions, and method of data collection can have a substantial impact on responses and hinder the ability to make accurate comparisons. Furthermore, the comprehension and analysis of data components may differ across cultural contexts. To ensure accurate comparisons, it is crucial to reduce the data collection workload for countries and regions with limited resources compared to wealthier Western countries. This will enable meaningful comparisons of health and aging data across various sources, including surveys, administrative data systems, and other data collection methods.

The implementation of the graduated minimum dataset could aid in the facilitation of health research and policy analysis pertaining to aging. This would be achieved by offering fundamental descriptive data on individuals, disease and disability metrics, long-term care programs and facilities, health service utilization, and other relevant data elements. An appropriate universal approach would involve a hierarchy of data collection modules, ranging from easily collected basic data elements to increasingly elaborate datasets, considering that not all nations can be expected to invest the same level of resources in data collection. This hierarchy could consist of five to ten levels, ranging from basic descriptive statistics to extensive and comprehensive data elements, similar to the ones found in the Health and Retirement Survey and the Medicare Current Beneficiary Survey. Each level would possess unambiguous definitions of components, exact phrasing, and specified categories for responses. The selection of data elements would be substantiated by reliability and validity studies that justify their inclusion. Each administrative authority has the discretion to determine the extent of its data collection. However, regardless of the chosen level, the collected data can be standardized to be comparable to data collected by other entities. The benefit of implementing such a system is that the administrative authority would have the ability to include any necessary data elements to fulfill local objectives, without compromising the consistency of data collection across different geographic areas. To evaluate this approach and address the implementation challenges, it would be beneficial to conduct a feasibility study on a limited set of measures about aging, particularly those related to disability.

6.5.1.3. Linking of Health Data

The compilation of data from a wide variety of sources is necessary to conduct an assessment of the health of older individuals. These sources include personal and family surveys, vital records, healthcare administrative records from a variety of providers, and other health-relevant sectors of society. It is also possible for older people to seek medical and social services from a variety of providers due to the fact that they frequently suffer from multiple conditions and impairments over the course of their lives. There is abundant evidence that demonstrates the significance of data linkage in terms of enhancing the formulation of policies (National Research Council, 1988). The use of primary institutional records not only serves to supplement information that can only be obtained through interviews, but it also helps to increase the accuracy of the information that is available for statistical analysis. On the other hand, there are many potential obstacles that could prevent the linkage of records. These obstacles include the costs involved, concerns regarding privacy, and the logistics involved in assembling data from a variety of sources.

6.6. Addressing Challenges in Conducting Cross-National Research on the Health Status of the Elderly

As previously mentioned, making cross-national comparisons can be advantageous in various ways when addressing concerns regarding the health status of elderly populations. A cross-national perspective allows for the examination of a wide range of variations that can provide valuable qualitative insights into different institutional arrangements, policies, and programmatic interventions. These insights are not possible to study within the confines of a single country. Comparisons between different countries can also offer insights into the extent to which observations made in specific national and cultural contexts can be applied more broadly. When similar patterns and trends are observed in nations with different social structures, cultures, and approaches to health and welfare, it increases confidence in the validity of formulated generalizations. Simultaneously, it is important to acknowledge the intricacy associated with comparing national health systems that have different historical backgrounds, organizational structures, cultural impacts, and statistical methodologies. When making comparisons, the analyst must have a thorough understanding of the contexts being compared and the unique measurement, definitional, and linguistic features of each system. This ensures that comparable units are being properly evaluated. Comparing concepts that may seem simple can be challenging when considering different systems. For instance, physicians have diverse roles in various national healthcare systems. In the United Kingdom and other European countries, general practitioners exclusively work in the community setting. However, in the United States, they usually also provide care to patients who are admitted to hospitals or other healthcare institutions.

Aside from cultural differences, there are numerous factors that can restrict or complicate cross-national research. These factors must be taken into account to ensure the validity of the study's findings. For instance, the overall health condition of the population may differ between countries, and this disparity can result in diverse consequences for the implementation of a particular health policy or intervention. Potential discrepancies in the characteristics, composition, inclusiveness, or comprehensiveness of population samples and health administration databases could result in misleading analytical discoveries. The inconsistency and incompleteness of clinical and vital records information can complicate cross-national comparisons as well. The definitions of health states, specific diseases and conditions, and disability can differ between nations and cultures. These differences may not be completely represented by international disease coding systems. The variations in clinical practice styles, healer-patient interaction, and the utilization of alternative practitioners may hinder the complete comparability of summary diagnostic information. The presence of different organizational modes, financing methods, and budgeting systems in health services can pose challenges in accurately measuring resource levels or allocations for comparable units of service delivery. Considering these discrepancies, the inability to detect specific impacts of national health systems on a particular health or programmatic outcome could be attributed to both the incomparability of the study units and the potential absence of any actual effect.

Simultaneously, there is a noticeable rise in the comparability of clinical/administrative and survey data collected across nations. Increased international exchange of scientific information, advancements in survey instruments and measurement techniques, improvements in healthcare evaluation methodology, advancements in clinical training and achievement norms, database computerization and management, and the establishment of regulatory standards for drugs, devices, and other medical interventions are expected to enhance cross-national research in the future. The progress will be amplified by the expansion of multinational corporations and industries that cater to the delivery of clinical services across various regions of the globe.

6.7. Recommendations

- Government-sponsored nationwide surveys should improve the collection of fundamental health data for elderly individuals and establish a stronger basis for standardized metrics that can be used to compare different countries. When it comes to the health status of older individuals, it is essential to have information that includes the frequency and rates of (1) deaths and their main causes; (2) significant acute and chronic medical conditions and their main symptoms; (3) measurements of important self-reported health status; (4) levels of physical, social, and mental function in the population; (5) behaviors related to prevention and health promotion; and (6) significant disabilities. Furthermore, comprehensive healthcare information for elderly individuals should encompass several key aspects. These include: (1) the frequency at which important health services, both institutional and home-based, are utilized; (2) the financial burden incurred by individuals and their families for formal health services; (3) the rates at which medications and medical devices are used; (4) the significant cultural factors that influence perceptions of health and the utilization of health services, such as gender, ethnicity, geographic location, and socioeconomic status; and (5) the utilization of informal, alternative, and complementary healthcare services, which encompass self-care practices and support from nonprofessional sources, including family members.

- Implementing a graduated minimum dataset would help to facilitate health research and policy analysis that is relevant to aging populations. Countries should implement systematic data collection procedures to gather fundamental descriptive data on individuals, disease and disability measures, long-term care programs and facilities, and health service utilization. Due to varying resource capacities, it is not feasible for all nations to allocate equal amounts of resources to data collection. Therefore, a hierarchical system of data collection modules, starting from easily obtainable basic data elements and progressing to more complex datasets, would be a suitable approach that can be universally implemented. A hierarchy of this nature could consist of five to ten levels, ranging from basic descriptive statistics to extensive and comprehensive data elements, similar to those observed in specific OECD countries.
- All nations must enable the integration of population-based and administrative health information with other crucial economic, social, and health service data. Despite the difficulties in coordinating and managing various aspects, integrating population survey data with medical, vital, administrative, and other social and economic records can enhance the usefulness of the data in assessing the health status of the population and facilitating programmatic and policy planning and evaluation. This integration can be particularly valuable in evaluating disability rates, estimating the impact of insurance coverage on healthcare costs, and providing additional insights into the functioning of medical programs.
- It is important to gather longitudinal data on the health of older individuals in order to accurately identify the risk factors, causes, and preventive measures for disease and disability. Panel (cohort) studies should incorporate economic, behavioral, and social aspects in order to identify specific groups and individuals who are at a higher risk of illness and their corresponding utilization of healthcare resources. Additionally, these studies can determine if there are variations in health outcomes based on different healthcare interventions, programs, and policies.
- Utilizing cross-national panel studies is necessary to elucidate the correlation between the organization, administration, and financing of health systems, and the resulting health status and outcomes. Longitudinal, population-based surveys that are linked to administrative records and have comparable questions across countries are crucial for comparing health outcomes between countries and determining the specific factors that contribute to changes in health. Furthermore, conducting comparative research can enhance our comprehension of how specific

diseases and conditions manifest as disability in different family, social, and residential settings. This can offer valuable insights into which policies and interventions are the most effective.

6.8. The Impact of Social Inequality on the Health of Older Individuals

Socioeconomic position is a determining factor for health and functioning in all societies. The extent of these disparities and their origins fluctuate over time, both within and between societies. To formulate effective policies that can mitigate these disparities, it is essential to comprehend their underlying causes. Policy interventions aimed at addressing socioeconomic disparities in health and functioning should ideally encompass a broad spectrum of factors, encompassing both medical care and social services. Socioeconomic disparities are expected to exist in the delivery, availability, and utilization of these services.

Health disparities based on social factors impact individuals across different age groups, including both older and younger populations. Figure 6.4 displays the mortality rates based on employment grade among British civil servants who participated in the initial Whitehall study conducted by Marmot and Shipley in 1996. The data clearly demonstrates that mortality rates exhibit a distinct pattern based on social stratification.

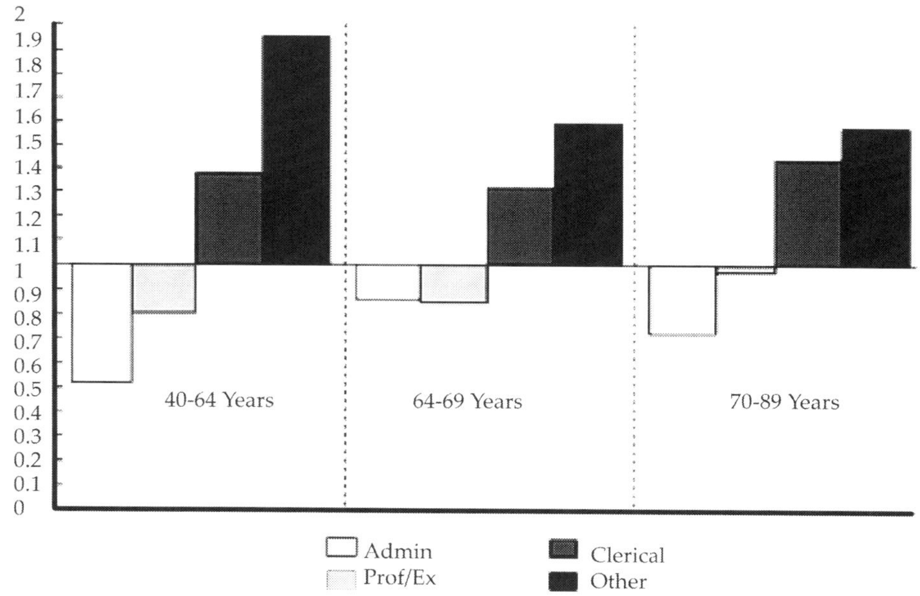

Figure 6.4. *Relative mortality (for all causes) based on employment grade, specifically for Whitehall men, over a 25-year period.*

Source: Marmot and Shipley (1996).

The implication for monitoring and policy is that the relationship between health and material deprivation is not straightforward. It is not simply a matter of poor health among the deprived and better health for everyone else. Instead, there is a social gradient in health that spans across all levels of society. Although Figure 6.4 focuses solely on mortality, it is important to note that social disparities in morbidity are significant among the elderly population. The policy implications in this area may be even more complex and demanding. An issue prevalent in numerous developed nations is the substantial population of elderly women who reside alone and face limitations due to disability. Their predicament is exacerbated by factors associated with their social status, which will be further discussed below.

Additionally, Figure 6.4 demonstrates that the disparity in mortality rates decreases as individuals age, with a smaller difference between the highest and lowest mortality rates observed in older age groups compared to younger ones. Two additional concerns arise from this: determining the suitable metric for quantifying the impact of disease and identifying the suitable metric for categorizing social groups. While the relative difference in mortality may decrease with age, the absolute difference becomes larger due to higher overall mortality rates. While relative differences are commonly used to gauge the influence of causal factors, absolute differences provide a more accurate measure of the societal significance of the overall burden of disease and suffering.

6.8.1. Classification of Socioeconomic Position

Several countries have a longstanding tradition of assessing socioeconomic status. The theoretical foundation for the different measures that have been employed is occasionally stated explicitly, more frequently implied, and occasionally absent. Indicators that rely on education, income, occupation, or a combination of these factors are widely used and frequently lack a theoretical foundation. Some have contended that a more solid theoretical foundation for socioeconomic classification would lead to a more comprehensive comprehension of the factors involved. An approach to achieve this goal is to conceptualize three distinct forms of social stratification: one predicated on the extent of material deprivation, another rooted in social power dynamics, and a third based on overall social status (Bartley & Marmot, 2000).

Measures of material deprivation are suitable for evaluating disparities in health among individuals living in conditions of extreme poverty. These measures are not as suitable in cases where health is influenced by social factors, as seen in the Whitehall studies (Marmot & Shipley, 1996; Marmot et al., 1991). In such instances, there exist evident disparities in health outcomes among individuals who are not experiencing material deprivation. Therefore, other concepts must be considered. Another approach that may be relevant to the overall social gradient is centered around power dynamics within the workplace. Occupations are categorized based on their level of authority and independence, a viewpoint that originates from the Marxist notion of social class. The Eriksson-Goldthorpe scheme serves as the foundation for this approach, which in turn establishes the framework for the new British socioeconomic classification that will be implemented nationwide for the 2001 census. The third approach, which is related to general social standing, shares similarities with Weber's notion of status, which is determined by consumption patterns and lifestyle. The status group is characterized by a shared level of prestige or esteem, as well as similar patterns of consumption and lifestyle. Furthermore, members of this group tend to restrict their interactions with individuals from other groups.

Providing a universal recommendation for the most suitable indicators of socioeconomic status across different cultures is not feasible. It would be beneficial to try to connect the developed and implemented measures with theoretical concepts, such as the three outlined above.

A metric that is suitable for categorizing individuals within the working-age population may be less suitable for those who are older and no longer in the workforce. Social classification in numerous countries is often based on occupation. The rationale for this approach is well-founded, as work plays a pivotal role in individuals' lives (Marmot & Feeney, 1996). One's occupation plays a significant role in determining their income, which subsequently impacts their opportunities and prospects in life. Furthermore, the professional trajectory plays a significant role in the process of social integration and the establishment of one's social identity beyond the confines of the familial context. It provides prospects for both achieving and hindering life's objectives. The occupational level has a significant impact on self-esteem, social approval, personal attitudes, and behavioral patterns. Ultimately, the nature of one's job and the environment in which they work can significantly contribute to social disparities in health.

The extent to which occupation remains a dependable indicator of these four elements in individuals beyond the working age will differ. Further techniques for social categorization will be required. This will particularly apply to older women, especially those who are single, widowed, or divorced. Additional socioeconomic indicators that have been utilized include educational attainment, income level, housing ownership, residential area characteristics, and, in the case of Britain, household car ownership. The matter of proper categorization pertains to the inquiry of why disparities in health between genders may be less pronounced in women compared to men. Historically, the social standing of married women was primarily determined by their husband's profession rather than their own. Although this situation may still exist in certain situations and populations, it is being questioned due to significant social changes (Bartley et al., 1999). It is crucial to carefully consider the most suitable methods that will enable the comparison of health disparities between genders, both within and across different populations.

6.8.2. Data Needs for Understanding Determinants of Social Inequalities in Health and Well-Being

Various aspects of social or personal life, biology, and services can impact social disparities in health. The International Center for Health and Society at University College London compiled research findings on the social determinants of health into 10 categories, as requested by the World Health Organization (Wilkinson & Marmot, 1998).

- Social gradient through the life course
- Stress
- Early life
- Social exclusion
- Work
- Unemployment
- Social support
- Addiction
- Food
- Transport

According to Marmot and Wilkinson (1999), these categories were presented with the intention of serving as a guide for policy makers; however, they could also be used as a template for research. From this list, there is one aspect that does not appear to be immediately obvious, and that is the quality of housing as well as the physical and social environment of neighborhoods. These may be considered to fall under the category of social exclusion; however, just like health in general, the quality of these things is likely to follow a social gradient. In most cases, longitudinal and representative population surveys are required to achieve a more comprehensive understanding of the factors that are responsible for socioeconomic differences in the health and functioning of individuals. The establishment of causal associations and the evaluation of the magnitude of causes operating in all directions are both essential for conducting such surveys. In other words, longitudinal data are essential for determining the extent to which levels of health and functioning determine social and economic position, as well as for determining the magnitude and nature of the social determinants of health. In addition, longitudinal data are essential for determining an individual's social and economic position.

6.8.3. An Inquiry Into Health Disparities in the United Kingdom: A Policy Response to the British Independent Office

With a government-sponsored investigation that eventually became known as the Black Report (Black et al., 1988), the United Kingdom took the initiative on a global scale in the late 1970s to compile various pieces of evidence concerning health disparities. Despite the fact that it had a significant impact on research on this topic both in Britain and internationally, the Black Report had very little discernible impact on policy. Under the leadership of Sir Donald Acheson, a former chief medical officer, the newly elected Labor government in Britain established an independent investigation into health disparities in 1997 (Acheson, 1998). This investigation was the subject of the investigation. The Acheson Inquiry provided a summary of the evidence regarding the factors that determine social inequalities in health and made a total of 39 recommendations. Noteworthy is the fact that these recommendations were arranged according to the stages of the life course, with a particular emphasis on older people as well as other age groups. At this very moment, the government is undertaking the process of putting these recommendations into action.

6.9. The Most Commonly Applied Measurements of Health Status

Clinical symptoms, signs, and syndromes; morbidity, or medical conditions that are discretely defined; self-rated health; functional status and disability; physiological and pathological measures; mortality data and derived measures; and aging and mental illness are the seven categories that can be used to classify the health status measurements that are typically utilized for survey questionnaires and administrative data collection. Following is a review of the measures that were utilized in each of these categories in its own order.

6.9.1. Symptoms, Signs, and Syndromes

The clinical definition of symptoms, signs, or syndromes refers to the observations and perceptions that are associated with an illness.

Symptoms refer to bodily perceptions that individuals interpret as abnormal. Various symptoms can manifest, including knee pain, headaches, fatigue, itchy skin, reduced joint mobility, insomnia, or a melancholic mood. Due to their inherent subjectivity, individuals may arrive at varying interpretations and subsequently exhibit different behaviors. For example, one person may decide to seek medical care for a specific symptom, while another person may opt not to do so. The symptoms are particularly common in older individuals, which, combined with the frequent lack of concrete evidence, makes medical diagnosis in this population challenging and complex. To enhance our understanding of the necessity for medical treatment, it is feasible to acquire a more comprehensive comprehension of the frequency rates of notable symptoms. Additional evaluation and therapy often require a substantial allocation of resources, regardless of whether symptoms are indicative of significant underlying medical conditions. Cross-cultural studies of symptoms aim to assess the variations and commonalities in the impact on healthcare delivery in specific areas, such as tooth pain (Moore et al., 1998) and jaw arthritis (Suvinen et al., 1997).

Signs are observable indications of an anomaly that can be perceived by both the individual and the healthcare practitioner. Examples encompass manifestations such as dermatological eruptions, elevated temperature or erythema of a specific anatomical region upon palpation, perceptible wheezing sounds, and maladaptive conduct within a specific sociocultural context. Signs are prevalent among older individuals. Regarding symptoms, they may or may not serve as an indication of a significant underlying medical issue and may or may not result in the decision to seek medical attention.

A syndrome refers to the occurrence of characteristic patterns, clusters, or signs and symptoms in an individual. An example would be a respiratory infection such as a cold or influenza, which typically presents with symptoms including cough, runny nose, headache, fever, muscle aches, and weakness. Typically, syndromes are frequently observed but do not necessarily indicate a specific underlying ailment. For instance, in some cases, the symptoms commonly associated with the flu may actually be indicative of tuberculosis or an immune deficiency. Significantly, syndromes play a crucial role in medical care, similar to signs and symptoms. The majority of cases of "flu syndromes" are a result of viral infections and result in a significant use of medical resources. Therefore, it is crucial to gather data on the prevalence of these syndromes in both geographical and patient populations to develop effective healthcare policies. Gaining knowledge about the frequency of their occurrence and their impact on healthcare resources in different cultures and countries can help in comprehending strategies for their effective administration.

6.9.2. Morbidity, or Discretely Defined Medical Conditions

In this context, "morbidity" refers to specific medical conditions that are used by health professionals, administrators, patients, and their families to define and communicate health information. The majority of pathological conditions, such as diabetes mellitus, stroke, lung cancer, and myocardial infarction (heart attack), have widely accepted definitions that are applicable in most cases. Nevertheless, there can be significant discrepancies in disease terminology and usage within a linguistic community or nation, as well as notable variations on an international scale. The consequence is a decrease in the precision and accuracy of information derived from medical records, which necessitates the standardized relabeling (coding) of diagnostic designations for both clinical and administrative purposes. Disease names offer valuable insights into the biological and clinical impact of a specific condition on individuals and populations. They provide information about the average level of bodily damage, typical treatment approaches, and prognosis, although the severity and scope of the condition may vary. The utilization of clinical care resources can be deduced based on the name of a disease within a specific country and healthcare system. Although there are currently limitations in the way diseases are designated and classified, it is crucial to know disease names and taxonomy to accurately gather and measure information for policy, research, and administrative purposes. Furthermore, precise and universally agreed upon disease names are crucial for evaluating clinical evidence, creating practice guidelines, and ensuring quality in healthcare activities. These applications are relevant on both national and international levels (Grimshaw & Russell, 1993; Muir Gray, 1997).

The significance of morbidity data for older individuals in terms of policy is evident. A detailed understanding of the prevalence, intensity, and functional consequences of different diseases is essential for the creation, upkeep, and assessment of programs aimed at preventing, treating, or rehabilitating these conditions. Healthcare data is a valuable source of information that can be easily obtained due to the computerization of clinical encounter records in both ambulatory and institutional settings. However, to accurately assess the occurrence of morbidity in a population, it may be necessary to conduct sample surveys that represent the entire population. This is because the coverage of the health system may not align with specific geographic regions and only applies to individuals who actually use the system. Population surveys can provide a crucial viewpoint, but data collected from elderly individuals in this way may be inadequate or only partially reliable. Certain individuals may lack a complete understanding or the ability to identify their own conditions, and certain conditions may not have undergone clinical evaluation. For instance, a significant proportion of older Americans have undiagnosed adult-onset, non-insulin-dependent diabetes. To ensure the highest level of accuracy and policy relevance, it is recommended to obtain morbidity rates from both population-based and institutional sources.

Elderly individuals frequently experience multiple medical conditions, any of which can potentially affect the characteristics of the others. Therefore, when comparing the diagnosis, treatment, or outcomes of a specific condition, whether it is within a country or region or across different countries, it is often necessary to account for other diseases and conditions, known as "comorbidity." For instance, the existence of additional medical conditions alongside the primary disease can impact the scores on quality-of-life scales (Xuan et al., 1999), accelerate the development of disability (Fried et al., 1999), improve the accuracy of predicting hospital stays (Roe et al., 1998), and generally modify health outcomes following hospitalization (Elixhauser et al., 1998). Comorbidity scales can be utilized for both population survey data and healthcare administrative datasets (Katz et al., 1996).

The International Classification of Diseases and Conditions (ICD) is the universally accepted method for organizing morbidity and clinical diagnoses into a taxonomy that is recognized internationally. The International Classification of Diseases (ICD), currently in its 10th edition, is disseminated by the World Health Organization (WHO). The database encompasses numerous medical conditions and rubrics, aiming to accurately represent the intricate nature of health and disease and the advancements made in their comprehension. The International Classification of Diseases (ICD) has been widely used in all Western-style health systems. It has been modified and translated for various general applications. Nevertheless, although the ICD is crucial for examining community disease data, it is important to acknowledge certain limitations:

The International Classification of Diseases (ICD) is a comprehensive framework that encompasses the study of anatomy, physiology, disease behavior, and causation. It serves as a representation of our current knowledge and understanding of diseases.

Certain clinical information, such as an individual's functional status or the physiological severity of a condition, cannot be found in disease names.

As previously mentioned, there is limited capacity to address the numerous coexisting medical conditions that commonly arise in older individuals (comorbidity) and how these conditions impact the specific disease under consideration.

The ICD often reflects political, economic, and intellectual controversy due to scientific uncertainty, limited understanding of many diseases, and the increasing connection between diagnostic guidelines and health system reimbursement.

The International Classification of Diseases (ICD) does not effectively address the preventive, legal, and administrative components of clinical practice.

Due to these and other restrictions, alternative and supplementary disease naming and classification systems have been created. An example of a system that uses a multiaxial approach to designate a specific medical condition is the Systematized Nomenclature of Medicine (SNOMED) system (Lussier et al., 1998). Information is categorized into different domains, including anatomical locale, physiological impact, and putative causes of the condition. Additionally, various other taxonomies have been created, including the ICD-O, which is a comprehensive inventory of different types of cancer, their severity, and the extent of the disease; E-Codes, a comprehensive coding system for environmental exposures linked to human diseases; and N-Coding, a detailed classification system for bodily injuries.

Collaborative international studies have been carried out to analyze the occurrence of morbidity to aid in the planning of health services programs. An exemplary instance is the World Health Organization (WHO) initiative known as the Multinational Monitoring of Trends and Determinants in Cardiovascular Disease (MONICA) program. Coronary disease is the leading cause of mortality among elderly individuals in the majority of countries. Since 1981, MONICA has been monitoring coronary disease events in 16 European countries, as well as Australia, Canada, China, New Zealand, and the United States. An extensive cross-national analysis (Tunstall-Pedoe et al., 2000) found a correlation between improvements in the quality of coronary care in different geographic regions and short-term survival rates for heart attacks, as measured by the "case-fatality ratio." The ecological analysis, conducted independently for both males and females, has provided evidence that a more significant enhancement in coronary care (measured by a higher "treatment score") is linked to a greater reduction in the case-fatality ratio, indicating improved chances of survival. Although additional evaluation is required, this cross-national study provides evidence for the importance of investing in enhanced coronary care facilities using various approaches to such care.

6.9.3. Self-Rated Health

Self-rated health measures are commonly included in various types of surveys. An illustration can be seen in a query that prompts participants to categorize their general health condition using options such as excellent, good, fair, or poor. These assessments may or may not align with the evaluations that a physician would give.

The inherent focus on the individual in these questions renders them highly valuable for various applications in health research. Self-related health is a term commonly used to assess health, psychological well-being, and health-related quality of life. These concepts are often vague but typically involve aspects of physical well-being and functioning. The individual is undoubtedly the most reliable source of information for these matters. Furthermore, self-rated health can serve as a valuable screening tool for identifying high-risk groups and risk factors. Numerous national and international studies have consistently shown that individuals with poor self-rated health tend to have low socioeconomic status and a higher prevalence of other illness risk factors. Furthermore, self-rated health can serve as an outcome measure in the assessment of medical interventions, providing valuable insights in addition to the conventional measures of mortality and morbidity. It is worth noting that treatments that have comparable impacts on life expectancy may have varying implications in terms of the overall quality of those years. Furthermore, self-rated health can serve as a reliable indicator for predicting illness behavior, retirement, and the prolonged utilization of medication and other healthcare services. In studies examining retirement decision-making, this measure has frequently been employed as the sole indicator of an individual's health status (Bjorner et al., 1996). Ultimately, the most convincing rationale for incorporating self-rated health in surveys lies in its evident ability to predict mortality. A study conducted in Canada in 1982 revealed that self-assessments of health provided by a representative group of elderly individuals living in Manitoba in 1971 were more accurate in predicting mortality by 1977 compared to their medical records or self-reported conditions. In a 1997 review, 27 published studies from 13 countries were examined. These studies analyzed self-rated health and mortality in representative samples. Out of the 23 studies, self-rated health was found to be a significant predictor of mortality for both males and females, even when considering other measures of health status (Idler & Benyamini, 1997). A subsequent review conducted after a span of 2 years discovered 19 studies that encompassed 4 more countries. Out of these studies, only 2 reported no significant correlation between self-rated health and the risk of mortality (Benyamini & Idler, 1999).

The impressive number of these studies and the consistent findings they have produced are noteworthy for several reasons. The proliferation of numerous studies within a relatively brief period (17 years, with a majority published after 1990) is remarkable on its own, particularly given that the data presented are derived from longitudinal studies, many of which were premeditated and initiated years prior. It appears that a question was included in the interviews for these studies that aimed to assess the overall health status. This question was initially considered useful for another purpose, but later it was discovered that it is also associated with the risk of mortality in additional analyzes. This extensive body of research also reveals two paradoxes. One limitation is that the interviews used in the analyzes were conducted in the language spoken by the respondents, and there were minimal efforts made to standardize the questions or response options. Another factor is the significant variation among countries in the percentage of respondents who rate their health in the lowest category ("poor," "bad," "extremely bad," "very sick," "worse health compared with others," or "not healthy"). The unexpected nature of these consistent findings is heightened by the fact that health perceptions, both in terms of cultural and linguistic meanings, vary significantly across countries, as do the more quantifiable measures of morbidity and mortality. Indeed, numerous studies have shown that individuals with poor self-perceived health have a similar risk of mortality as smokers, as indicated by effect sizes and significance levels. These findings emphasize the validity of lay perspectives on health and the value of a holistic approach in defining health, in a way that few other findings could. Survey respondents are providing their own interpretations of health, which may encompass various aspects of the World Health Organization's comprehensive definition of human health, including physical, mental, and social well-being. Self-assessments of health offer a straightforward and cost-effective method of measuring one's perception of health, allowing individuals to define their own criteria as broadly or inclusively as they desire.

6.9.4. Functional Status and Disability

When it comes to directing health policy, the functional characterization of older people along physical, cognitive, and social dimensions is of the utmost importance. There is a significant amount of potential for the prevention of functional disability, which is a condition that is particularly prevalent among older people. Chronic medical conditions, such as heart disease, stroke, vascular disease, arthritis, Parkinson's disease, cancers, and dementia, are frequently the direct cause of age-related increases in physical and cognitive disability. These conditions contribute to the progression of age-related disability. They are, however, also connected to social and environmental factors. There are many factors that can lead to a decline in social interaction and engagement, including changes in both physical and cognitive abilities, the loss of friends and family due to death or migration, and a decline in social roles, including the loss of productive work. The outcomes of physical disability and cognitive impairment can become even more severe when there is a decrease in social engagement.

6.9.4.1. Physical Disability

A physical disability leads to a reduction in the ability to carry out tasks that are necessary for maintaining one's independence and productivity as well as for keeping one's home in order. More than 20% of older adults in the United States are estimated to have limitations in their ability to perform major daily activities as a result of an underlying disease (Manton et al., 1997). This prevalence is estimated to be higher in the United States. The aspects of physical disability that are most frequently considered are the ability to perform tasks that are essential to living independently in the home (such as preparing meals or paying bills) or to perform tasks that are necessary for self-care (such as bathing and dressing). On the other hand, a wide range of activities that require more effort, such as paid work, activities that are done not for compensation, and recreational pursuits, are also impacted.

The prevalence of disability and dependence among older adults, as well as the utilization of long-term care, varies significantly across regions and cultures, as well as according to socioeconomic status and social structure characteristics. To provide a foundation for planning for future chronic care requirements, it is helpful to have an understanding of the rates of disability both within and between countries and regions, as well as the health, health care, social, and economic factors that may have an impact on these populations. In addition, disabled older adults have the greatest need for the most intensive and expensive general healthcare as well as community organizations. In light of this, the size of the disabled population has a significant bearing on the requirements for healthcare in the present and in the future as a whole.

To reiterate, there is a growing body of evidence indicating that there is the potential to prevent disability. Among these measures are the primary prevention of diseases that are incapacitating and the tertiary prevention of diseases to reduce the progression and impact of these diseases. There is also the possibility of reducing disability through social approaches (e.g., by modifying the social factors that have an effect on function) and through modifications to the environment. It is also possible to use recently developed methods to screen for people who are at risk of developing a disability or the progression of an existing disability, which will allow for the implementation of appropriate interventions. It is important to note that the potential for all of these different approaches to reduce disability argues for continuous national tracking of disability levels through representative surveys and other methods related to the topic.

6.9.4.2. Cognitive Impairment

In every population that was investigated, the decline in cognitive function corresponds to an increase in age. This cognitive decline, in turn, leads to significant clinical and functional consequences that are more commonly referred to as dementia. Alzheimer's disease is the most prevalent form of dementia in the majority of industrialized nations where it is prevalent.

As is the case with physical function, the prevalence rates of dementia differ from community to community, culture to culture, and nation to nation (Jorm & Jolley, 1998). There is a possibility that the rates among people aged 85 and older in industrialized countries could reach over 50%. A loss of independence in one or more aspects of day-to-day function is a significant factor that is associated with dementia. This association between functional impairment and subsequent dementia suggests that cognitive impairment mediates certain age-related transitions in physical function (Carlson et al., 1999). They found that functional impairment was associated with dementia.

6.9.4.3. Social Function

Social function is a term that describes the degree to which an individual interacts with their family, friends, and society. Interactions with other people can vary in terms of their nature, quality, and frequency, depending on the social network in question. Participation in social, religious, and political institutions, as well as paid and volunteer work, are all examples of different ways in which individuals and groups can become engaged with society. People who participate in activities like these frequently report feeling productive and like they are making a positive contribution to society. Research conducted by Glass et al. (1999) and Musick et al. (1999) has demonstrated that the risk of mortality can be reduced through continuous participation in structured activities. These activities include paid or volunteer work, as well as the management of a household. There is a correlation between having positive social networks and a lower risk of disability in relation to activities of daily living (also known as basic self-care activities), in addition to other health outcomes. In contrast, research conducted by Bassuk et al. in 1998 demonstrated that social disengagement is a reliable indicator of cognitive decline and disability. On the other hand, it is important to recognize that a better health status may also make it possible to engage in more productive and active social functions.

6.9.4.4. Assessment of Functional Status

Whether an individual can perform the tasks of daily life or has limitations in doing so, it is common practice to evaluate their ability to do so through self-reports or through functional performance testing in the clinic or at home. It is possible to use functional measures to describe specific limitations in discrete areas, such as the ability to remember numbers or the use of a spoon. The cumulative impact on an individual of one or more chronic conditions, cognitive impairments, and physiological changes associated with aging, as well as the social, environmental, and psychological modifiers of these conditions, can be described using other measures. These measures can be used to describe the cumulative impact. Therefore, functional status and disability measures serve two purposes: first, they evaluate the overall impact that disease and aging have had on the individual, and second, they express the individual's capacity to care for themselves and to manage a household.

Rather than describing a single or multiple specific diseases, disability measures essentially describe a syndrome. For instance, a person may have difficulty walking across a room due to arthritis, a neurological condition, cardiopulmonary disease, or a variety of other factors. Even though chronic diseases have a significant influence on functional levels, not all people who have a particular disease experience measurable functional declines, and not all people will become disabled as a result of their disease.

It is common practice to evaluate a person's physical function by referring to activities in which physical movement is the predominant activity. These activities include basic self-care activities, such as bathing, dressing, and using the restroom; more complex, instrumental activities, such as cooking, shopping, and recreational exercise; mobility, which involves moving from one location to another; and other fundamental physical movements, such as reaching, kneeling, and fine hand movements. In this context, it is important to note that the living environments and social role expectations of individuals can have a significant impact on the outcomes of these measures in certain situations.

In most cases, cognitive function is evaluated employing specialized cognitive-psychological testing of fundamental cognitive processes carried out by the human brain. These processes include memory, calculation, visuo-spatial abilities, and reasoning. However, impairment can sometimes be inferred from declines in the performance of instrumental activities. It is generally not possible to diagnose a specific disease based on the measurement of a decline in particular cognitive functions; rather, for this to be possible, a comprehensive clinical evaluation is required. In addition, formal psychological testing is utilized as a means of assisting in the diagnosis of mental illness.

The last step in the evaluation of social function is to ask questions of individuals, families, and other people to ascertain the nature of social networks, including the type of network, its quality, whether it is positive or negative, and the frequency of interaction. It is also possible to determine the various types of social engagement, which refers to the frequency with which individuals participate in social or productive activities.

It is becoming increasingly common for clinical practice to collect functional status measurements. The information on such measures, on the other hand, is frequently not coded or easily retrieved from administrative datasets or clinical records. This contrasts with the information on morbidity, which refers to diseases that are associated with the healthcare system. Although it is difficult to draw such inferences, it is possible to infer functional status from a variety of diagnostic rubrics (e.g., dementia) or from clinical interventions (e.g., physical rehabilitation). More and more population surveys with health and economic objectives are including functional status measures. These surveys frequently take a longitudinal perspective and offer a significant amount of analytical potential for policy applications.

There are a great number of functional status measurements, and while they can be utilized in international research to gain an understanding of the factors that contribute to the varying levels and changes that occur among the elderly population of a variety of countries, the number of comparisons that can be made could be quite substantial. Application of summary measures of several individual functional attributes, using survivorship methods or "health expectancy measures" (Robine et al., 1999) to create a disability profile employing the time to onset of disability among the population of each age in the context of general survivorship is one approach to addressing this issue. An additional approach is to use survivorship methods. The application of this method is illustrated in a schematic form in Figure 6.5 which provides an example of its application. In many countries, age-specific prevalence rates have been determined for representative population samples. These rates provide valuable information and have been determined for a variety of countries. Presented in Figure 6.6 are the prevalence rates for severe disability in four different countries, broken down according to gender and age. It is interesting to note that there are distinct differences between countries in terms of trends according to age, which calls for further investigation. Such differences between countries present unique opportunities to investigate the environmental, cultural, and biological factors that may be responsible for that difference. As a result of the fact that studies that investigate decreases in age-specific levels of physical disability (Manton et al., 1993; Crimins et al., 1997; Freedman & Martin, 1998) do not go very far in explaining such trends, there is an obvious requirement for international comparisons to provide and test hypotheses regarding the causes of these trends. The extent to which the more recent epidemiological transition in less developed countries will lead to different patterns of disability change as the decline in mortality continues is another topic that is of interest.

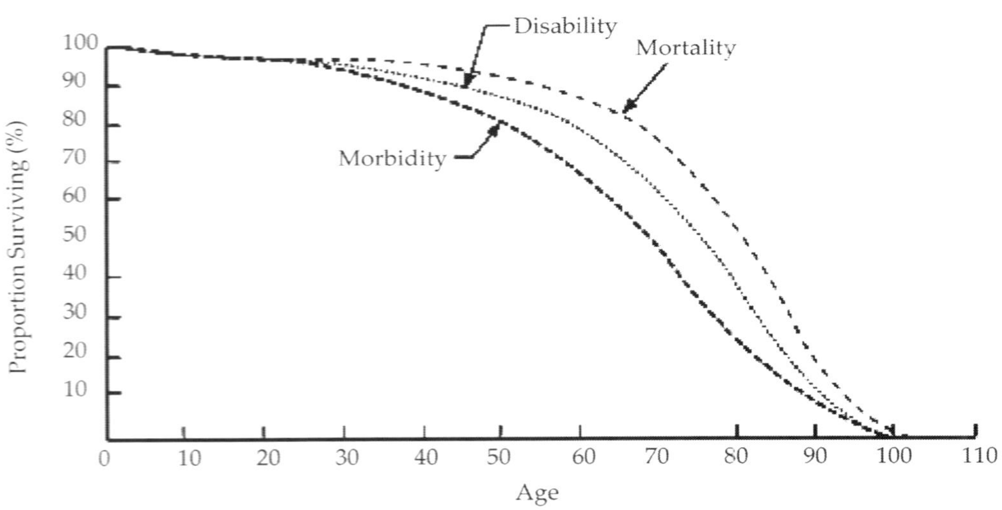

Figure 6.5. *A comprehensive framework depicting the overall condition and progression of health (including recorded death rates and theoretical curves illustrating the persistence of illness and disability) among females in the United States in the year 1980.*

Source: World Health Organization (1984). Reprinted with permission.

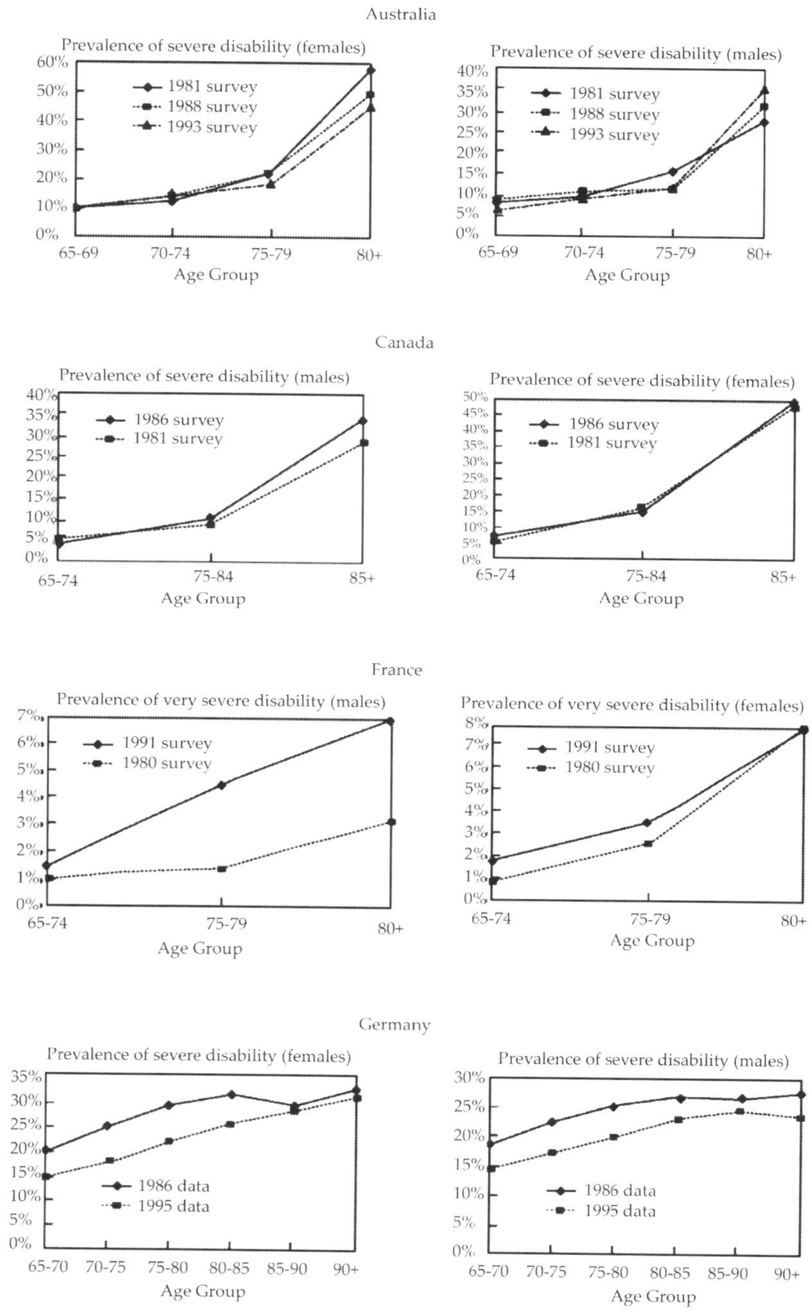

Figure 6.6. *An analysis of the occurrence of severe disability among the elderly in four countries. Notes: Australia: severe handicap, households and institutions; Canada: HALS survey, households and institutions, severe disability; France: households, confined to bed.*

Source: *(Jacobzone, 1998)*

6.9.5. Physiological and Pathological Measures

For a minimum of 150 years, the collection of bodily materials and the evaluation of human physiological functions have been integral to medical practice to diagnose and evaluate the effectiveness of treatment. The progress in implementing these measures in clinical practice has been constrained solely by the availability of required resources and the patient's willingness to bear the diagnostic responsibility. In Western tertiary care settings, a wide range of technologically advanced tests and procedures are conducted.

These include intricate metabolic investigations, noninvasive imaging of body organs, and evaluation of complex organ functions such as those of the brain and heart. Genetic determinations are gaining significance in clinical practice. Additionally, numerous conventional and regular blood and urine tests are highly prevalent. These tests offer a wide range of specific measurements to assess various disease processes.

These laboratory assessments give rise to several significant policy questions that are relevant to older individuals. Does the growing accessibility of these advanced measures contribute to enhanced health outcomes among older individuals? What strategies can be implemented to optimize the application of these intricate and costly tests, both in terms of geographical distribution and individual patient selection? Do their utilization result in secondary medical interventions that enhance health outcomes? Are there any long-term negative health consequences resulting from incorrect medical decision-making based on these tests? Many of these questions can be explored through cross-national investigations, as there are significant differences in access to, funding for, and implementation of these procedures at regional and national levels. This allows for valuable and significant outcome studies. Nevertheless, to conduct a cross-national evaluation of the outcomes of different medical tests and procedures, it is essential to ensure that these tests and procedures possess comparable properties and interpretations, enabling comparative studies.

A crucial concern is the implementation of laboratory testing protocols for surveys conducted on geographically defined elderly populations. The adoption of this application has been limited due to challenges in making the tests portable for community studies, lower acceptance of testing among individuals without obvious clinical conditions, and limited access to individuals with significant functional impairment or living in institutional settings. Several strategies have been developed to address this issue, such as inviting survey participants to regional clinical testing centers, creating more convenient portable testing and specimen-collection devices, and implementing various limitations on testing. These limitations may include focusing on tests for risk factors related to important chronic conditions in older individuals, such as blood pressure, blood cholesterol, or blood sugar levels. Additionally, simpler physical testing devices, like those for respiratory function or muscle strength, can be used, as well as physical performance tests that assess common functions like self-care activities. Furthermore, tests can be conducted to measure blood determinants that reflect more complex factors, such as levels of environmental contaminants or genetic determinations. It is important to acknowledge that ongoing evaluations of new testing procedures for population health assessments are taking place and should always be taken into consideration.

6.10. Mortality Data and Derived Measures

Mortality data, although they may have some inaccuracies and limitations as indicators of population health, have been extensively utilized to inform health policy, primarily due to their widespread accessibility from developed nations. Significant progress in both the socioeconomic and health domains, coupled with shifts in individual and collective lifestyles, have led to a remarkable rise in the life expectancy of older adults. An individual who is 60 years old and from Europe, North America, or Japan can anticipate a remaining lifespan of approximately 20–25 years for women and 18–20 years for men of the same age group. Until just two decades ago, individuals of the same age, regardless of gender, had a life expectancy that was 2 to 4 years shorter. A significant portion of the recent increase in the number of people surviving can be attributed to reductions in death rates caused by heart disease. Survivorship among older individuals, especially those in the oldest age group, is projected to rise, potentially leading to increased health and welfare expenses. Expenses may rise specifically for the prevention and treatment of chronic degenerative illnesses, support for individuals with disabilities, and care related to other debilitating diseases that affect the elderly population. These potential changes necessitate the gathering of data required to estimate future trends in overall mortality and specific diseases.

Although mortality rates have generally been declining, there are notable disparities among different groups within industrialized nations. Women, married individuals, and those of higher social status tend to have lower mortality rates. Furthermore, significant disparities exist at both regional and national levels, which require the gathering of health data specific to each region and the development of adaptable health and social policies to effectively address these variations. In order to analyze the mortality and survival patterns among the elderly, it is necessary to gather data on overall mortality (deaths from all causes) as well as specific causes, categorized based on specific characteristics. Additionally, data is required to describe the population that is at risk of dying.

Mortality data are commonly derived from death certificates obtained from national vital record systems. Presently, there is significant disparity in the quality of the data, and there may be a lack of information for specific geographic areas, which hinders the comprehension of mortality patterns for policy-related objectives. The impact of this variability in quality on analytical studies is contingent upon the objectives and policy inquiries at hand. Table 6.4 provides a summary of the different options available for comparing mortality rates among different older populations, either by looking at them at a specific point in time or by observing them over a period. The options presented include both group or collective mortality data and individually tracked mortality data, which encompass the entire lifespan's health and disease history.

Table 6.4. Options for Comparing Mortality Rates

Type of Data	Approaches	Data Needs	Measures and Methods
Collective	Cross-sectional	Deaths by age, gender, and calendar year; population at risk Deaths by cause and year, population at risk, and competing events	Rates by age, age-standardized cancer ratio, proportional mortality ratio, standardized mortality rates, probability, life table by cause
	Longitudinal (by cohort)	Deaths by age and year of birth, population at risk	Rates by age and cohort, probability and life tables by cohort
Individual	Longitudinal biographies	Death records, data on individual survival, linkage data	Survival analyzes, Kaplan-Meier models, Cox models, etc.
		Follow-up data	Analysis of life histories, biographies (hazard models)

Source: *Principles of Epidemiology. (n.d.). https://archive.cdc.gov/www_cdc_gov/csels/dsepd/ss1978/lesson3/section3.html*

6.10.1. Availability of General Mortality Information

Since World War II, mortality data categorized by gender and age have been accessible for 48 countries, both European and non-European. Only a select few countries have longer time series. Certain central statistical offices provide data that are categorized based on year of birth, making it easier to analyze mortality rates for various age groups. Typically, deaths and the proportion of the population at risk of dying are categorized by specific ages up to 99 years old, and as a single group for those aged 100 and above. However, many countries have recently made efforts to also provide data for specific ages in this older population segment. Kannisto (1994) has created a database that includes a collection of mortality data for individuals aged 80 and above from a group of developed countries that release this information on a yearly basis. The data have undergone several tests to determine their credibility and internal coherence. Based on these tests, countries have been categorized into four quality tiers: those with high-quality data (Czechoslovakia, Denmark, England and Wales, Finland, France, Germany, Hungary, Iceland, Italy, Japan, Luxembourg, the Netherlands, Norway, Scotland, Sweden, and Switzerland); those with data of acceptable quality (Australia, New Zealand-non Maori, and Portugal); those with data of acceptable quality under specific conditions (Estonia, Ireland, Latvia, Poland, and Spain); and those whose data should be used cautiously (Canada, New Zealand-Maori, and the United States). The database was created using mortality data organized into cohort survival histories. Once data on mortality rates by age are obtained, life tables can be created and analyzes of survival among the elderly can be conducted. The combination of data on life expectancy, diseases, and disabilities will enable the calculation of measures that include both the duration of healthy life and the duration of life with disabilities.

6.10.2. Quality of Vital Records

Mortality estimates for elderly individuals may encounter obstacles due to various issues, as documented by Coale and Kisker (1986, 1990), Kannisto (1994, 1996), and Thatcher et al. (1998). Age misreporting is commonly observed in death registration, censuses, and other surveys. The primary indications of the data quality issue include improbable fluctuations in mortality rates across different age groups and unusually low estimates of mortality among older individuals (Preston et al., 1997). Two prevalent issues include the inclination to express age in whole numbers (such as multiples of 5 or 0) and the tendency to overstate one's age among the elderly population. Additional issues regarding the accuracy of data about occupation, education, and surviving relatives have been documented.

6.10.3. Causes of Death

Although records of causes of death have been kept in industrialized countries since the early 1900s, it is only in recent times that specific improvements have been made to standardize the registration process. Medical doctors are responsible for issuing death certificates, as per the guidelines set by the World Health Organization (WHO). The certificate is partitioned into two sections. The first list enumerates fatal diseases, while the second provides information on additional conditions, known as associated causes, that may have played a role in the occurrence of death. In the initial section, the doctor is required to enumerate the primary reason for death, referred to as the immediate cause. This is followed by the pathology that immediately preceded it, known as the intermediate cause. Lastly, the doctor must specify the originating or main cause of death. A death certificate may contain indications regarding more than one cause, thus making it possible to trace back the whole process leading to death, at least in theory. Death is commonly regarded as the ultimate outcome of a series of illnesses, which may be connected to other preexisting medical conditions. When analyzing mortality data, the focus is usually on the primary cause of death, which can be challenging to determine, especially when dealing with older individuals. In order to develop effective policies for the prevention and treatment of specific diseases, it would be extremely beneficial to have access to the complete information recorded on death certificates. Acquiring this data is essential for identifying specific diseases, such as diabetes, that may not be listed as the main causes on death certificates but significantly contribute to mortality rates. If the required data is available, it is possible to define indicators of mortality by multiple causes, as stated by Nam (1990).

Multiple sources of error can arise during the certification process for determining the causes of death. Physician certifiers may commit diagnostic errors, or there may be insufficient clinical information accessible. Occasionally, vague terms like "senility" or "heart attack" are used to describe older individuals when there is a lack of specific clinical information. Additionally, coding errors in the reporting of death events by vital registrars may occur. Nevertheless, the implementation of quality control measures in this field is on the rise, resulting in a reduction of errors originating from this source.

6.10.4. Individual Data and Mortality Differentials

The study of mortality differentials has provided many explanatory hypotheses and offered the possibility of moving from the description of the differences observed to the identification of their root causes. Many studies have involved analyzing mortality differences according to socioeconomic status, usually encompassing cross-sectional analyzes of older populations (e.g., Mare, 1990; Martelin, 1995). However, the impact of social status may be cumulative throughout the life course. Mortality in old age can depend on living conditions during childhood, adolescence, and adulthood, and thus a longitudinal approach may be valuable. Such an approach involves a more complete overview of the entire process as it occurred during the individual's lifetime (Sahli et al., 1995). Death is considered the final event in a life history composed of a succession of various passages spanning a variety of situations and experiences, gradually culminating in an illness (or accident) and then death (Caselli et al., 1987). Data from health, census, and other sources are linked to derive a lifetime picture of social, economic, medical, and other influences.

6.10.5. Cross-National Mortality Contrasts

Cross-national comparisons of the mortality of older persons can be instructive. Figure 6.7 shows the probabilities of death for men and women aged 80–99 (the oldest old) in five countries—Sweden, Japan, France, Italy, and Australia—during the last half of the 20th century. In addition to the clear decline over the study interval and the almost universal finding of higher mortality probabilities in men than in women, three observations stand out. One is that gains in survivorship are happening even among the oldest segments of the world's elders. Another is that the relative survivorship gains among women have been greater than those among men. Finally, the dispersion of the gains is greater among women than among men. The latter two findings should prompt cross-national research into national differences in changing survivorship.

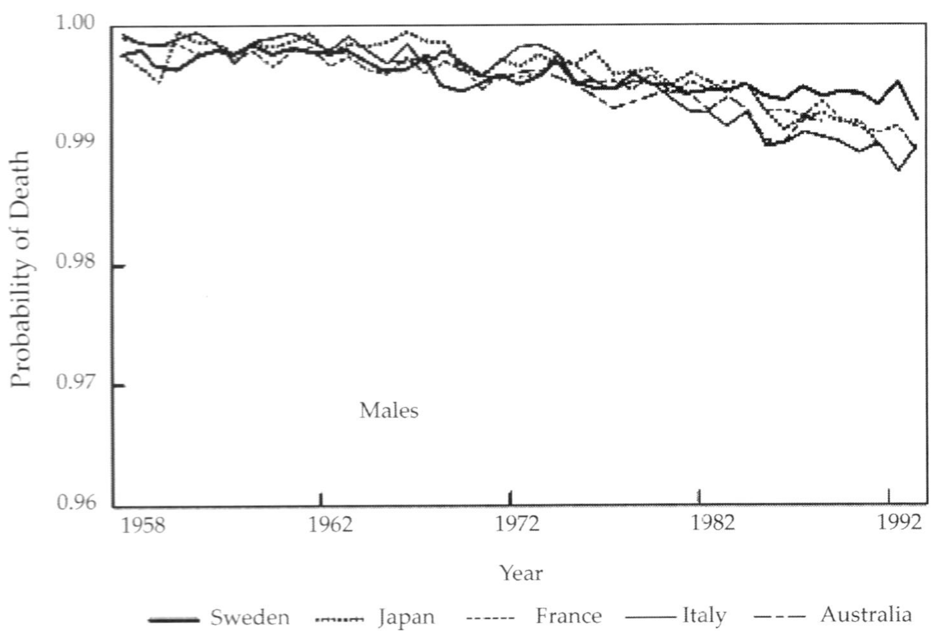

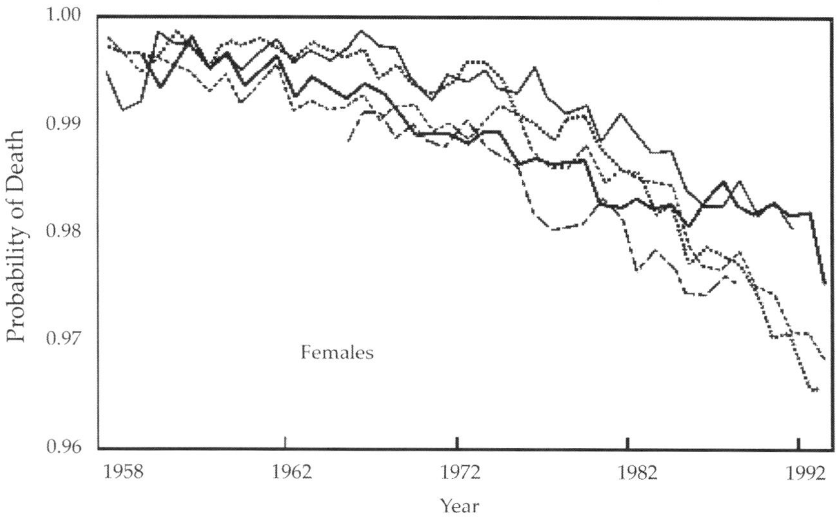

Figure 6.7. *Probability of death at ages 80–99 in five countries: 1952 to 1994.*

Source: Prepared by the panel based on data from the Max Planck Institute for Demographic Research, Rostock, Germany.

6.11. Aging and Mental Illness

Psychiatric disorders are significant contributors to physical, social, and emotional dysfunction and disability among the elderly, but it is only recently that such problems have drawn significant attention (Wells et al., 1989). All of the important mental conditions of young adulthood and middle age, including depression, mania, schizophrenia, personality disorders, addictions (including alcoholism), phobias, anxiety, and panic disorders, occur in older persons. Moreover, with increased survivorship and longevity among older persons, dementia and Alzheimer's disease have become quite common. The dementing illnesses themselves are often accompanied by additional psychiatric symptoms that require medical treatment. These symptoms are among the most important reasons for institutionalization or community-based long-term care.

A particularly important and common condition of older persons is depression, a disorder that illustrates the difficulties of determining the population burden and health service needs associated with psychiatric illness. Early epidemiological studies of mental illness indicated lower rates of depression among the elderly than among younger population subgroups, but there is much reason to doubt the validity of such estimates. Older people are more reluctant to admit to depressive symptoms than younger persons and are more likely to express their symptoms in somatic terms. Most of the instruments measuring depression in community settings, however, depend substantially on psychological items that elderly persons are less likely to endorse. Prevalence estimates of depression among the elderly can vary as much as 15-fold depending on the definitions used, populations studied, and research approaches (Gurland et al., 1996). An important difficulty in assessing and treating depression among older persons involves their different life circumstances as compared with younger persons. Elders have more physical illness and take more medications, making it more difficult to differentiate depression from other health states. In addition, older persons who suffer decrements in function and who lose spouses and friends experience depressive symptoms that they and health professionals commonly view as part of the aging process itself. Researchers often have difficulty differentiating reactions to the losses of normal aging from depression per se. Depression among the elderly is common in primary care practice, and doctors caring for this population tend to be skeptical of psychologically oriented epidemiological instruments. New efforts are being made to derive valid measures of depression in elderly populations and to provide more appropriate treatment (Unutzer et al., 1999).

Depression exemplifies the problems of determining the care burden of mental illness among older persons. Among elders, mental conditions are often associated with important medical illnesses but receive lower priority in clinical diagnosis and treatment. In addition, as noted, many mental problems are mistakenly considered to be part of normal aging and not given appropriate attention, particularly in the primary care setting. Also, administrative and clinical records related to treating mental illness, while sometimes in the mainstream of medical systems, are often kept in separate locations with separate access restrictions. Thus, population rates of mental illness may not be attainable from clinical or administrative records, and the use of population surveys for this purpose should be considered. It is ironic that surveying for mental illness requires a substantial participant burden, as the instruments are often long and detailed. This constraint has limited the number of community- and population-based assessments available for planning and evaluation. Thus, it is not surprising that even among industrialized countries, clinical services for the prevention and treatment of mental illness are often lacking because of their costs and competing clinical priorities. There are also substantial differences among cultures in the behavioral manifestations and lay and professional interpretations of mental symptoms and conditions. This variation makes international comparisons particularly hazardous and necessitates extreme care and documentation of clinical events when conducting such research studies (Yang et al., 2017).

A Closer Look

The Social Factors Impacting Older Health

Social determinants such as socioeconomic status, social support networks, education, and living conditions play pivotal roles. Older adults with lower socioeconomic status often face barriers to accessing quality healthcare, nutritious food, and safe living environments. Financial instability can lead to stress and anxiety, exacerbating health issues and reducing life expectancy.

Social support networks, including family, friends, and community connections, are crucial for maintaining mental and physical health. Isolation and loneliness, common among older adults, are associated with higher risks of depression, cognitive decline, and chronic diseases. Conversely, strong social ties provide emotional support, encourage healthy behaviors, and facilitate access to healthcare services. Engaging in social activities and maintaining relationships can significantly enhance life satisfaction and overall health.

Education also impacts older health by shaping health literacy and behaviors. Those with higher education levels are more likely to engage in preventive health measures, understand medical advice, and manage chronic conditions effectively. Educational opportunities throughout life contribute to better cognitive function in older age, reducing the risk of dementia and other cognitive impairments.

Living conditions, including housing quality and neighborhood safety, influence health outcomes. Older adults living in substandard housing or unsafe neighborhoods face increased risks of accidents, stress, and limited mobility. Access to transportation and amenities like parks and community centers also affects the ability to stay active and socially connected.

Addressing these social determinants through policies and programs aimed at reducing inequalities, enhancing social support, improving education, and ensuring safe living conditions is essential for promoting healthy aging. Comprehensive approaches that consider the multifaceted nature of these factors are vital for improving the health and well-being of older adults, ultimately leading to longer, healthier lives.

Summary

- This chapter explores the unique health challenges faced by the elderly and provides strategies for maintaining and enhancing their well-being.
- It emphasizes the importance of preventive care, lifestyle modifications, and access to quality healthcare services.
- It addresses common age-related issues such as chronic diseases, mental health concerns, and social isolation, offering practical advice on managing these conditions effectively.
- Through a holistic approach that considers physical, mental, and social aspects of aging, this chapter aims to empower older adults to lead healthier and more fulfilling lives.

References

1. Aaron, D. J., Storti, K. L., Robertson, R. J., Kriska, A. M., & LaPorte, R. E. (2002). Longitudinal study of the number and choice of leisure time physical activities from mid to late adolescence: Implications for school curricula and community recreation programs. *Archives of Pediatrics & Adolescent Medicine, 156*(11), 1075–1080. https://doi.org/10.1001/archpedi.156.11.1075.
2. Abt, G., Boreham, C., Davison, G., Jackson, R., Nevill, A., Wallace, E., & Williams, M. (2020). Power, precision, and sample size estimation in sport and exercise science research. *Journal of Sports Sciences, 38*(17), 1933–1935. https://doi.org/10.1080/02640414.2020.1741301.
3. Amaro, H., Reed, E., Rowe, E., Picci, J., Mantella, P., & Prado, G. (2010). Brief screening and intervention for alcohol and drug use in a college student health clinic: Feasibility, implementation, and outcomes. *Journal of American College Health, 58*(4), 357–364. https://doi.org/10.1080/07448481.2010.502192.
4. Amuthavalli Thiyagarajan, J., Mikton, C., Harwood, R. H., Gichu, M., Gaigbe-Togbe, V., Jhamba, T., & Steffan, G. S. (2022). The UN Decade of healthy ageing: Strengthening measurement for monitoring health and wellbeing of older people. *Age and Ageing, 51*, afac147. https://doi.org/10.1093/ageing/afac147.
5. Angelini, L., Caon, M., Carrino, S., Bergeron, L., Nyffeler, N., Jean-Mairet, M., & Mugellini, E. (2013). Designing a desirable smart bracelet for older adults. In *Association for Computing Machinery* (pp. 425–434). Zurich, Switzerland. [Google Scholar].
6. Arai, H., Ouchi, Y., Yokode, M., Ito, H., Uematsu, H., Eto, F., & Sasaki, H. (2012). Toward the realization of a better aged society: Messages from gerontology and geriatrics. *Geriatrics & Gerontology International, 12*(1), 16–22. https://doi.org/10.1111/j.1447-0594.2011.00779.x.
7. Ashe, M. C., Miller, W. C., Eng, J. J., & Noreau, L. (2009). Older adults, chronic disease and leisure-time physical activity. *Gerontology, 55*(1), 64–72. https://doi.org/10.1159/000140087.
8. Assari, S., Smith, J. L., Zimmerman, M. A., & Bazargan, M. (2019). Cigarette smoking among economically disadvantaged African-American older adults in South Los Angeles: Gender differences. *International Journal of Environmental Research and Public Health, 16*(7), 1208. https://doi.org/10.3390/ijerph16071208.
9. Baylina, P., Barros, C., Fonte, C., Alves, S., & Rocha, Á. (2018). Healthcare workers: Occupational health promotion and patient safety. *Journal of Medical Systems, 42*(9), 159. https://doi.org/10.1007/s10916-018-1036-2.

10. Bobo, J. K., & Husten, C. (2000). Sociocultural influences on smoking and drinking. *Alcohol Research & Health, 24*(4), 225–232. [Google Scholar].

11. Böhm, A. W., Mielke, G. I., da Cruz, M. F., Ramirez, V. V., & Wehrmesister, F. C. (2016). Social support and leisure-time physical activity among the elderly: A population-based study. *Journal of Physical Activity and Health, 13*(6), 599–605. https://doi.org/10.1123/jpah.2015-0510.

12. Brawley, L. R., Rejeski, W. J., & King, A. C. (2003). Promoting physical activity for older adults: The challenges for changing behavior. *American Journal of Preventive Medicine, 25*(3 Suppl 2), 172–183. https://doi.org/10.1016/s0749-3797(03)00182-x.

13. Bromell, L., & Cagney, K. A. (2014). Companionship in the neighborhood context: Older adults' living arrangements and perceptions of social cohesion. *Research on Aging, 36*(2), 228–243. https://doi.org/10.1177/0164027513502087.

14. Brooks, R. D., Grier, T., Dada, E. O., & Jones, B. H. (2019). The combined effect of cigarette smoking and fitness on injury risk in men and women. *Nicotine & Tobacco Research, 21*(12), 1621–1628. https://doi.org/10.1093/ntr/ntz108.

15. Caetano, S. C., Silva, C. M., & Vettore, M. V. (2013). Gender differences in the association of perceived social support and social network with self-rated health status among older adults: A population-based study in Brazil. *BMC Geriatrics, 13*, 122. https://doi.org/10.1186/1471-2318-13-122.

16. Chen, M. Y., Chou, C. C., Shiau, H. S., Wang, E. K., Chiou, H. J., & Liao, J. C. (1997). The development of Chinese version health promoting lifestyle profile. *Chang Gung Nursing, 8*, 14–24. [Google Scholar].

17. Childs, E., & de Wit, H. (2014). Regular exercise is associated with emotional resilience to acute stress in healthy adults. *Frontiers in Physiology, 5*, 161. https://doi.org/10.3389/fphys.2014.00161.

18. Choi, H. (2021). Giving or receiving spouse care and marital satisfaction among older Korean individuals. *Social Science & Medicine, 272*, 112071. https://doi.org/10.1016/j.socscimed.2021.112071

19. Churchill, R., Riadi, I., Kervin, L., Teo, K., & Cosco, T. (2021). Deciphering the role of physical activity in stress management during a global pandemic in older adult populations: A systematic review protocol. *Systematic Reviews, 10*, 140. https://doi.org/10.1186/s13643-021-01688-8.

20. Cohen, J. (1988). *Statistical Power Analysis for The Behavioral Sciences* (2nd ed.). Lawrence Erlbaum Associates.

21. Conner, M., & Norman, P. (2017). Health behavior: Current issues and challenges. *Psychology & Health, 32*(8), 895–906. https://doi.org/10.1080/08870446.2017.1327912.

22. Coswig, V. S., Barbalho, M., Raiol, R., Del Vecchio, F. B., Ramirez-Campillo, R., & Gentil, P. (2020). Effects of high vs moderate-intensity intermittent training on functionality, resting heart rate and blood pressure of elderly women. *Journal of Translational Medicine, 18*, 88. https://doi.org/10.1186/s12967-020-02294-7.

23. Cunningham, C., O'Sullivan, R., Caserotti, P., & Tully, M. A. (2020). Consequences of physical inactivity in older adults: A systematic review of reviews and meta-analyses. *Scandinavian Journal of Medicine & Science in Sports, 30*(5), 816–827. https://doi.org/10.1111/sms.13622.

24. de Souto Barreto, P. (2014). Direct and indirect relationships between physical activity and happiness levels among older adults: A cross-sectional study. *Aging & Mental Health, 18*(7), 861–868. https://doi.org/10.1080/13607863.2014.899978.

25. Del Pozo Cruz, B., Ahmadi, M., Naismith, S. L., & Stamatakis, E. (2022). Association of daily step count and intensity with incident dementia in 78,430 adults living in the UK. *JAMA Neurology, 79*(8), 1059–1063. https://doi.org/10.1001/jamaneurol.2022.1525.

26. Dobarrio-Sanz, I., Ruiz-González, C., Fernández-Sola, C., Roman, P., Granero-Molina, J., & Hernández-Padilla, J. M. (2021). Healthcare professionals' perceptions of loneliness amongst older adults: A qualitative study. *International Journal of Environmental Research and Public Health, 18*(4), 2071. https://doi.org/10.3390/ijerph18042071.

27. Donovan, N. J., & Blazer, D. (2020). Social isolation and loneliness in older adults: Review and commentary of a National Academies report. *The American Journal of Geriatric Psychiatry, 28*(11), 1233–1244. https://doi.org/10.1016/j.jagp.2020.07.008.

28. Đošić, A., Živković, D., Milanović, Z., Živković, M., Bjelaković, L., Bratić, M., & Pantelić, S. (2021). The association between level of physical activity and body mass index, and quality of life among elderly women. *Frontiers in Psychology, 12*, 804449. https://doi.org/10.3389/fpsyg.2021.804449.

29. Elliot, C. A., & Hamlin, M. J. (2018). Combined diet and physical activity are better than diet or physical activity alone at improving health outcomes for patients in New Zealand's primary care intervention. *BMC Public Health, 18*, 230. https://doi.org/10.1186/s12889-018-5136-8.

30. Evenson, K. R., & Spade, C. L. (2020). Review of validity and reliability of Garmin activity trackers. *Journal of Measurement in Physical Behavior, 3*(3), 170–185. https://doi.org/10.1123/jmpb.2019-0056.

31. Faller, E. M., Bin Miskam, N., & Pereira, A. (2018). Exploratory study on occupational health hazards among healthcare workers in the Philippines. *Annals of Global Health, 84*(2), 338–341. https://doi.org/10.29024/aogh.20.

32. Fang, B., Sun, F., Quan, Z., Liu, H., & Shan, J. (2021). Smart bracelet system for temperature monitoring and movement tracking analysis. *Journal of Healthcare Engineering, 2021*, 8347261. https://doi.org/10.1155/2021/8347261.

33. Feng, Z., Cramm, J. M., & Nieboer, A. P. (2019). A healthy diet and physical activity are important to promote healthy ageing among older Chinese people. *Journal of International Medical Research, 47*(12), 6061–6081. https://doi.org/10.1177/0300060519878220.

34. Ferreira, R., Baixinho, C. L., Ferreira, Ó. R., Nunes, A. C., Mestre, T., & Sousa, L. (2022). Health promotion and disease prevention in the elderly: The perspective of nursing students. *Journal of Personalized Medicine, 12*(3), 306. https://doi.org/10.3390/jpm12030306.

35. Fong, S. S., Ng, S. S., Cheng, Y. T., Zhang, J., Chung, L. M., Chow, G. C., Chak, Y. T., Chan, I. K., & Macfarlane, D. J. (2016). Comparison between smartphone pedometer applications and traditional pedometers for improving physical activity and body mass index in community-dwelling older adults. *Journal of Physical Therapy Science, 28*(6), 1651–1656. https://doi.org/10.1589/jpts.28.1651.

36. Gao, X., Wang, L., Shen, F., Ma, Y., Fan, Y., & Niu, H. (2019). Dynamic walking stability of elderly people with various BMIs. *Gait & Posture, 68*, 168–173. https://doi.org/10.1016/j.gaitpost.2018.12.036.

37. Gardiner, C., Geldenhuys, G., & Gott, M. (2018). Interventions to reduce social isolation and loneliness among older people: An integrative review. *Health & Social Care in the Community, 26*(2), 147–157. https://doi.org/10.1111/hsc.12367.

38. Gast, J., Peak, T., & Hunt, A. (2020). Latino health behavior: An exploratory analysis of health risk and health protective factors in a community sample. *American Journal of Lifestyle Medicine, 14*(1), 97–106. https://doi.org/10.1177/1559827619835672.

39. Glebova, E., & Desbordes, M. (2021). Chapter 5: Technology innovations in sports: Typology, nature, courses and impact. In *Innovation and Entrepreneurship in Sport Management*. Edward Elgar Publishing.

40. Goh, S. L., Persson, M. S. M., Stocks, J., Hou, Y., Welton, N. J., Lin, J., Hall, M. C., Doherty, M., & Zhang, W. (2019). Relative efficacy of different exercises for pain, function, performance and quality of life in knee and hip osteoarthritis: Systematic review and network meta-analysis. *Sports Medicine, 49*(5), 743–761. https://doi.org/10.1007/s40279-019-01083-2.

41. Golinowska, S., Groot, W., Baji, P., & Pavlova, M. (2016). Health promotion targeting older people. *BMC Health Services Research, 16*(Suppl. 5), 345. https://doi.org/10.1186/s12913-016-1550-6.

42. Gomes, M., Figueiredo, D., Teixeira, L., Poveda, V., Paúl, C., Santos-Silva, A., & Costa, E. (2017). Physical inactivity among older adults across Europe based on the SHARE database. *Age and Ageing, 46*(1), 71–77. https://doi.org/10.1093/ageing/afw166.

43. Gretebeck, K. A., Sabatini, L. M., Black, D. R., & Gretebeck, R. J. (2017). Physical activity, functional ability, and obesity in older adults: A gender difference. *Journal of Gerontological Nursing, 43*(3), 38–46. https://doi.org/10.3928/00989134-20170215-02.

44. Haase, M. (2022). Working out only on weekends is just as effective as daily exercise, study finds. *Prevention*. Retrieved from: https://www.prevention.com/fitness/workouts/a40542944/working-out-only-on-weekends-as-effective-as-daily-exercise-study-finds/ (accessed on 11 July 2024).

45. Han, A., Kim, J., & Kim, J. (2021). A study of leisure walking intensity levels on mental health and health perception of older adults. *Gerontology & Geriatric Medicine, 7*, 2333721421999316. https://doi.org/10.1177/2333721421999316.

46. Harooni, J., Hassanzadeh, A., & Mostafavi, F. (2014). Influencing factors on health promoting behavior among the elderly living in the community. *Journal of Education and Health Promotion, 3*, 40. https://doi.org/10.4103/2277-9531.131913.

47. Harris, J. C., Mereish, E. H., Faulkner, M. L., Assari, S., Choi, K., Leggio, L., & Farokhnia, M. (2022). Racial differences in the association between alcohol drinking and cigarette smoking: Preliminary findings from an alcohol research program. *Alcohol and Alcoholism, 57*(3), 330–339. https://doi.org/10.1093/alcalc/agab050.

48. Harris, T., Limb, E. S., Hosking, F., Carey, I., DeWilde, S., Furness, C., Wahlich, C., Ahmad, S., Kerry, S., Whincup, P., et al. (2019). Effect of pedometer-based walking interventions on long-term health outcomes: Prospective 4-year follow-up of two randomized controlled trials using routine primary care data. *PLOS Medicine, 16*(4), e1002836. https://doi.org/10.1371/journal.pmed.1002836.

49. Haugan, G., & Eriksson, M. (2021). *Health Promotion in Health Care—Vital Theories and Research*. Springer International Publishing.

50. Henriksen, A., Haugen Mikalsen, M., Woldaregay, A. Z., Muzny, M., Hartvigsen, G., Hopstock, L. A., & Grimsgaard, S. (2018). Using fitness trackers and smartwatches to measure physical activity in research: Analysis of consumer wrist-worn wearables. *Journal of Medical Internet Research, 20*(10), e110. https://doi.org/10.2196/jmir.9857.

51. Hong, K. L., & Glover, B. M. (2018). The impact of lifestyle intervention on atrial fibrillation. *Current Opinion in Cardiology, 33*(1), 14–19. https://doi.org/10.1097/HCO.0000000000000466.

52. Izquierdo, M., Merchant, R. A., Morley, J. E., Anker, S. D., Aprahamian, I., Arai, H., & Cesari, M. (2021). International exercise recommendations in older adults (ICFSR): Expert consensus guidelines. *The Journal of Nutrition, Health & Aging, 25*(8), 824–853. https://doi.org/10.1007/s12603-021-1685-9.

53. Joshi, A., Kale, S., Chandel, S., & Pal, D. (2015). Likert scale: Explored and explained. *British Journal of Applied Science & Technology, 7*(4), 396–403. https://doi.org/10.9734/BJAST/2015/18086.

54. Kelley, K., & Rausch, J. R. (2006). Sample size planning for the standardized mean difference: Accuracy in parameter estimation via narrow confidence intervals. *Psychological Methods, 11*(4), 363–385. https://doi.org/10.1037/1082-989X.11.4.363.

55. Koehler, K., & Drenowatz, C. (2019). Integrated role of nutrition and physical activity for lifelong health. *Nutrients, 11*(6), 1437. https://doi.org/10.3390/nu11061437.

56. Kong, H., Wang, X. Q., & Zhang, X. A. (2022). Exercise for osteoarthritis: A literature review of pathology and mechanism. *Frontiers in Aging Neuroscience, 14*, 854026. https://doi.org/10.3389/fnagi.2022.854026.

57. Kouvelioti, R., Vagenas, G., & Langley-Evans, S. (2014). Effects of exercise and diet on weight loss maintenance in overweight and obese adults: A systematic review. *Journal of Sports Medicine and Physical Fitness, 54*(4), 456–474. [Google Scholar].

58. Langhammer, B., Bergland, A., & Rydwik, E. (2018). The importance of physical activity exercise among older people. *BioMed Research International, 2018*, 7856823. https://doi.org/10.1155/2018/7856823.

59. Lao, C., Wang, B., Wang, R. S., & Chang, H. (2021). The combined effects of sports smart bracelet and multi-component exercise program on exercise motivation among the elderly in Macau. *Medicina, 57*(1), 34. https://doi.org/10.3390/medicina57010034.

60. Laroche, D. P., Marques, N. R., Shumila, H. N., Logan, C. R., Laurent, R. S., & Gonçalves, M. (2015). Excess body weight and gait influence energy cost of walking in older adults. *Medicine & Science in Sports & Exercise, 47*(5), 1017–1025. https://doi.org/10.1249/MSS.0000000000000505.

61. Larson, N. I., Story, M., Perry, C. L., Neumark-Sztainer, D., & Hannan, P. J. (2007). Are diet and physical activity patterns related to cigarette smoking in adolescents? Findings from Project EAT. *Preventing Chronic Disease, 4*(2), A51. https://doi.org/10.5888/pcd4.020181.

62. Lee, I. M., Shiroma, E. J., Kamada, M., Bassett, D. R., Matthews, C. E., & Buring, J. E. (2019). Association of step volume and intensity with all-cause mortality in older women. *JAMA Internal Medicine, 179*(8), 1105–1112. https://doi.org/10.1001/jamainternmed.2019.0899.

63. Levant, R., Wimer, D., & Williams, C. (2011). An evaluation of the Health Behavior Inventory20 (HBI-20) and its relationships to masculinity and attitudes towards seeking psychological help among college men. *Psychology of Men & Masculinity, 12*(1), 26–41. https://doi.org/10.1037/a0020927.

64. Li, Y., Pan, A., Wang, D. D., Liu, X., Dhana, K., Franco, O. H., & Willett, W. C. (2018). Impact of healthy lifestyle factors on life expectancies in the US population. *Circulation, 138*(4), 345–355. https://doi.org/10.1161/CIRCULATIONAHA.117.032047.

65. Lim, K. H., Jasvindar, K., Cheong, S. M., Ho, B. K., Lim, H. L., Teh, C. H., & Ambigga, D. (2016). Prevalence of smoking and its associated factors with smoking among elderly smokers in Malaysia: Findings from a nationwide population-based study. *Tobacco Induced Diseases, 14*(1), 8. https://doi.org/10.1186/s12971-016-0070-7.

66. Lindsay Smith, G., Banting, L., Eime, R., O'Sullivan, G., & van Uffelen, J. G. Z. (2017). The association between social support and physical activity in older adults: A systematic review. *International Journal of Behavioral Nutrition and Physical Activity, 14*(1), 56. https://doi.org/10.1186/s12966-017-0510-0.

67. Lombardo, M., Aulisa, G., Padua, E., Annino, G., Iellamo, F., Pratesi, A., & Caprio, M. (2020). Gender differences in taste and foods habits. *Nutrition & Food Science, 50*(2), 229–239. https://doi.org/10.1108/NFS-02-2019-0045.

68. Luo, X., Zhao, H., & Chen, Y. (2022). Research on user experience of sports smart bracelet based on fuzzy comprehensive appraisal and SSA-BP neural network. *Computational Intelligence and Neuroscience, 2022*, 5597662. https://doi.org/10.1155/2022/5597662.

69. MacIntosh, B. R., Murias, J. M., Keir, D. A., & Weir, J. M. (2021). What is moderate to vigorous exercise intensity? *Frontiers in Physiology, 12*, 682233. https://doi.org/10.3389/fphys.2021.682233.

70. Mauldin, R. L., Fujimoto, K., Wong, C., Herrera, S., & Anderson, K. A. (2021). Social networks in an assisted living community: Correlates of acquaintance and companionship ties among residents. *The Journals of Gerontology, Series B: Psychological Sciences and Social Sciences, 76*(7), 1463–1474. https://doi.org/10.1093/geronb/gbaa210.

71. McPhee, J. S., French, D. P., Jackson, D., Nazroo, J., Pendleton, N., & Degens, H. (2016). Physical activity in older age: Perspectives for healthy ageing and frailty. *Biogerontology, 17*(3), 567–580. https://doi.org/10.1007/s10522-015-9631-7.

72. Mehri, A., Solhi, M., Garmaroudi, G., Nadrian, H., & Sighaldeh, S. S. (2016). Health promoting lifestyle and its determinants among university students in Sabzevar, Iran. *International Journal of Preventive Medicine, 7*, 65. https://doi.org/10.4103/2008-7802.183619.

73. Messier, S. P., Mihalko, S. L., Beavers, D. P., Nicklas, B. J., DeVita, P., Carr, J. J., ... & Hunter, D. J. (2021). Effect of high-intensity strength training on knee pain and knee joint compressive forces among adults with knee osteoarthritis: The START randomized clinical trial. *JAMA, 325*(6), 646–657. https://doi.org/10.1001/jama.2020.25553.

74. Mihailovic, N., Szőllősi, G. J., Rancic, N., János, S., Boruzs, K., Nagy, A. C., & Reshetnikov, V. (2020). Alcohol consumption among the elderly citizens in Hungary and Serbia–Comparative assessment. *International Journal of Environmental Research and Public Health, 17*(4), 1289. https://doi.org/10.3390/ijerph17041289.

75. Niemiro, G. M., Rewane, A., & Algotar, A. M. (2022). Exercise and fitness effect on obesity. In *StatPearls*. StatPearls Publishing. Retrieved from: https://www.ncbi.nlm.nih.gov/books/NBK539826/ (accessed on 11 July 2024).

76. Notthoff, N., & Carstensen, L. L. (2014). Positive messaging promotes walking in older adults. *Psychology and Aging, 29*(2), 329–341. https://doi.org/10.1037/a0036834.

77. Nuttall, F. Q. (2015). Body mass index: Obesity, BMI, and health: A critical review. *Nutrition Today, 50*(3), 117–128. https://doi.org/10.1097/NT.0000000000000092.

78. O'Sullivan, B., Scully, P., Curtin, R. J., & Plant, B. J. (2021). A study to assess smoking habits and smoking exposure in sportspeople. *QJM: An International Journal of Medicine, 114*(5), 306–310. https://doi.org/10.1093/qjmed/hcab009.

79. Ong, R. H. S., Chow, W. L., Cheong, M., Lim, G. H., Xie, W., Baggs, G., & Tan, N. C. (2021). Associations between socio-demographics, nutrition knowledge, nutrition competencies and attitudes in community-dwelling healthy older adults in Singapore: Findings from the SHIELD study. *Journal of Health, Population, and Nutrition, 40*, 52. https://doi.org/10.1186/s41043-021-00242-7.

80. Paavola, M., Vartiainen, E., & Haukkala, A. (2004). Smoking, alcohol use, and physical activity: A 13-year longitudinal study ranging from adolescence into adulthood. *Journal of Adolescent Health, 35*(3), 238–244. https://doi.org/10.1016/j.jadohealth.2003.12.013.

81. Philip, K. E., Bu, F., Polkey, M. I., Brown, J., Steptoe, A., Hopkinson, N. S., & Fancourt, D. (2022). Relationship of smoking with current and future social isolation and loneliness: 12-year follow-up of older adults in England. *The Lancet Regional Health – Europe, 14*, 100302. https://doi.org/10.1016/j.lanepe.2022.100302.

82. Piercy, K. L., Troiano, R. P., Ballard, R. M., Carlson, S. A., Fulton, J. E., Galuska, D. A., & Olson, R. D. (2018). The Physical Activity Guidelines for Americans. *JAMA, 320*(19), 2020–2028. https://doi.org/10.1001/jama.2018.14854.

83. Quadir, S. G., Santos, J. R., Campbell, R. R., Wroten, M. G., Singh, N., Holloway, J. J., & Szumlinski, K. K. (2016). Homer2 regulates alcohol and stress cross-sensitization. *Addiction Biology, 21*(3), 613–633. https://doi.org/10.1111/adb.12244.

84. Rababa, M., Al Ali, N., & Alshaman, A. (2021). Health promoting behaviors, health needs and associated factors among older adults in Jordan: A cross-sectional study. *International Journal of Community Based Nursing and Midwifery, 9*(2), 106–116. https://doi.org/10.30476/IJCBNM.2021.89876.1111.

85. Raptou, E., & Papastefanou, G. (2018). An empirical investigation of the impact of smoking on body weight using an endogenous treatment effects model approach: The role of food consumption patterns. *Nutrition Journal, 17*(1), 101. https://doi.org/10.1186/s12937-018-0414-2.

86. Reeder, B., & David, A. (2016). Health at hand: A systematic review of smart watch uses for health and wellness. *Journal of Biomedical Informatics, 63*, 269–276. https://doi.org/10.1016/j.jbi.2016.09.018.

87. Reichardt, C. S., & Little, T. D. (2019). *Quasi-Experimentation: A Guide to Design and Analysis*. The Guilford Press.

88. Resnick, B., D'Adamo, C., Shardell, M., Orwig, D., Hawkes, W., Hebel, J. R., ... & Yu-Yahiro, J. (2008). Adherence to an exercise intervention among older women post hip fracture. *Journal of Clinical Sport Psychology, 2*(1), 41–56. https://doi.org/10.1123/jcsp.2.1.41.

89. Rivera-Torres, S., Fahey, T. D., & Rivera, M. A. (2019). Adherence to exercise programs in older adults: Informative report. *Gerontology and Geriatric Medicine, 5*, 2333721418823604. https://doi.org/10.1177/2333721418823604.

90. Rondón García, L. M., & Ramírez Navarrro, J. M. (2018). The impact of quality of life on the health of older people from a multidimensional perspective. *Journal of Aging Research, 2018*, 4086294. https://doi.org/10.1155/2018/4086294.

91. Rounds, S., Lu, Q., & Siamwala, J. (2022). Cigarette smoking increases the risk of acute respiratory distress syndrome. *Transactions of the American Clinical and Climatological Association, 132*, 224–235.

92. Rovniak, L. S., Kong, L., Hovell, M. F., Ding, D., Sallis, J. F., Ray, C. A., & Chinchilli, V. M. (2016). Engineering online and in-person social networks for physical activity: A randomized trial. *Annals of Behavioral Medicine, 50*(6), 885–897. https://doi.org/10.1007/s12160-016-9816-8.

93. Rudnicka, E., Napierała, P., Podfigurna, A., Męczekalski, B., Smolarczyk, R., & Grymowicz, M. (2020). The World Health Organization (WHO) approach to healthy ageing. *Maturitas, 139*, 6–11. https://doi.org/10.1016/j.maturitas.2020.06.001.

94. Schrempft, S., Jackowska, M., Hamer, M., & Steptoe, A. (2019). Associations between social isolation, loneliness, and objective physical activity in older men and women. *BMC Public Health, 19*, 74. https://doi.org/10.1186/s12889-018-6364-x.

95. Sharon-David, H., & Tenenbaum, G. (2017). The effectiveness of exercise interventions on coping with stress: Research synthesis. *Studies in Sport Humanities, 22*, 19–29.

96. Shin, G., Jarrahi, M. H., Fei, Y., Karami, A., Gafinowitz, N., Byun, A., & Lu, X. (2019). Wearable activity trackers, accuracy, adoption, acceptance and health impact: A systematic literature review. *Journal of Biomedical Informatics, 93*, 103153. https://doi.org/10.1016/j.jbi.2019.103153.

97. Sinha, R. (2008). Chronic stress, drug use, and vulnerability to addiction. *Annals of the New York Academy of Sciences, 1141*, 105–130. https://doi.org/10.1196/annals.1441.030.

98. Sjöberg, A., Hallberg, L., Höglund, D., & Hulthén, L. (2003). Meal pattern, food choice, nutrient intake and lifestyle factors in The Göteborg Adolescence Study. *European Journal of Clinical Nutrition, 57*, 1569–1578. https://doi.org/10.1038/sj.ejcn.1601710.

99. Strasser, B., & Schobersberger, W. (2011). Evidence for resistance training as a treatment therapy in obesity. *Journal of Obesity, 2011*, 482564. https://doi.org/10.1155/2011/482564.

100. Stults-Kolehmainen, M. A., & Sinha, R. (2014). The effects of stress on physical activity and exercise. *Sports Medicine, 44*(1), 81–121. https://doi.org/10.1007/s40279-013-0090-5.

101. Sullivan, A. N., & Lachman, M. E. (2016). Behavior changes with fitness technology in sedentary adults: A review of the evidence for increasing physical activity. *Frontiers in Public Health, 4*, 289. https://doi.org/10.3389/fpubh.2016.00289.

102. Suni, E., & Singh, A. (2022). How much sleep do we really need? Sleep Foundation. Retrieved from: https://www.sleepfoundation.org/how-sleep-works/how-much-sleep-do-we-really-need (accessed on 11 July 2024).

103. Tabrizi, J. S., Behghadami, M. A., Saadati, M., & Söderhamn, U. (2018). Self-care ability of older people living in urban areas of northwestern Iran. *Iranian Journal of Public Health, 47*(12), 1899–1905.

104. Takahashi, P. Y., Quigg, S. M., Croghan, I. T., Schroeder, D. R., & Ebbert, J. O. (2016). Effect of pedometer use and goal setting on walking and functional status in overweight adults with

multimorbidity: A crossover clinical trial. *Clinical Interventions in Aging, 11*, 1099–1106. https://doi.org/10.2147/CIA.S110220.

105. Taylor, G., McNeill, A., Girling, A., Farley, A., Lindson-Hawley, N., & Aveyard, P. (2014). Change in mental health after smoking cessation: Systematic review and meta-analysis. *BMJ, 348*, g1151. https://doi.org/10.1136/bmj.g1151.
106. Team, J. (2022). Amsterdam, The Netherlands; Version 0.12.2 Computer Software. Retrieved from: https://jasp-stats.org/previous-versions/ (accessed on 11 July 2024).
107. Tedesco, S., Sica, M., Ancillao, A., Timmons, S., Barton, J., & O'Flynn, B. (2019). Validity evaluation of the Fitbit Charge2 and the Garmin vivosmart HR+ in free-living environments in an older adult cohort. *JMIR mHealth and uHealth, 7*(4), e13084. https://doi.org/10.2196/13084.
108. Thomeer, M. B., Hernandez, E., Umberson, D., & Thomas, P. A. (2019). Influence of social connections on smoking behavior across the life course. *Advances in Life Course Research, 42*, 100294. https://doi.org/10.1016/j.alcr.2019.100294.
109. Torres-Berrio, A., Cuesta, S., Lopez-Guzman, S., & Nava-Mesa, M. O. (2018). Interaction between stress and addiction: Contributions from Latin-American neuroscience. *Frontiers in Psychology, 9*, 2639. https://doi.org/10.3389/fpsyg.2018.02639.
110. Tsirtsakis, A. (2022). Regular exercise can improve brain function by up to 15%: Study. *RACGP NewsGP*. Retrieved from: https://www1.racgp.org.au/newsgp/clinical/regular-exercise-can-improve-brain-function-by-up (accessed on 11 July 2024).
111. Tudor-Locke, C., Craig, C. L., Aoyagi, Y., Bell, R. C., Croteau, K. A., De Bourdeaudhuij, I., & Lutes, L. D. (2011). How many steps/days are enough? For older adults and special populations. *International Journal of Behavioral Nutrition and Physical Activity, 8*, 80. https://doi.org/10.1186/1479-5868-8-80.
112. Turcotte, P.-L., Carrier, A., Roy, V., & Levasseur, M. (2018). Occupational therapists' contributions to fostering older adults' social participation: A scoping review. *British Journal of Occupational Therapy, 81*(8), 427–449. https://doi.org/10.1177/0308022618762431.
113. Valenti, G., Bonomi, A. G., & Westerterp, K. R. (2016). Walking as a contributor to physical activity in healthy older adults: 2-week longitudinal study using accelerometry and the doubly labeled water method. *JMIR mHealth and uHealth, 4*(2), e56. https://doi.org/10.2196/mhealth.4978.
114. Van Hoecke, A. S., Delecluse, C., Bogaerts, A., & Boen, F. (2014). Effects of need-supportive physical activity counseling on well-being: A 2-year follow-up among sedentary older adults. *Journal of Physical Activity and Health, 11*(7), 1492–1502. https://doi.org/10.1123/jpah.2012-0313.
115. Vozzi, F., Palumbo, F., Ferro, E., Kreiner, K., Giugni, F., Dutton, R., & Riso, P. (2022). Nutritional and physical improvements in older adults through the DOREMI remote coaching approach: A real-world study. *Intelligent Medicine, 2*, 187–192. https://doi.org/10.1016/j.inmed.2022.100156.
116. Weber, M., Belala, N., Clemson, L., Boulton, E., Hawley-Hague, H., & Becker, C. (2018). Feasibility and effectiveness of intervention programmes integrating functional exercise into daily life of older adults: A systematic review. *Gerontology, 64*(2), 172–187. https://doi.org/10.1159/000485816.

117. West, R. (2017). Tobacco smoking: Health impact, prevalence, correlates and interventions. *Psychology and Health, 32*(8), 1018–1036. https://doi.org/10.1080/08870446.2017.1346756.

118. Westcott, W. L. (2012). Resistance training is medicine: Effects of strength training on health. *Current Sports Medicine Reports, 11*(4), 209–216. https://doi.org/10.1249/JSR.0b013e31825dabb8.

119. World Health Organization. (2011). Global health and aging. Department of health and human services, national institute on aging, national institutes of health. Retrieved from: https://www.nia.nih.gov/sites/default/files/2017-06/global_health_aging.pdf (accessed on 11 July 2024).

120. World Health Organization. (2018). Global action plan on physical activity 2018–2030. World Health Organization. Retrieved from: https://apps.who.int/iris/bitstream/handle/10665/272722/9789241514187-eng.pdf (accessed on 11 July 2024).

121. World Health Organization. (2019). Typhoid vaccines: WHO position paper, March 2018—Recommendations. *Vaccine, 37*(2), 214–216. https://doi.org/10.1016/j.vaccine.2018.09.056.

122. Yang, S. C., Luo, Y. F., & Chiang, C. H. (2017). The associations among individual factors, eHealth literacy, and health-promoting lifestyles among college students. *Journal of Medical Internet Research, 19*(2), e15. https://doi.org/10.2196/jmir.6651.

123. Yannakoulia, M., Mamalaki, E., Anastasiou, C. A., Mourtzi, N., Lambrinoudaki, I., & Scarmeas, N. (2018). Eating habits and behaviors of older people: Where are we now and where should we go? *Maturitas, 114*, 14–21. https://doi.org/10.1016/j.maturitas.2018.05.004.

124. Yuenyongchaiwat, K., Pipatsitipong, D., & Sangprasert, P. (2018). Increasing walking steps daily can reduce blood pressure and diabetes in overweight participants. *Diabetology International, 9*(2), 75–79. https://doi.org/10.1007/s13340-017-0355-4.

125. Zaitsu, T., Kanazawa, T., Shizuma, Y., Oshiro, A., Takehara, S., Ueno, M., & Kawaguchi, Y. (2017). Relationships between occupational and behavioral parameters and oral health status. *Industrial Health, 55*(5), 381–390. https://doi.org/10.2486/indhealth.2016-0221.

126. Zhang, Y., Liu, Z., Zhang, L., Zhu, P., Wang, X., & Huang, Y. (2019). Association of living arrangements with depressive symptoms among older adults in China: A cross-sectional study. *BMC Public Health, 19*, 1017. https://doi.org/10.1186/s12889-019-7345-4.

127. Zheng, Z., & Chen, H. (2020). Age sequences of the elderly' social network and its efficacies on well-being: An urban-rural comparison in China. *BMC Geriatrics, 20*, 372. https://doi.org/10.1186/s12877-020-01763-w

Chapter

7

NUTRITION DISORDERS IN COMMUNITY: STRATEGIES FOR PREVENTION AND MANAGEMENT

Contents

Introduction

The discipline of dietetics, as outlined by Swinburn et al. (2019), focuses on the strategic development and implementation of dietary practices to prevent diseases and promote health across communities. In the field of community health nutrition, as described by Hwalla et al. (2018), the goal is to establish environments that encourage healthy lifestyles and dietary choices by addressing the entire spectrum of food production, distribution, and consumption.

There is a broad category of diseases known as nutrition disorders. These diseases manifest themselves when an individual's dietary intake does not provide the necessary amount of nutrients required for healthy bodily function, or when the body experiences difficulties in properly absorbing nutrients from the foods that are consumed. Several dietary imbalances, such as undernutrition, overnutrition, or an incorrect proportion of nutrients, can give rise to these disorders. The term "undernutrition," as defined by the World Health Organization (WHO, 2020), refers to the condition in which the body does not receive an adequate amount of nutrients. This can result in a variety of health problems, including stunted growth in children, impaired immune function, and an increased risk of contracting diseases. On the opposite end of the spectrum, overnutrition, which refers to the consumption of an excessive amount of particular nutrients, can result in a variety of health complications, including an increased risk of obesity, cardiovascular disease, and type 2 diabetes. One more factor that can contribute to nutrition-related disorders is an imbalance of nutrients. This can occur when the diet contains an adequate amount of energy but is deficient in certain nutrients, such as vitamins and minerals, or vice versa. Because of this imbalance, conditions such as micronutrient deficiencies or excesses can arise, each of which is associated with its own unique set of health risks.

It is important to note that the interplay between undernutrition, overnutrition, and an imbalanced nutrient intake highlights the complexity of nutrition disorders and emphasizes the critical role that community health nutrition plays in addressing these challenges. Community health nutrition professionals put in a lot of effort to reduce the prevalence of nutrition disorders and pave the way for communities that are healthier and more resilient. They do this by employing comprehensive strategies that include education, policymaking, and community-based interventions. Community health initiatives and the prevalence of nutrition-related disorders are the subject of this chapter, which focuses on the critical relationship between the two.

Orientation and Directional Terms

Term	Definition	Illustration
Malnutrition	A condition resulting from inadequate or unbalanced intake of nutrients, which can lead to various health issues such as stunted growth, weakened immune system, and increased susceptibility to disease.	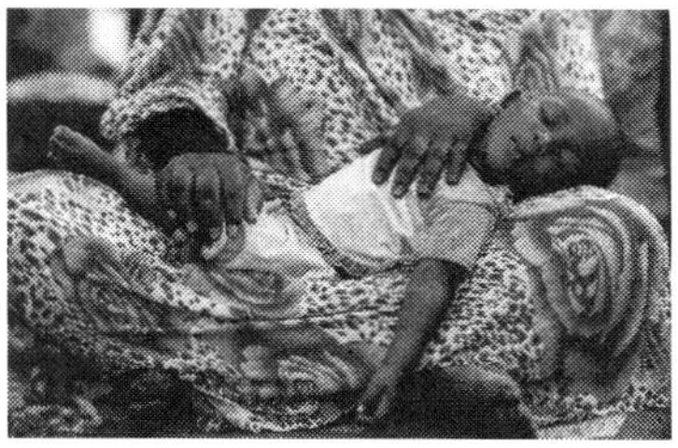
Cardiovascular Disease	A group of disorders affecting the heart and blood vessels, including conditions such as coronary artery disease, heart attacks, and stroke, often linked to risk factors like high blood pressure and cholesterol levels.	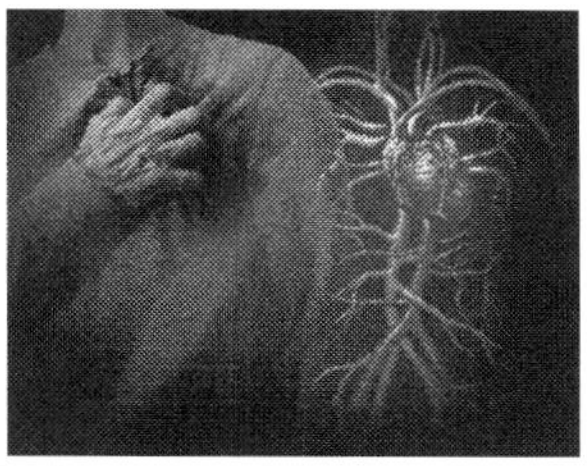
Hypertension	A chronic medical condition where the blood pressure in the arteries is persistently elevated, increasing the risk of heart disease, stroke, and kidney damage. It is also known as high blood pressure.	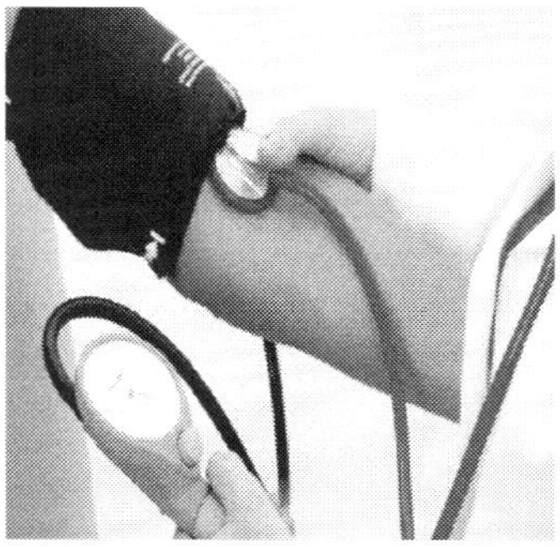
Cancer	A broad term for a range of diseases characterized by abnormal cell growth with the potential to invade or spread to other parts of the body. Types include breast cancer, lung cancer, and prostate cancer.	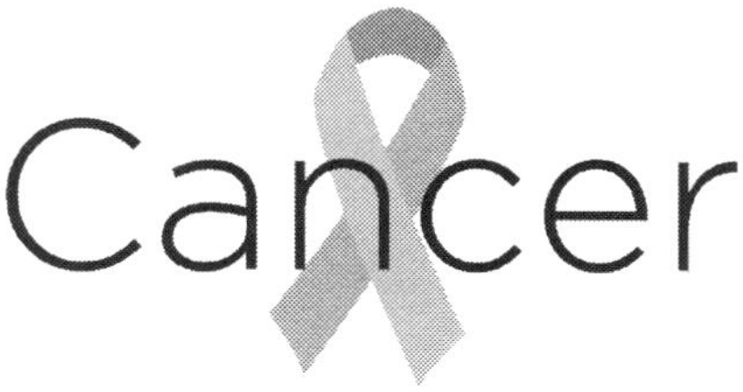
Diabetes Mellitus	A metabolic disorder characterized by high blood sugar levels over a prolonged period due to defects in insulin production, insulin action, or both. Types include Type 1 diabetes (autoimmune) and Type 2 diabetes (related to lifestyle factors).	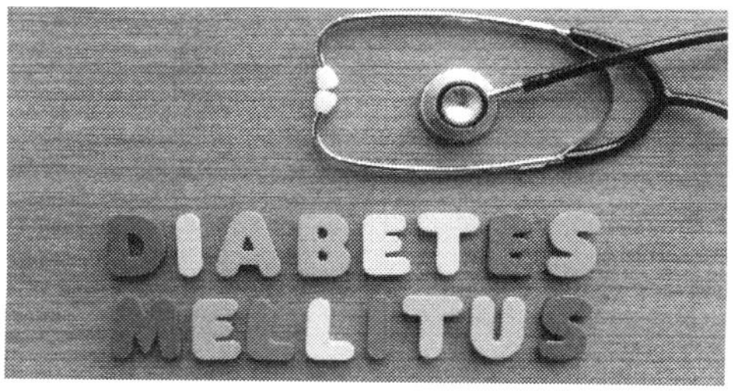

7.1. Nutritional Well-Being

Food is the primary source of essential nutrients that are required to maintain human life and health (Smith, 2018). Human nutrition, as a field, is concerned with the provision of these nutrients. Inadequate nutrition is a persistent issue that is frequently associated with impoverishment, a lack of food security, or an inadequate understanding of nutrition and dietary practices (Jones & Brown, 2019). Internationally, malnutrition and its consequences are major contributors to the number of deaths and disabilities that occur (World Health Organization, 2020). A healthy diet is essential for the physical development of children as well as for the normal biological development of humans (Johnson et al., 2017).

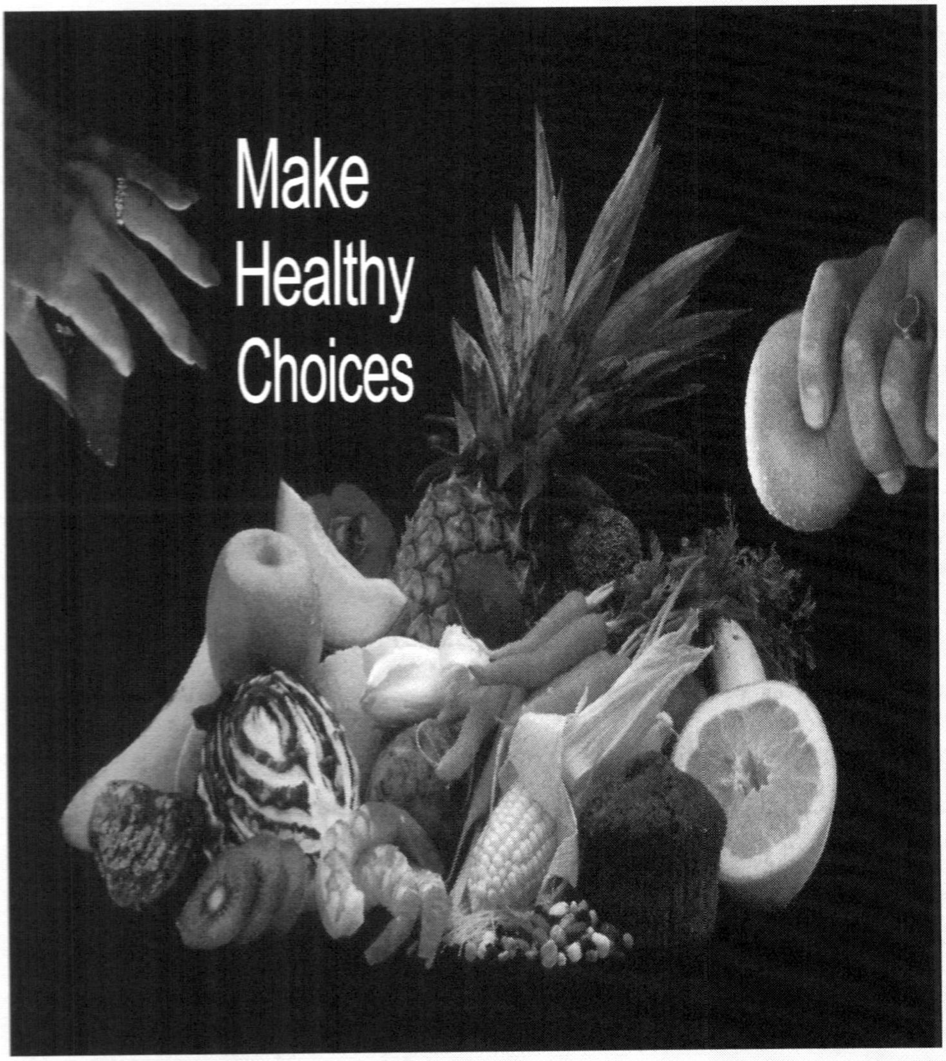

Figure 7.1. *Diet can benefit mental health.*

Source: By Unknown photographer – This image was released by the National Cancer Institute, an agency part of the National Institutes of Health, with the ID 8048 (image) (next)., Public Domain, https://commons.wikimedia.org/w/index.php?curid=24048856.

Carbohydrates, fats, fiber, minerals, proteins, vitamins, and water are the seven components that make up the seven primary categories of nutrients (Adams, 2016). Micronutrients are those that are required in very small amounts, while macronutrients are those that are required in large quantities (Brown & Smith, 2020). The macronutrients that are responsible for providing energy are carbohydrates, fats, and proteins (Adams, 2016). Although they are macronutrients, water and fiber do not contribute to the production of energy. Both minerals and vitamins are considered micronutrients (Jones & Brown, 2019).

The field of study known as human nutrition is a scientific discipline that focuses on the availability and utilization of food and nutrients to maintain life, health, growth, development, and overall contentment (Smith, 2018). Biological and metabolic nutrition, whole-body nutrition, clinical nutrition, and the massive community health nutrition issues of national nutrition programs, as well as the global prevention, control, and elimination of malnutrition and nutritional disorders, are all examples of the extent to which human nutrition encompasses a wide range of practices (World Health Organization, 2020). Food, care, health, and environment are the factors that have the most significant impact on a person's nutritional well-being (Johnson et al., 2017) (Figure 7.1).

7.1.1. Food and Nutrient Security

It is the goal of food and nutrient security to ensure that all individuals, regardless of age or season, have access to the food, diet, and nutrients that are necessary for them to live a healthy life. From the point of view of the World Health Organization (WHO), this entails taking measures to ensure, among other things, that pregnant women are provided with the additional food they require to fulfill their nutritional requirements during pregnancy; and that infants are breastfed exclusively for the first four to six months of their lives, and that they continue to be breastfed after complementary feeding has begun; that infants and young children consume a safe and balanced diet to ensure optimal growth and development; that iodine requirements of the entire population are met through the consumption of iodized salt; that the requirements for vitamin A are met through a balanced diet, fortified foods, and supplementation if necessary; that iron requirements are met through a balanced diet, fortified foods, and supplementation if necessary; and that folate requirements of adolescents are met.

7.1.2. Caring for the Vulnerable

The provision of care for nutritionally vulnerable individuals involves the provision of the necessary time, attention, and behavior (in addition to the requirements for household food security) to guarantee healthy nutrition (FAO, 2021). Support for mothers during pregnancy and lactation; the time and support required to meet the nutritional needs of older persons; and improvements in education, literacy, social security, employment opportunities, and the rights of women are all examples of caring behaviors (WHO, 2019). Breastfeeding and complementary feeding are two types of feeding that are appropriate for infants and young children (UNICEF, 2020).

7.1.3. Health for All

The maintenance of healthy growth and development is dependent upon proper nutrition, and good health is just as important to nutritional wellbeing as it is to good health (Smith, 2018). For optimal nutrition, it is essential to take measures to prevent infections and manage infectious diseases, intending to reduce the frequency, duration, and severity of these conditions (Jones & Brown, 2019). It is necessary to ensure that everyone has access to adequate healthcare services to guarantee priority interventions (Garcia et al., 2020). Immunization, early diagnosis and management of infectious diseases, particularly diarrhea, respiratory disease, measles, malaria, and tuberculosis, education on health and nutrition, and growth monitoring are some of the things that fall under this category (Chen et al., 2017).

7.1.4. A Safe Environment

There is a significant relationship between the physical and biological environments and health, and it is necessary to have policies that are sustainable to address the major environmental conditions that influence food and nutrition. When combined with the daily struggle of the poor to maintain their subsistence, population pressures in developing countries are having a significant impact on the natural resources that are essential to human survival.

There is a significant impact that environmental degradation has on nutrition. A good example of this would be the loss of approximately 5 to 7 million hectares of agricultural land each year. Desertification poses a security risk to 27 million hectares of irrigated land, 170 million hectares of rain-fed cropland, and 3,000 million hectares of rangeland in regions that are characterized as arid and semi-arid.

In addition to contributing to an energy crisis, deforestation also has a direct impact on the capacity of families to provide care for their children and nutrition. Pollution and contamination of soil and water are increasingly putting a strain on the production of food and the safety of food in many regions of the world. Microbial contaminants are responsible for 90% of all foodborne illnesses that occur in developing countries. These illnesses include typhoid fever, cholera, dysentery, and hepatitis A. Even though the prevalence of these diseases has decreased in industrialized nations, the contamination of food with salmonella and other pathogens of a similar nature continues to increase.

To address issues such as soil degradation, erosion, deforestation, overgrazing, and other practices that are not suitable for land use, as well as to conserve fuel and energy sources and to protect habitat, it is necessary to have environmental policies that are sustainable (sustainable). Policy and action initiatives about urbanization, pollution, and the quality of food and water are of particular concern to the World Health Organization (WHO). A growing number of nations are becoming increasingly concerned about the contamination of food and water from agricultural production methods that are both unsafe and excessively intensive.

Several areas that require action include the creation of environmentally sustainable methods for enhancing food, nutrition, and health. It is necessary to ensure that low-income households have access to sufficient resources to reduce the likelihood of any negative impact on the environment. It is necessary to take action to reduce environmental health hazards, particularly those that are transmitted through food and water, and to encourage lifestyles that do not pose a threat to either the environment or health over the course of an extended period.

7.2. Malnutrition

When the body does not receive an adequate amount of nutrients, malnutrition can develop (Smith, 2015). This could mean that you are not getting enough food in general, which can result in starvation. Alternatively, it could mean that you are lacking a single nutrient, such as vitamin C deficiency, which can result in scurvy (Jones, 2017). Several factors can lead to malnutrition, including a lack of sufficient food to consume, an inability to consume a well-balanced diet, the presence of medical conditions that hinder the proper absorption of food, and psychological issues, such as anorexia nervosa (Brown, 2019).

The severity of the problem and the type of malnutrition both play a role in determining the symptoms that are present. A person may not exhibit any symptoms at all if their condition is considered to be mild. Dizziness, fatigue, and a loss of weight are some of the general symptoms that may be associated with this condition. In the event that an individual experiences both fainting and hair loss, it is imperative that they seek medical attention (Smith, 2015). Moreover, a woman should get in touch with her physician if she experiences a cessation of her menstrual cycle, and parents should get in touch with a pediatrician if they notice that their child is not developing normally (Jones, 2017).

When there is widespread poverty or famine in an area, the problem becomes more difficult to solve. It is possible that there is an insufficient amount of food supplies. Second, it's possible that people don't have the financial means to buy the available food. Thirdly, there is a possibility that there is an inadequate number of medical professionals available to treat not only malnutrition but also any underlying causes that go beyond a lack of food that may be contributing to this condition (Brown, 2019).

When children are growing, they need to receive adequate nutrition. If there is a severe lack of food available, children may develop a condition known as marasmus, which is characterized by the child's growth being stunted and the child's body being thinner than it should be. A condition known as kwashiorkor is another one that can affect children. This condition is known as Kwashiorkor, and it occurs when a child consumes an adequate amount of calories but not enough protein. Apathy, delayed development, and an enlarged liver are some of the symptoms that are associated with kwashiorkor (Smith, 2015). Elderly people can develop malnutrition, although they do not require as much food as they did when they were younger. There are some elderly people who experience a loss of their sense of smell, which can make eating unpleasant. Some elderly people produce less stomach acid than younger people, which can make it more difficult for them to absorb nutrients. Moreover, the physical activity required to prepare and consume nutritious meals may be more challenging (Jones, 2017).

7.2.1. Spectrum of Malnutrition

Hunger and malnutrition continue to be among the most devastating problems that the majority of the world's poor and needy are confronted with, and they continue to dominate the health of the nations that are the nation with the lowest standard of living. There are numerous types of malnutrition, and nearly 30% of the world's population, including infants, children, adolescents, adults, and older people living in developing countries, are currently suffering from one or more of these symptoms. In spite of the fact that the world possesses the resources and the knowledge necessary to put an end to this catastrophe, this continues to be a travesty of the fundamental human right to adequate food and nutrition, as well as freedom from hunger and malnutrition.

Several tragic outcomes are associated with malnutrition, including death, disability, and stunted mental and physical growth, which ultimately leads to a retardation in the socioeconomic development of the nation. Malnutrition is responsible for approximately 49% of the 10.7 million deaths that occur annually among children under the age of five in developing countries because of malnutrition. Iodine deficiency is the single most preventable cause of brain damage and mental retardation across the entire world. A deficiency in vitamin

A continues to be the single most preventable cause of blindness in children that is considered to be unnecessary.

At the same time, a massive global epidemic of obesity is emerging in children, adolescents, and adults. This epidemic is affecting more than half of the adult population in some countries, which has led to an increase in the number of deaths caused by cardiovascular disease, hypertension, stroke, and diabetes. This epidemic is particularly prevalent in countries that are rapidly industrializing and industrializing. Diet is also a major contributor to the problems that post-menopausal women experience, as well as to the development of many different types of cancer.

Other significant nutrition problems that affect large populations include the following: only 35% of infants are ever breastfed exclusively between the ages of 0 and 4 months; poor complementary feeding practices are extremely widespread, which is a major cause of childhood malnutrition; scurvy, beriberi, and rickets in severely deprived populations and refugee populations; folate deficiency in women of childbearing age and adolescent girls, which causes 3-quarters of the cases of anemia and neural tube defects; zinc deficiency in deprived populations, which contributes to growth retardation, diarrhea, immune deficiencies, and skin lesions; selenium deficiency, which is widespread in China and the Russian Federation and causes Keshan disease and Kashin-Beck disease.

7.2.2. Malnutrition Across the Life Span

The condition of malnutrition affects people of all ages and throughout their entire lives. It is important to note that intrauterine nutrition has a significant impact on growth, development, morbidity, and mortality beginning at the time of conception and continuing through the fetal period and into early infancy. As a result of the reduced physical and mental capacity in childhood, there is an increased risk of developing diet-related noncommunicable diseases later in life. These health implications range from intrauterine brain damage and growth failure to a reduction in the potential for physical and mental development.

7.2.3. Maternal Malnutrition

A low gestational weight gain, a low pre-pregnancy body mass index, and a short maternal stature are all indicators that maternal malnutrition is the primary factor in the development of intrauterine growth retardation (IUGR) in developing countries. Several other important etiological factors include maternal anemia, infections of the gastrointestinal and respiratory tracts, malaria, and smoking cigarettes during pregnancy.

In addition to the significantly increased risks that it poses for infants and young children (such as increased malnutrition, morbidity, mortality, and poor cognitive and neurological development), IUGR requires immediate attention. This is just one of the many reasons why it is so important to address this issue. Several diseases, including cardiovascular disease, high blood pressure, obstructive lung disease, diabetes, and renal disease, may be more likely to manifest themselves later in adulthood as a consequence of this.

Rather than simply being an indicator of a high risk of malnutrition, morbidity, and mortality for the newborn, high rates of IUGR should be interpreted as an urgent community health warning of the high risk of malnutrition and morbidity in women of childbearing age. When it comes to human and socioeconomic development potential, IUGR also contributes to the perpetuation of the intergenerational cycle of malnutrition, poverty, and disease, which results in enormous costs.

7.2.4. Protein-Energy Malnutrition

Protein-energy malnutrition (PEM), which is the most prevalent form of malnutrition in the world, is the primary manifestation of chronic undernutrition. In the continuum of PEM, which is also known as protein-calorie malnutrition, individuals, and children in particular, consume an insufficient amount of either protein or energy. The condition known as kwashiorkor, which is characterized by a severe protein deficiency, is located at one end of the continuum, and marasmus, which is an absolute food deprivation with grossly inadequate amounts of both energy and protein, is located at the other end.

In addition to being extremely underweight, an infant who has marasmus has lost the majority of or all of their subcutaneous fat. Although a child's body appears to be made up of "skin and bones," the child is extremely fragile and highly susceptible to infections. Because of poverty, the cause is a diet that is extremely low in calories from all sources, including protein. This low-calorie diet is often the result of early weaning to a bottled formula that is prepared with unsafe water and diluted. Due to a lack of proper hygiene and ongoing depletion, a vicious cycle of gastroenteritis and deterioration of the lining of the gastrointestinal tract occurs. This impedes the absorption of nutrients from the limited available food, which further reduces the individual's resistance to infection. In the absence of treatment, marasmus can lead to death due to starvation or heart failure.

The disease known as Kwashiorkor, which is a Ghanaian word that means "the disease that the first child gets when the new child comes," is typically observed in situations where a child is transitioning from high-protein breast milk to a carbohydrate food source that contains insufficient amounts of protein from the breast milk. Children who suffer from this condition, which is characterized by a bloated abdomen as a result of edema (fluid retention), are weak, grow poorly, and are more susceptible to infectious diseases, which can lead to diarrhea that is fatal. Other signs and symptoms of kwashiorkor include apathy, discoloration of the hair, dry, peeling skin, and wounds that do not heal properly. The presence of edema, an enlarged fatty liver, and intestinal parasites can make it appear as though the individual is losing weight. In addition, there may be a slight loss of muscle and body fat to conceal the weight loss.

It is also possible for kwashiorkor and marasmus to occur in hospitalized patients who are receiving intravenous glucose for an extended period of time, such as when they are recovering from surgery, or in patients who are suffering from illnesses that cause them to lose their appetite or have difficulty absorbing nutrients. It is possible for individuals who suffer from eating disorders, cancer, AIDS, and other illnesses that cause a loss of appetite or hinder the absorption of nutrients to experience a loss of muscle and organ tissue in addition to fat tissue stores.

PEM treatment consists of three different components. The resolution of life-threatening conditions, such as fluid and electrolyte imbalances, as well as infections, is required. A child who is starving may experience rapid weight gain within one to two weeks. It is important to restore the child's nutritional status as quickly and safely as possible. (3) If nutritional rehabilitation is to be successful over the long term, the treatment will then shift its focus to that. It is dependent on the severity of malnutrition, the timeliness of treatment, and the sufficiency of ongoing support whether or not recovery will be successful and how quickly it will occur. A reduction in brain growth and intellectual functioning that cannot be fully restored can be the result of starvation, particularly during the first year of a person's life.

7.2.5. Micronutrient Malnutrition

In the context of nutrition, the term "micronutrient malnutrition" is used to describe diseases that are brought on by a lack of vitamins or minerals in the diet. There is a possibility that micronutrient malnutrition influences the lives of more than 2 billion people around the world today. There are several types of micronutrient malnutrition, the most common of which are deficiencies in vitamin A, iron deficiency anemia, and iodine deficiency disorders. There is a possibility that micronutrient malnutrition will affect people from all different population groups and in every region of the world.

In addition to being a significant barrier to socioeconomic development, micronutrient malnutrition is a contributor to a vicious cycle of underdevelopment, which is to the detriment of groups that are already at a disadvantage. It has far-reaching implications for issues of health, learning capacity, and productivity. Due to the high rates of illness and disability, micronutrient malnutrition results in a tragic loss of human potential, as well as high social and public costs. It also reduces the work capacity of populations. When it comes to ensuring rapid and appropriate development, overcoming micronutrient malnutrition is a prerequisite.

Several factors contribute to micronutrient malnutrition, including but not limited to poverty, a lack of access to a diverse range of foods, an absence of knowledge regarding the most effective dietary practices, and a high prevalence of infectious diseases. There is a need for the development of policies and programs that will guarantee the availability of and access to a sufficient quantity and variety of nutritious foods that are safe for consumption by all people across the globe.

7.2.5.1. Iodine Deficiency Disorders (IDD)

The body needs to have iodine to produce thyroid hormones in the correct manner.

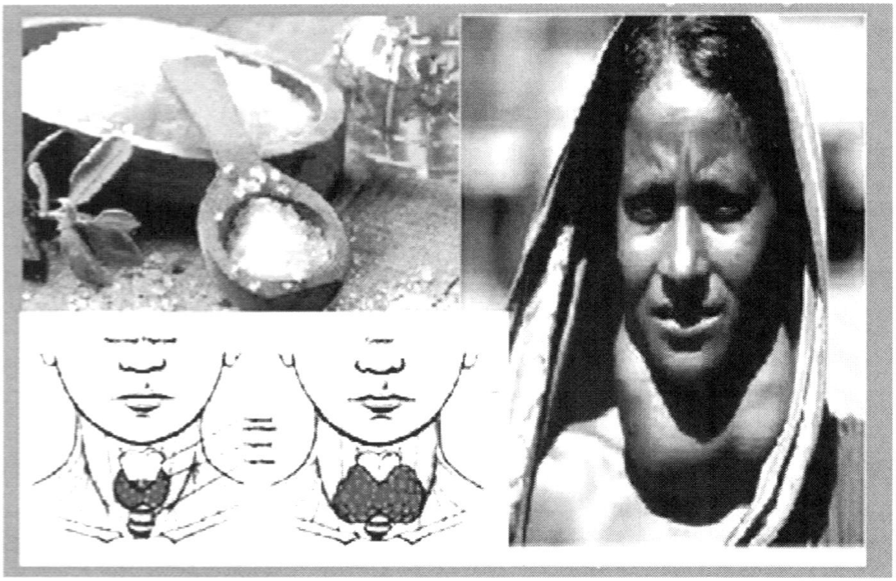

Figure 7.2. *Iodine deficiency disorders (IDD) constitute the single greatest cause of preventable brain damage in the fetus and infant, and of retarded psychomotor development in young children.*

Source: https://img.jagranjosh.com/.

It is not possible for the human body to produce it, and iodine is an absolutely necessary nutrient. The fact that iodine is not easily accessible in a great number of foods makes it challenging for a great number of people to acquire it. Ocean water is one particular source that one can find in large quantities, despite the fact that it is not an effective source for dietary purposes. Iodine deficiency diseases (IDDs) have the potential to manifest themselves prior to birth; consequently, it is of the utmost importance for all populations to possess adequate levels of the micronutrient to forestall the onset of similar diseases at an earlier stage (Figure 7.2).

IDD continues to be a significant risk to the health and development of populations all over the world, but it is especially prevalent among preschool-aged children and pregnant women in countries located in low-income regions.

Goitre, stillbirth, and miscarriages are some of the unintended consequences of this condition; however, the most devastating consequences include mental retardation, deaf-mutism, and impaired education. Even though cretinism is the most extreme manifestation, the more subtle degrees of mental impairment that lead to poor academic performance, decreased intellectual ability, and impaired work capacity are of significantly greater significance.

7.2.5.2. Vitamin A deficiency (VAD)

It is a major problem in the developing world, particularly in Africa and Southeast Asia; in the poorest countries, hundreds of thousands of children become blind each year due to a deficiency of the vitamin. Vitamin A deficiency is the leading cause of preventable blindness in children and is a concern in the developing world. A deficiency of any severity can have a negative impact on immune function, which in turn can lower disease resistance. Night blindness is an early indicator of vitamin A deficiency, which is then followed by abnormal dryness of the eye and, ultimately, scarring of the cornea, which is a condition known as xerophthalmia. Dry skin, the hardening of epithelial cells in other parts of the body (such as mucous membranes), and impaired growth and development are some of the additional symptoms this condition can cause. The practice of administering a single, substantial dose of vitamin A to children once every six months is helping to reduce the prevalence of vitamin A deficiency in many regions where the condition is widespread. The use of a genetically modified form of rice that contains beta-carotene, which is a precursor to vitamin A, has the potential to significantly reduce the number of people who are deficient in vitamin A; however, the use of this so-called golden rice is controversial.

7.2.5.3. Iron Deficiency and Anemia (IDA)

Not only does iron deficiency affect industrialized countries, but it also affects developing countries. It is the most widespread nutritional disorder in the world. Within the former, the most common reason for anemia is a lack of iron in the body. Iron deficiency is associated with other micronutrient deficiencies (folic acid, vitamins A and B12), parasitic infestations such as malaria and hookworm, and chronic infections such as HIV, which all contribute to an increased risk of anemia in developing countries. This factor makes the risk of anemia even more severe. The typical diet of the poorest populations is not only monotonous, but it is also based on cereals, which are low in iron and contain high levels of absorption inhibitors. They are also the most common source of iron. Iron stores are typically low in these cases, particularly in young children and pregnant women. This is especially true in the case of adolescents.

The detrimental effects of iron deficiency on human health and development are numerous and extensive. The consequences of this condition include a reduction in the extent of physical activity levels, as well as impaired psychomotor development, coordination, and academic achievement in infants and young children. Iron deficiency is associated with a reduction in work capacity and a decrease in resistance to fatigue in adults of both boys and girls. Iron deficiency causes anemia in pregnant women, which is linked to an increased risk of maternal mortality and morbidity, fetal morbidity and mortality, and intrauterine growth retardation. Anemia is associated with an increased risk of all three of these outcomes.

A comprehensive plan to manage anemia should include preventative measures to prevent iron deficiency as one of its components. This strategy ought to be based on a combination of iron supplementation, dietary approaches, food fortification, and more general community health measures to address the other factors that contribute to anemia. To this day, the most effective method for preventing iron deficiency and anemia in the majority of countries is to administer iron supplements to pregnant women and, on a less frequent basis, to young children. There is a lack of inclusion of dietary improvement strategies in IDA control programs, which is a major concern. Since increasing the amount of bioavailable iron in the diet requires ensuring access to foods that are typically unaffordable or even frequently unavailable to population groups that are at risk of iron deficiency, their practical implementation is not always an easy task. Animal foods and fresh fruits and vegetables are two examples of the types of foods that fall under this category. As a consequence of this, it is heartening to observe that an increasing number of nations are initiating iron fortification programs.

7.2.5.4. Other Micronutrient Deficiencies

Several other forms of malnutrition, or nutrition deficiency disorders, affect large and often vulnerable population groups worldwide. Action is urgently required on the following:

7.2.5.4.1. Folate Deficiency

Which frequently exacerbates iron deficiency anemia that was already present in the mother, causing widespread megaloblastic anemia associated with pregnancy. Folate deficiency is recognized as an independent risk factor for coronary heart disease and stroke because it is also associated with elevated plasma homocysteine levels. Folate deficiency is also associated with this increase. There is also a correlation between it and the occurrence of neural tube defects, such as anencephaly and spina bifida, in high-risk population groups all over the world, including in China, Europe, and the Middle East. There is also a correlation between low folate status and cancer, particularly cancer of the colon.

7.2.5.4.2. Zinc Deficiency

In addition to causing growth retardation or failure, diarrhea, immune deficiencies, skin and eye lesions, changes in behavior, and delayed sexual maturation, it also causes skin and eye lesions. Zinc plays an important part in the structure and function of biomembranes, as well as in the stabilization of DNA, RNA, and ribosomal structures. Zinc is involved in more than 200 biochemical reactions due to its involvement in enzyme reactions. The administration of zinc supplements to malnourished infants and young children who have growth retardation has led to an improvement in their growth. Other functions that have responded to zinc supplementation include immune functions in older people and complications of pregnancy such as prematurity, prolonged labor, pregnancy-induced hypertension, and intrapartum hemorrhage. Zinc supplementation has made a positive impact on these functions. There is a growing body of evidence suggesting that this mild zinc deficiency may be significantly more prevalent than was previously believed. For instance, there is evidence that zinc deficiency can cause intrauterine growth retardation and even neural tube defects in the fetus. Additionally, there is evidence that zinc deficiency can affect taste acuity and that it can cause dermatitis and impaired immune function in the elderly.

7.2.5.4.3. Calcium deficiency and Osteoporosis

Inadequate calcium intake from the diet has been linked to several prevalent and persistent medical conditions all over the world. These conditions include osteoporosis, osteoarthritis, cardiovascular disease (hypertension and stroke), diabetes, dyslipidemias, hypertensive disorders of pregnancy, obesity, and cancer of the colon.

- **Calcium:** For normal growth and the development of the skeleton, which is a significant component of mineralized tissues, is necessary. To maximize and maintain peak adult bone mass and minimizing bone loss among older individuals, two of the most important factors in lowering the risk of osteoporosis, it is essential to consume an adequate amount of calcium. Requirements for calcium can vary. In the later stages of adulthood, during pregnancy and lactation, and during the period of rapid growth that occurs during adolescence, the greatest needs are the most important. Calcium requirements are largely determined by skeletal requirements. This is because bone tissue contains 99% of the total calcium found in the body.
- **Osteoporosis:** The relative significance of calcium in the diet is not entirely clear, but it is the result of a complicated chain of events that led to this. When it comes to the effectiveness of calcium supplementation in preventing and mitigating osteoporosis, the research literature contains a great deal of research that contradicts itself. Further complicating matters is the hypothesis that a calcium intake in the diet that is not all that dissimilar to the levels that are proposed for the diet can result in a variety of unfavorable biological effects. However, when viewed from a global perspective, the situation becomes even more perplexing. The relationship between calcium intake and the incidence of osteoporosis is not always as strong as this theory predicts it to be, even though trends generally suggest that there is an inverse relationship between the two. Because of this, there are some nations in which relatively low calcium intakes do not lead to significant increases in the prevalence of osteoporosis. It is possible that the role of other factors, such as hormone levels and exercise, may be more important than the role of dietary calcium alone. This could be a contributing factor to the problem.
- **Selenium Deficiency:** Selenium is an important mineral. It's necessary for many processes, such as:
  - thyroid hormone metabolism
  - DNA synthesis
  - reproduction
  - protection from infection

Selenium deficiency is a condition in which the body does not contain an adequate amount of selenium. This can lead to several different health issues. There is a strong correlation between the quality of the soil used to cultivate food sources and the amount of selenium that is present in those sources. Rainfall, evaporation, and pH levels are all factors that influence the concentration of selenium in soil. Because of this, selenium deficiency is more prevalent in certain regions of the world's population. Due to the fact that it is essential to the operation of several different systems, selenium is an especially important mineral. Among these are the cardiovascular system, the immune system, and the endocrine system. The organ that contains the highest concentration of selenium in relation to the total weight of organ tissue is the thyroid, which is a component of the endocrine system.

7.3. Diet and Chronic Disease

The relationship between diet and chronic disease, which is defined as a disease that worsens over a prolonged period and does not go away on its own, is a complicated one (Smith et al., 2018). This is not only because many diseases take years to develop, but also because it is extremely challenging to pinpoint a specific dietary cause. Several prospective epidemiologic studies try to circumvent this challenge by carefully monitoring the participants over the course of several years (Jones & Brown, 2020). Despite this, it is difficult to establish a causal relationship between the diet and chronic diseases due to the sheer complexity of the diet and the multifactorial origins of chronic diseases (Adams, 2017) (Figure 7.3).

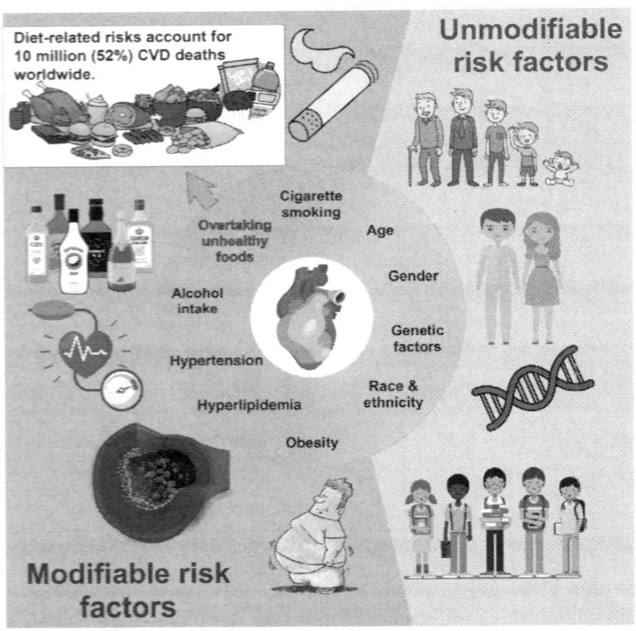

Figure 7.3. *Diet and chronic diseases: CVD.*

Source: *Chen W, Zhang S, Hu X, Chen F, & Li D. (2023). A review of healthy dietary choices for cardiovascular disease: from individual nutrients and foods to dietary patterns. Nutrients, 15(23), 4898. https://doi.org/10.3390/nu15234898.*

To put it simply, a poor diet is one of the primary factors that contributes to the leading causes of death and chronic illness. Diets that are healthy and physical activity are both essential components of good nutrition and are required for a life that is both long and healthy. At every stage of life, it is essential to maintain a healthy weight by eating foods that are high in nutrients, balancing the amount of energy that one consumes with the amount of physical activity that is required. Consuming foods that are high in energy (sugar, starch, and/or fat) but low in essential nutrients is a contributing factor in the development of energy excess, as well as for being overweight and obese. The amount of energy that is consumed in relation to physical activity, as well as the quality of the food that is consumed, are important factors that determine nutrition with chronic disease.

7.3.1. Cardiovascular Disease

The leading cause of death in developed countries is cardiovascular disease, which is a broad term that encompasses diseases that affect both the heart and the blood vessels. Ischemic heart disease, also known as coronary artery disease, is the most prevalent form of cardiovascular disease, and it is also the form that results in the greatest number of fatalities. As a result of the narrowing and obstruction of the arteries that carry blood to the heart and, consequently, oxygen and nutrients, coronary heart disease (CHD) develops. Atherosclerosis, a condition in which fibrous plaques (deposits of lipid and other material) build up on the inner walls of arteries, causes these arteries to become stiff and less responsive to changes in blood pressure. This narrowing is typically the result of atherosclerosis. A myocardial infarction, also known as a heart attack, is a condition that can occur when there is a disruption in the flow of blood in the coronary arteries that surround the heart. A cerebrovascular accident, also known as a stroke, can be caused by a restriction in blood flow to the brain, which can be caused by a blood clot or a hemorrhage. Peripheral arterial disease can be caused by a narrowing of the abdominal aorta, its major branches, or the arteries of the legs. In the majority of cases, the cause of heart attacks and strokes is not the complete obstruction of the arteries by plaque, but rather the formation of blood clots, which occurs more frequently in areas where small plaques are already partially blocking the arteries.

This disease may actually begin in childhood, with the appearance of fatty streaks, which are precursors to plaque. Although it typically takes decades for atherosclerosis to manifest in the form of a heart attack or stroke, the disease may actually begin in childhood. Plaque formation is, in essence, an inflammatory response that is directed toward repairing injuries in the arterial wall during the process of plaque deposition. Among the many factors that are associated with vessel injury, cigarettes, high blood pressure, diabetes, and elevated levels of low-density lipoprotein (LDL) cholesterol in the blood are among the most prominent. Infection with particular bacteria or viruses may also be a factor in the development of inflammation and damage to blood vessels. People who are middle-aged men, particularly those who have a family history of coronary heart disease, as well as people who have hereditary conditions such as familial hypercholesterolemias, are especially susceptible to developing coronary heart disease at an earlier age.

High levels of low-density lipoprotein (LDL) cholesterol, high levels of high-density lipoprotein (HDL) cholesterol, high blood pressure, and diabetes are the four major risk factors for coronary heart disease (CHD). Diet and weight loss are influential in modifying these risk factors. Diet, on the other hand, does not appear to play as significant of a role in influencing the established risk factors as the risk factors themselves do in coronary heart disease cases. When combined with other methods, such as quitting smoking and engaging in regular physical activity, dietary strategies are most effective in achieving the desired results. Pharmacological treatment may involve the administration of cholesterol-lowering medications like statins, bile acid sequestrants, and niacin, as well as anticoagulants or aspirin to prevent the formation of blood clots and antihypertensive medication to reduce blood pressure. Recent studies have called into question the efficacy of hormone therapy in lowering the risk of coronary heart disease in women who have gone through menopause. This is even though it is believed that endogenous estrogen, which is estrogen that is produced by the body, protects against coronary heart disease in premenopausal women.

7.3.1.1. Blood Lipoproteins

A lipoprotein (a) test is a method that determines the amount of lipoprotein (a) that is present in your blood. Proteins and fats combine to form lipoproteins, which are substances that transport cholesterol through the bloodstream. Two primary categories of cholesterol are as follows:

- HDL, also known as "good" cholesterol stands for high-density lipoprotein.
- LDL cholesterol, also known as "bad" cholesterol, is a type of cholesterol.

Lipoprotein (a) is a subtype of LDL cholesterol, also known as "bad" cholesterol. If your lipoprotein (a) level is high, it may indicate that you are at risk for developing heart disease.

When determining whether an individual is at risk for a stroke, heart attack, or other heart diseases, a lipoprotein (a) test is necessary. Neither is it a typical examination. People who have certain risk factors, such as a history of heart disease in their family, are typically the only ones qualified to receive it.

7.3.1.1.1. Why Do Need a Lipoprotein (a) Test?

You may need this test if you have:

- Heart disease, despite normal results on other lipid tests
- High cholesterol, despite maintaining a healthy diet
- A family history of heart disease, especially heart disease that has occurred at an early age and/or sudden deaths from heart disease

7.3.1.2. Dietary Fat

There is a consensus among experts that a diet low in fat can reduce cholesterol levels in the blood and protect against cardiovascular disease. In addition, a high-fat diet is frequently associated with obesity, although this is not always the case. Obesity, in turn, can bring about an increased risk of cardiovascular disease. However, the situation is made more complicated by the fact that different lipoproteins that carry cholesterol are affected differently by the various fatty acids that are included in the equation. In addition, eliminating certain fats from the diet may result in the substitution of other components that are associated with an increased risk of adverse health effects. In the case of certain individuals, such as those who are predisposed to metabolic syndrome or type 2 diabetes, diets that are high in carbohydrates, for instance, may actually increase the risk of cardiovascular disease. Within the context of an individual's reaction to specific dietary manipulations, heredity is also a factor.

7.3.1.2.1. Unhealthy Fats

There are two main types of potentially harmful dietary fats:

1. **Saturated Fat:** This type of fat comes mainly from animal sources of food, such as red meat, poultry and full-fat dairy products. Saturated fats raise high-density lipoprotein (HDL or "good") cholesterol and low-density lipoprotein (LDL or "bad") cholesterol levels, which may increase your risk of cardiovascular disease.
2. **Trans Fat:** This type of fat occurs naturally in some foods in small amounts. However, most trans fats are made from oils through a food processing method called partial hydrogenation. These partially hydrogenated trans fats can increase total blood cholesterol, LDL cholesterol and triglyceride levels, but lower HDL cholesterol. This can increase your risk of cardiovascular disease.

When the temperature is at room temperature, most fats that contain trans-fat or that have a high percentage of saturated fat are solid. Solid fats are the term that is most used to refer to them. The following are some examples of these: beef fat, pork fat, butter, coconut oil, stick margarine, and shortening.

7.3.1.2.2. Healthier Fats

The potentially helpful types of dietary fat are primarily unsaturated fats:

1. **Monounsaturated Fatty Acids:** This type of fat is found in a variety of foods and oils. Studies show that eating foods rich in monounsaturated fatty acids instead of saturated fats improves blood cholesterol levels, which can decrease your risk of heart disease and may also help decrease the risk of type 2 diabetes.
2. **Polyunsaturated Fatty Acids:** This type of fat is found mostly in plant-based foods and oils. Evidence shows that eating foods rich in polyunsaturated fatty acids instead of saturated fats improves blood cholesterol levels, which can decrease your risk of heart disease and may also help decrease the risk of type 2 diabetes.
3. **Omega-3 Fatty Acids:** One type of polyunsaturated fat is made up of mainly omega-3 fatty acids and may be especially beneficial for heart health. Omega-3, found in some types of fatty fish, appears to decrease the risk of coronary artery disease. There are plant sources of omega-3 fatty acids. However, it hasn't yet been determined whether replacements for fish oil—plant-based or krill—have the same health effects as omega-3 fatty acids from fish.

Canola oil, olive oil, safflower oil, peanut oil, sunflower oil, and corn oil are examples of foods that are liquid at room temperature and are composed primarily of monounsaturated and polyunsaturated fats.

For example, salmon, tuna, trout, mackerel, sardines, and herring are all examples of fish that are rich in omega-3 fatty acids. The ground form of flaxseed, oils (canola, flaxseed, and soybean), nuts and other seeds (walnuts, butternuts, and chia seeds), and flaxseed meal are all examples of plant-based sources of omega-3 fatty acids.

7.3.1.3. Dietary Cholesterol

Cholesterol in the blood and cholesterol in the food are two separate entities, but people frequently get them confused with one another. The only foods that contain cholesterol in the diet are those that come from animals, and the egg yolk and organ meats contain the highest levels of cholesterol. The consumption of cholesterol elevates LDL cholesterol, but not to the same extent as the consumption of saturated fatty acids. There is a possibility that the consumption of additional cholesterol will not further raise blood cholesterol levels due to feedback control mechanisms if the cholesterol levels in the diet are already too high. Additionally, the response of individuals to cholesterol in their diets varies greatly from person to person. Those who are in good health should consume an average of less than 300 milligrams of cholesterol on a daily basis. However, because the body is capable of producing cholesterol on its own, there is no need to consume any cholesterol in the diet.

7.3.1.4. Other Dietary Factors

Additionally, the consumption of soluble fiber, which is a component of dietary fiber (indigestible plant material), has been associated with a reduction in the levels of LDL and total blood cholesterol, as well as a reduction in mortality from cardiovascular disease. Psyllium and other fiber supplements may also be recommended in addition to whole oats, barley, legumes, certain vegetables, and fruits, particularly apples, plums, apricots, blueberries, strawberries, and citrus fruits. Soluble fiber can be found in these foods. There is a lack of clarity regarding the mechanism by which soluble fiber reduces cholesterol levels; however, it is likely associated with its capacity to bind with cholesterol and bile acids in the digestive tract, thereby removing them from circulation. Additionally, there are additional factors that could be contributing, such as the fermentation of fiber by bacteria in the colon, which results in compounds that inhibit the synthesis of cholesterol.

Due to its ability to raise HDL cholesterol levels and possibly because it helps prevent blood clot formation, alcohol consumption that is light to moderate (up to two drinks per day for men and one drink per day for women) is associated with a reduced risk of coronary heart disease (CHD). The consumption of alcohol may help explain the so-called French paradox, which states that the rates of coronary heart disease in France are low despite having a risk profile that is comparable to that of the United States, where the rates are relatively high. Several antioxidant compounds, including resveratrol derived from grape skins, are found in wine. These compounds have the potential to inhibit the oxidation of LDL, but it is likely that the beneficial effect of these substances is significantly less than that of alcohol itself.

Only in individuals who are overweight, who may have a greater sensitivity to dietary sodium, is there a significant association between the amount of sodium (salt) an individual consumes in their diet and the risk of death from cardiovascular disease and stroke. Additionally, it appears that sodium consumption has a direct impact on the risk of stroke, in addition to the effect that it has on blood pressure, which in turn has an impact on the risk of stroke. On the other hand, there is a correlation between diets that are high in potassium and a lower risk of stroke.

There is a correlation between the consumption of soy foods and lower levels of both LDL and total blood cholesterol, in addition to other vascular effects that are associated with a lower risk of coronary heart disease. Tofu, tempeh, miso, soy flour, soy milk, and soy nuts are some examples of soy foods that contain isoflavones. Isoflavones are estrogen-like compounds that are believed to be responsible for the beneficial effects that soy foods have on the cardiovascular system.

Vitamin C, vitamin E, and beta-carotene, which come from plants and are precursors to vitamin A, are all examples of antioxidant substances that can be found in food and also taken as dietary supplements. Although clinical trials have not yet provided evidence to support this hypothesis, dietary antioxidants may reduce the risk of coronary heart disease (CHD).

7.3.2. Hypertension

The condition known as hypertension, also known as high blood pressure, is one of the most prevalent health issues in developed nations. It is a significant risk factor for several other diseases, including coronary heart disease, congestive heart failure, stroke, aneurysm, and kidney disease, among others. The majority of people who have high blood pressure have essential hypertension, also known as primary hypertension, which is characterized by the absence of a specific cause. In addition to the role that heredity plays in the development of the disease, modifiable factors such as being overweight, not being physically active, drinking a lot of alcohol, and eating a diet that is high in salt also play a role. African Americans have some of the highest rates of hypertension in the world, and the reasons behind this are not entirely clear.

In most cases, hypertension is defined as a blood pressure that is equal to or higher than 140/90 mm Hg. This is equivalent to the pressure that would be exerted by a column of mercury that is 140 mm high during the contraction of the heart (systole) and 90 mm high during the relaxation of the heart (diastole). In hypertension, either the systolic or diastolic blood pressure, or both, may be elevated. It is possible for people who have hypertension to go years without experiencing any symptoms, and then all of a sudden, they suffer a fatal stroke or heart attack. By taking preventative measures and managing hypertension, one can significantly reduce the likelihood of experiencing complications. to begin making changes to one's lifestyle as soon as possible, it is essential to identify hypertension at an early stage.

People who are overweight, particularly those who have excess abdominal fat, have a significantly higher risk of developing hypertension (high blood pressure) than lean people. When it comes to lowering high blood pressure, weight loss alone can be very effective. Sometimes, as little as 4.5 kilograms (10 pounds) should be sufficient. As a matter of course, increasing one's level of physical activity can be beneficial for weight control, but it also appears to be able to lower blood pressure on its own.

Large-scale research projects that investigated the relationship between salt consumption and blood pressure in communities all over the world have unequivocally demonstrated that there is a positive correlation between blood pressure and the amount of sodium (salt) that humans consume through their diet. There is a very low prevalence of hypertension in primitive societies because sodium consumption is low. Additionally, the rise in blood pressure that is typically associated with advancing age in industrialized societies does not take place in these societies. On the other hand, hypertension is prevalent in nations that consume an excessive amount of salt, and stroke is the leading cause of death in these nations. In addition, there is evidence from experimental studies that reducing sodium consumption can bring about a reduction in blood pressure.

There is a correlation between heavy alcohol consumption (more than two drinks per day) and hypertension. Eaters of meat are more likely to have higher blood pressure than vegetarians, and vegans, in particular, who do not consume any foods derived from animals, including milk and eggs, tend to have lower blood pressure. The diet that is recommended for lowering blood pressure, which will also be beneficial to cardiovascular health, places an emphasis on fruits, vegetables, and dairy products with a low fat content; it also includes whole grains, poultry, fish, and nuts; and it contains only small amounts of red meat and sugary foods and beverages. If you cut back on your salt consumption, you should see an even greater improvement in the effectiveness of the diet.

The treatment of hypertension involves the use of a wide range of medications, some of which have adverse effects on one's diet. Thiazide diuretics, for instance, cause an increase in the amount of potassium that is lost from the body. As a result, it is typically necessary to consume additional potassium, which is particularly abundant in foods like bananas, citrus fruits, vegetables, and potatoes. Under no circumstances is it recommended to use potassium-based salt substitutes without the supervision of a medical professional.

7.3.3. Cancer

Cancer is the leading cause of death among adults aged 45 and older, and it is the second leading cause of death in many parts of the world, behind only cardiovascular disease. In addition to the location in the body and the type of cells that are affected, the various types of cancer differ not only in the progression of the disease, the treatments that are administered, and the factors that are thought to be either the cause or a contributor.

The majority of substances that cause cancer, also known as carcinogens, are likely to enter the body through the alimentary canal due to the presence of food and beverages. In spite of the fact that certain foodborne toxins, pesticides, and food additives have the potential to cause cancer if consumed in sufficient quantities, the foods themselves are the primary reason for the development of cancer. Several dietary patterns or components have the potential to either promote or inhibit the development of cancer.

Substances in the diet or other environmental factors can have an effect at any stage of the multistage process of cancer development (carcinogenesis). These stages include initiation, in which DNA, the genetic material found in a cell, is altered; promotion, in which cells with altered DNA multiply; and progression, in which cancer cells spread to surrounding tissue and distant sites (metastasis).

There has been a lack of consistency in the studies that have attempted to establish a connection between total fat or particular types of fat and a variety of cancers. A high consumption of fat in the diet may increase the risk of developing cancer; however, this may be at least partially attributable to the additional energy (calories) that fat supplies. There is a correlation between obesity and several different types of cancer, including colorectal, prostate, uterine, pancreatic, and breast cancers. Increased levels of estrogen, insulin, and other hormones in the bloodstream are associated with increased body fat, which may be a possible mechanism for this effect. Additionally, several studies have demonstrated that being physically active consistently lowers the risk of developing breast and colon cancers. In laboratory animals, the most effective method for reducing the risk of cancer is to restrict the amount of energy that is consumed; chronic underfeeding inhibits the growth of many spontaneous tumors as well as the majority of tumors that are induced through experimentation.

High alcohol consumption is another factor that has been linked to the development of a variety of cancers, particularly those of the mouth, throat, liver, and esophagus (where it acts synergistically with tobacco), and most likely those of the breast, colon, and rectum as well. The fact that drinking alcohol in moderation has a positive impact on cardiovascular disease is illustrative of how complicated and potentially perplexing the relationship between food and health can be.

Additionally, foods typically contain substances that provide some degree of protection against cancer. Examples of foods that inhibit the production of nitrosamine include fresh fruits and vegetables, as well as vitamins C and E when consumed at the same time as foods that contain nitrates, such as ham, bacon, sausages, frankfurters, and luncheon meats. This helps to protect against stomach cancer. There have been several 100 studies that have found a strong association between diets that are high in vegetables and fruits and a lower risk for a variety of cancers. However, it has been more difficult to identify specific protective factors in diets including vegetables and fruits. The antioxidant systems of the body are responsible for preventing DNA damage caused by reactive molecules known as free radicals. Vitamin C, vitamin E, carotenoids such as beta-carotene (a plant precursor of vitamin A), and the trace mineral selenium interact with these antioxidant systems to accomplish this. In animal studies, it has been demonstrated that certain vegetables, particularly cruciferous vegetables (broccoli, cauliflower, Brussels sprouts, kale, and other members of the cabbage family), contain sulforaphane and other compounds known as isothiocyanates. These compounds induce enzymes that detoxify carcinogens and have been shown to protect against cancer. Because it dilutes potential carcinogens, binds to them, and speeds up transit time through the gut, dietary fiber found in plant foods may also be protective. This is because it reduces the amount of exposure to the carcinogens. There is a significant amount of phytochemicals, which are biologically active plant substances, found in fruits and vegetables. These phytochemicals are currently being researched for their potential anticarcinogenic activity. There is evidence from studies conducted on animals that the antioxidant compounds known as polyphenols, which are present in both black and green tea, may be protective against the development of cancer. There has been a correlation between regular consumption of tea and a reduced risk of various cancers, particularly stomach cancer; however, the evidence has been contradictory. This is especially true in Japan and China, where green tea is the preferred type of tea.

The dietary approach that is most likely to reduce the risk of cancer is abundant in foods derived from plant sources, such as fruits, vegetables (especially cruciferous ones), whole grains, beans, and nuts; has a limited intake of fat, particularly animal fat; includes a balance of energy intake and physical activity to maintain a healthy body weight; and includes alcohol in moderation, if one consumes it at all. Trimming fat and removing burned portions from meat before eating are two additional ways to cut down on the consumption of carcinogenic compounds.

7.3.3.1. Colorectal Cancer

One of the factors that is associated with a slight increase in the risk of colorectal cancer is the consumption of meat, particularly red meat and processed meat. Carcinogenic substances, such as heterocyclic amines and polycyclic aromatic hydrocarbons, are produced during high-temperature grilling and broiling, particularly of fatty muscle meats. However, it is not clear whether this effect is related to a particular component of meat; to the fact that other nutrients, such as fiber, may be in short supply in a diet that is high in meat; or to the fact that diet may be lacking in fiber. In addition, there is a correlation between an increased rate of colorectal cancer and factors such as high alcohol consumption, low calcium intake, and low folic acid intake.

Numerous studies have shown that foods high in fiber also appear to be protective against colorectal cancer. However, the attempts to demonstrate a specific protective effect of dietary fiber, which is distinct from the non-fiber constituents of vegetables and fruits, have been inconclusive. The presence of obesity is a significant risk factor for colorectal cancer in both men and women who have not yet reached menopause. On the other hand, a low to moderate level of physical activity is strongly associated with a reduced risk of colon cancer.

7.3.3.2. Prostate Cancer

The concept that a diet that is low in fat and animal products and high in fruits and vegetables, including those of the cruciferous variety, is protective against prostate cancer is gaining more and more support. The presence of pectin, a type of fiber that can be found in fruits and vegetables and has been demonstrated to possess anticancer properties, may assist in providing some explanation for this protection. There is a correlation between the consumption of tomatoes and tomato products, which are abundant sources of the carotenoid antioxidant lycopene, and a reduced risk of developing prostate cancer. Although there is a low incidence of prostate cancer in countries like Japan, which consumes a lot of soy foods, there is no direct evidence to suggest that soy can protect against the disease. This study is looking into whether or not vitamin E and the mineral selenium have any potential protective effects against prostate cancer.

7.3.3.3. Breast Cancer

There is a lack of clarity regarding the connection between diet and breast cancer. Based on international correlations between fat intake and breast cancer rates, as well as studies conducted on animals, it has been hypothesized that diets that are high in fat may play a role in the development of breast cancer. On the other hand, large prospective studies have not confirmed this connection, although a diet that is high in fat might not be the best choice for other reasons entirely. To a similar extent, a diet that is abundant in fruits and vegetables is unquestionably beneficial to one's health, but it does not offer any known protection against breast cancer. Although there is a correlation between drinking alcohol and breast cancer, the increased risk appears to be only associated with extremely heavy drinking. There is a possibility that engaging in regular exercise throughout one's entire life may offer protection against breast cancer. This could be because exercise assists in maintaining a healthy weight, which is a risk factor for postmenopausal breast cancer. Hereditary factors and estrogen levels over the course of a lifetime are the primary factors that have been known to influence the likelihood of developing breast cancer.

In the industrialized world, there has been a growing interest in the consumption of soy foods and products as a means of protecting against breast cancer in recent years. The situation of Japanese women, who have a low breast cancer rate, is not necessarily comparable to the situation of Western women who supplement with soy isoflavones (compounds that are similar to estrogen) in their midlife. This is because Japanese women have lifelong exposure to high levels of soy foods. Isoflavones appear to compete with estrogen (e.g., in premenopausal women), and as a result, they reduce the effect of estrogen. On the other hand, when they are present in an environment with low estrogen levels (e.g., in postmenopausal women), they have a weak estrogenic effect. The effects of dietary soy once cancer has already begun are unknown (estrogen is a cancer promoter), and there is no evidence that soy in the diet offers protection against breast cancer or any other type of cancer. As of yet, there is no consistent evidence that soy in the diet would offer such protection. Consumption of isolated soy constituents such as isoflavones, which have unknown risks, is not warranted, despite the fact that ongoing research on the benefits of soy is encouraging and that the consumption of soy foods such as tofu is encouraged.

7.3.4. Diabetes Mellitus

Diabetes mellitus (DM) is characterized by inadequate insulin secretion and varying degrees of peripheral insulin resistance, both of which contribute to elevated blood sugar levels. Several early symptoms are associated with hyperglycemia. These symptoms include blurred vision, polydipsia, polyphagia, and polyuria. Nephropathy, peripheral neuropathy, and vascular disease are some of the later complications that can arise. Additionally, there is an increased risk of infection. Measuring plasma glucose is the diagnostic method. Treatment consists of a change in diet, physical activity, and medications that lower glucose levels. These medications include insulin and oral antihyperglycemic drugs. It is possible to delay or prevent complications by maintaining adequate glycemic control; however, heart disease continues to be the leading cause of death in the diabetic population.

Type 1 diabetes and type 2 diabetes are the two primary types of diabetes mellitus, and they can be differentiated from one another based on a combination of characteristics.

1. **Type 1 Diabetes** can occur at any age but often begins in late childhood with the pancreas failing to secrete adequate amounts of insulin. The majority of cases of type 1 diabetes are caused by an autoimmune disorder, which may be triggered by a viral infection, a foreign protein, or an environmental toxin. However, there is a strong genetic link between each of these conditions. However, despite the fact that diabetes is characterized by high blood sugar levels, the presence of sugar or carbohydrates in the diet is not the root cause of the disease. The management of type 1 diabetes involves administering insulin injections, as well as eating a series of small meals and snacks at regular intervals. This helps to distribute glucose consumption throughout the day and reduces fluctuations in blood glucose levels.
2. **Type 2 diabetes** is the more common type of diabetes, constituting 90 to 95% of cases. This condition is characterized by insulin resistance, which prevents cells from taking in glucose, which ultimately leads to glucose accumulation in the blood. Although type 2 diabetes typically begins in middle age, there is a growing trend of reporting cases of the condition in children, particularly among children who are obese. There is a possibility that a person's genetic predisposition to this type of diabetes will not manifest itself unless they have excess body fat, particularly abdominal obesity. In addition to the use of oral antidiabetic agents, weight loss is frequently helpful in normalizing the regulation of blood glucose levels.

In individuals who are at a high risk for developing type 2 diabetes, engaging in lifestyle interventions such as diet and exercise has proven to be highly effective in delaying or preventing the disease.

7.3.5. Eating Disorders

Anorexia nervosa and bulimia nervosa are two examples of eating disorders that are associated with an unhealthy preoccupation with one's body weight. These disorders are serious health issues. Girls and young women are the most susceptible to the pressures that society places on them to be thin. However, boys and men are also susceptible to developing these disorders, which can have far-reaching consequences throughout their lives and even be fatal.

Anorexia nervosa is characterized by a low body weight, a tendency for drastic undereating, an intense fear of gaining weight or becoming fat (despite being underweight), and a distorted body image. These symptoms are all associated with the disorder. In addition to a diminished digestive function, the consequences include a compromised immune system and anemia. A state of semi-starvation that is comparable to marasmus may develop if there is no intervention, necessitating hospitalization and possibly even the use of force feeding to prevent death. In most cases, treatment necessitates a coordinated approach, which includes the participation of a physician, a psychiatrist, a dietitian, and possibly other medical professionals.

There is a prevalent belief that bulimia nervosa is more prevalent than anorexia nervosa, and it is even possible for a single individual to suffer from both disorders. A form of purging, such as self-induced vomiting, fasting, excessive exercise, or the use of laxatives, enemas, or diuretics, followed by recurrent episodes of "binge eating" is a characteristic feature of bulimia nervosa. During treatment, a structured eating plan is typically an integral component.

To conform the weight guidelines and body-image expectations of their sport, young athletes frequently limit the amount of energy they consume. This condition is most prevalent in female athletes, but male athletes, including gymnasts, wrestlers, boxers, and jockeys, are also susceptible to it. When young female athletes engage in strenuous training as well as restrict their food intake, they frequently experience amenorrhea, which is defined as the absence of menstruation for a period of at least three months in a row, as well as bone loss that is comparable to that which occurs during menopause. It is possible that calcium supplementation is necessary.

7.3.6. Tooth Decay

Dental caries, also known as tooth decay, is an oral infectious disease that occurs when bacteria in the dental plaque that are primarily *Streptococcus mutans* metabolize simple sugars and other fermentable carbohydrates into acids that dissolve tooth enamel. Dental plaque, which should not be confused with the lipid-containing plaque that can be found in arteries, is a mass of bacteria and sticky polymers that protects the tooth from saliva and the tongue, which in turn makes decay more likely to occur between the teeth. Honey, molasses, brown sugar, and corn syrup are all examples of dietary sugars that have the potential to cause tooth decay. Additionally, fermentable carbohydrates found in crackers, breads, cereals, and other grain products, as well as milk, fruits, and fruit juices, can cause tooth decay. Between meals, eating foods that are high in sugar or starch, particularly foods that are sticky and remain on the teeth for a longer period of time, increases the amount of time that teeth are exposed to acids that are harmful to them. Some chewing gums contain xylitol, a sugar alcohol that is cariostatic. This means that it reduces the amount of new tooth decay that occurs by inhibiting plaque and suppressing bacteria that cause decay. Artificial sweeteners are not cariogenic. It is possible to cause a condition known as "baby bottle tooth decay" by putting an infant to sleep with a bottle, particularly if the bottle contains juice or other sweetened beverages, milk, or infant formula. Particularly during the period in which enamel is being formed in the jaws before the eruption of permanent teeth, fluoride is an extremely effective and efficient method of protecting tooth enamel from decay. An approach to community health that is both safe and effective is the fluoridation of water in areas where fluoride levels are not naturally high. While water containing fluoride at a concentration of approximately one part per million protects against dental caries, it does not cause the mottling of teeth that can occur when fluoride concentrations are higher. In regions where fluoride is not added to the water supply, it is recommended that children take fluoride supplements. Fluoride can be found in significant amounts in a variety of foods, including seaweed, brewed tea, and marine fish cooked with bones.

Important preventative measures against periodontal disease (also known as gum disease) and dental caries include brushing and flossing the teeth and gums consistently, as well as rinsing the mouth after eating meals and snacks. The health of your gums is also dependent on having a correctly functioning immune system and having a healthy diet overall. Some of the most important nutrients include vitamin C, which helps prevent gingivitis (inflammation of the gums), as well as calcium and vitamin D, which contribute to the development of a robust jawbone and teeth.

7.3.7. Heartburn and Peptic Ulcer

Heartburn is a burning sensation that occurs when the contents of the stomach, which contain hydrochloric acid, flow backward from the stomach. This causes the lining of the esophagus to become inflamed, with the result being a burning sensation. The occurrence of occasional heartburn, which is also referred to as acid indigestion, is quite common and is typically brought on by the consumption of particular foods. Despite this, some individuals suffer from gastroesophageal reflux disease (GERD), which is characterized by persistent heartburn. It is recommended that people who suffer from gastroesophageal reflux disease (GERD) reduce their consumption of alcohol and caffeine, both of which relax the lower esophageal sphincter and actually cause reflux, as well as their consumption of fat, which causes the stomach to empty more slowly. Certain foods, such as chocolate, citrus fruits and juices, tomatoes and tomato products, peppermint and spearmint oils, and certain spices, have the potential to aggravate heartburn; however, it does not appear that these foods are the cause of the condition.

People who are overweight or obese and suffer from gastroesophageal reflux disease (GERD) may find that losing weight mitigates their symptoms. Several factors may help improve the condition, including eating smaller meals, chewing food thoroughly, eating more slowly, avoiding clothes that are too tight, not smoking, and not lying down until approximately three hours after eating. Antacids and acid controllers are medications that should be used only infrequently if they are not under the supervision of a medical professional.

In contrast to what was once believed, a peptic ulcer, which is a sore on the lining of the stomach or duodenum, is not caused by stress or eating spicy foods. Instead, the majority of peptic ulcers are caused by the infectious bacterial agent Helicobacter pylori, and they can be treated with a straightforward course of antibiotics. Stress and dietary factors, such as coffee, and other beverages containing caffeine, and alcohol, can, on the other hand, make an ulcer that is already present worse.

7.3.8. Bowel Conditions and Diseases

Insufficient dietary fiber (roughage) or other dietary factors, such as taking calcium or iron supplements, in addition to daily routines that prevent relaxation, can be the cause of constipation (Smith, 2018). Constipation is a condition that can last for a long time. In addition, straining during defecation can be a contributing factor in the development of diverticulosis, which is characterized by the presence of small outpouchings in the colonic wall (Jones & Brown, 2019). Diverticulitis, which involves inflammation of the colonic wall, can lead to serious complications. Stretching can also result in hemorrhoids, which are swollen veins of the rectum and anus that typically cause pain, itching, and bleeding (Williams et al., 2020). Hemorrhoids are another potential consequence of straining. Consuming foods that are high in fiber, such as cereals and breads made with whole grains, drinking an adequate amount of water, and engaging in regular physical activity are typically some of the most effective ways to treat constipation. Fiber, particularly the insoluble variety, contributes to the formation of a stool that is soft and bulky by transporting water into the large intestine (colon). Not only does the consumption of dried fruits like prunes, which are rich in fiber and contain a natural laxative substance called dihydroxyphenyl isatin, help stimulate the bowels, but it also helps stimulate the digestive system. Even though laxatives and enemas might be helpful, using them frequently can throw off the balance of fluids, minerals, and electrolytes (salt), and they can also interfere with the body's ability to absorb vitamins. If there is a persistent change in bowel habits, it is important to consult a physician.

The condition known as diarrhea, which is characterized by loose, watery stools and possibly an increased frequency of bowel movements, can be a cause for immediate concern, in contrast to constipation. Diarrhea of bacterial origin that is acute is relatively common and frequently resolves on its own. Infections caused by viruses, parasites, food intolerances or allergies, medications, medical or surgical treatments, and even stress are some of the other common causes of acute diarrhea (Miller, 2017). If you are experiencing a temporary bout of diarrhea, it is essential to drink fluids, regardless of the cause of the diarrhea. Diarrhea, on the other hand, can cause potentially dangerous dehydration and electrolyte imbalances if it is severe and continues for an extended period of time. This condition requires immediate medical attention, particularly in individuals who are infants or children. The risks associated with prolonged vomiting are comparable.

Depending on which part of the gastrointestinal tract is affected, inflammatory bowel disease (IBD), which includes conditions such as Crohn's disease (regional ileitis) and ulcerative colitis, can lead to a reduction in the body's ability to absorb a wide variety of nutrients when it is present. Children who have inflammatory bowel disease may not develop normally. As a general rule, treatment consists of a diet that is devoid of lactose (milk sugar), low in fat and fiber, high in protein, and easy-to-digest carbohydrates. It may be recommended to increase the intake of certain nutrients, such as iron, calcium, and magnesium, as well as to supplement with fat-soluble vitamins. Additionally, it may be recommended to consume additional fluid and electrolytes to compensate for the losses that are caused by diarrhea. Irritable bowel syndrome, also known as IBS, is a common gastrointestinal disorder that is characterized by a disruption in the peristalsis of the intestinal tract. Excessive gas, abdominal discomfort, and cramping are some of the symptoms, along with alternating bouts of diarrhea and constipation. Even though it can be very uncomfortable, irritable bowel syndrome does not cause any damage to the intestinal tract. Identification and avoidance of "problem" foods, particularly legumes and other vegetables and dairy products that produce gas, as well as possible reductions in caffeine consumption, are all components of the dietary treatment. A low-fat diet, smaller meals, and a gradual increase in fiber intake are helpful for the majority of people who suffer from irritable bowel syndrome (IBS) (Brown et al., 2021).

7.3.9. Food-Drug Interactions

Medications have the potential to either hinder or improve the utilization of nutrients, which can occasionally result in imbalances (Gibney et al., 2009). In the treatment of high blood pressure, the use of certain diuretics can lead to an increase in the loss of potassium, which is a common example (Williams & Nesse, 1991). Drugs that alter the acidity of the gastrointestinal tract, alter the function of the digestive system, or actually bind to nutrients can also have an effect on the absorption of nutrients (Gibney et al., 2009). Take, for instance, the use of laxatives, antacids, or mineral oil regularly; these substances can reduce the absorption of nutrients, which can eventually result in a deficiency (Whitney & Rolfes, 2019). People of advanced age who take several different medications are especially at risk of having their nutritional status compromised (Whitney & Rolfes, 2019).

On the other hand, foods have the potential to alter the absorption of drugs or interact with drugs in unfavorable ways, which can lead to the ineffectiveness or toxicity of the drug under consideration (Gibney et al., 2009). An example of this would be the fact that levodopa, which is used to treat Parkinson's disease, is rendered less effective when protein and vitamin B6 are present (Whitney & Rolfes, 2019). Individuals who are being treated for depression with monoamine oxidase (MAO) inhibitors may experience hypertension as a result of the presence of tyramine, which is a derivative of amino acids that can be found in certain aged cheeses and red wines (Williams & Nesse, 1991). Unique substances found in grapefruit juice can inhibit the breakdown of certain medications, which in turn can have an impact on how well they are absorbed and how effective they are (Whitney & Rolfes, 2019). In addition to psychiatric medications, these medications include certain statins that lower cholesterol, calcium channel blockers, anticonvulsant agents, estrogen, antihistamines, protease inhibitors, immunosuppressants, antifungal drugs, and antifungal drugs (Gibney et al., 2009). Consuming grapefruit or grapefruit juice within a few hours or even a few days of taking these medications may result in unintended consequences. Grapefruit juice may also have additional adverse effects.

Interactions between medications and herbal products, vitamin and mineral supplements, and other products can also occur (Gibney et al., 2009). One or more of the supplemental antioxidants evaluated, such as vitamin C, vitamin E, beta-carotene, and selenium, have the potential to reduce the efficacy of certain medications (for instance, high-dose niacin, when used in conjunction with statins) in terms of elevating HDL cholesterol levels and enhancing cardiovascular health (Whitney & Rolfes, 2019).

A Closer Look

Overnutrition

Overnutrition is a form of malnutrition arises from the excessive intake of nutrients, particularly calories, leading to a spectrum of health issues. Unlike undernutrition, overnutrition is often a consequence of an imbalance where the body's energy intake surpasses its expenditure, resulting in weight gain and associated health complications. This condition is increasingly prevalent in both developed and developing countries, driven by lifestyle changes, urbanization, and the availability of high-calorie, nutrient-poor foods.

One prominent example of overnutrition is the rising prevalence of obesity. Obesity is a complex disorder characterized by an excessive accumulation of body fat, posing significant risks to health. In the United States, for instance, over 40% of adults are classified as obese. This condition is linked to a higher risk of developing chronic diseases such as type 2 diabetes, cardiovascular diseases, and certain cancers. The availability and consumption of fast food, sugary beverages, and processed snacks contribute significantly to this epidemic. A diet high in saturated fats, sugars, and refined carbohydrates leads to the excessive accumulation of fat in the body, often resulting in obesity.

In addition to obesity, overnutrition can manifest in micronutrient toxicities. For example, excessive vitamin A intake, often due to overuse of supplements, can lead to hypervitaminosis A. Symptoms of this condition include dizziness, nausea, and even more severe health problems like liver damage and central nervous system disorders. Similarly, overconsumption of iron supplements without medical supervision can cause iron overload, leading to conditions such as hemochromatosis, which damages organs and can be fatal if untreated.

Addressing this challenge requires comprehensive strategies, including public health initiatives to promote balanced diets, regulation of food marketing, and education to raise awareness about the risks of excessive nutrient intake. By tackling overnutrition, societies can mitigate the associated health burdens and promote overall well-being.

Summary

- Community health initiatives and the prevalence of nutrition-related disorders are the subject of this chapter, which focuses on the critical relationship between the two.
- It describes how inadequate nutrition, whether occurring as a result of excesses or deficiencies, can result in a wide variety of health problems that have an effect on community health in many different ways. This chapter examines several different nutrition disorders, such as malnutrition, obesity, deficiencies in vitamins and minerals, and eating disorders. It also investigates the causes of these disorders, the effects they have, and the demographic groups that are most at risk for them.
- The chapter emphasizes the significance of effective community health policies and programs in the prevention of these disorders. It highlights various strategies, including nutritional education, food fortification, and access to healthy foods, as examples of these strategies.
- To address the underlying causes of nutritional disorders and to improve the overall outcomes of public health, it is necessary to take a multidisciplinary approach that includes the participation of government agencies, healthcare providers, and communities respectively.

References

1. Agostoni, C., Baselli, L., & Mazzoni, M. B. (2013). Early nutrition patterns and diseases of adulthood: A plausible link? *European Journal of Internal Medicine, 24*(1), 5–10. https://doi.org/10.1016/j.ejim.2012.10.005.
2. Alzaheb, R., & Alzaheb, A. R. (2016). Factors associated with the early introduction of complementary feeding in Saudi Arabia. *International Journal of Environmental Research and Public Health, 13*(7), 702. https://doi.org/10.3390/ijerph13070702.
3. Austrian Ministry of Labour, Social Affairs, Health and Consumer Protection. (2014). *Austrian Foodbased Dietary Guidelines for 1- to 3-Year-Old Toddlers*. Viena, Austria: Austrian Ministry of Labour, Social Affairs, Health and Consumer Protection.
4. Baldassarre, M., Di Mauro, A., Pedico, A., Rizzo, V., Capozza, M., Meneghin, F., Lista, G., & Laforgia, N. (2018). Weaning time in preterm infants: An audit of Italian primary care paediatricians. *Nutrients, 10*(5), 616. https://doi.org/10.3390/nu10050616.
5. Barrera, C. M., Hamner, H. C., Perrine, C. G., & Scanlon, K. S. (2018). Timing of introduction of complementary foods to US infants, national health and nutrition examination survey 2009–2014. *Journal of the Academy of Nutrition and Dietetics, 118*(3), 464–470. https://doi.org/10.1016/j.jand.2016.10.013.
6. Bell, S., Yew, S., Devenish, G., Ha, D., Do, L., & Scott, J. (2018). Duration of breastfeeding, but not timing of solid food, reduces the risk of overweight and obesity in children aged 24 to 36 months: Findings from an Australian cohort study. *International Journal of Environmental Research and Public Health, 15*(4), 599. https://doi.org/10.3390/ijerph15040599.

7. Braid, S., Harvey, E. M., Bernstein, J., & Matoba, N. (2015). Early introduction of complementary foods in preterm infants. *Journal of Pediatric Gastroenterology and Nutrition, 60*(6), 811–818. https://doi.org/10.1097/MPG.0000000000000743.

8. Brekke, H. K., Ludvigsson, J. F., van Odijk, J., & Ludvigsson, J. (2005). Breastfeeding and introduction of solid foods in Swedish infants: The All Babies in Southeast Sweden study. *British Journal of Nutrition, 94*(3), 377–382. https://doi.org/10.1079/BJN20051494.

9. Burgess, J. A., Dharmage, S. C., Allen, K., Koplin, J., Garcia-Larsen, V., Boyle, R., Waidyatillake, N., & Lodge, C. J. (2019). Age at introduction to complementary solid food and food allergy and sensitization: A systematic review and meta-analysis. *Clinical and Experimental Allergy, 49*(6), 754–769. https://doi.org/10.1111/cea.13383.

10. Burke, R. M., Leon, J. S., & Suchdev, P. S. (2014). Identification, prevention and treatment of iron deficiency during the first 1000 days. *Nutrients, 6*(10), 4093–4114. https://doi.org/10.3390/nu6104093.

11. Butte, N. F., Lopez-Alarcon, M. G., & Garza, C. (2001). *Nutrient Adequacy of Exclusive Breastfeeding for the Term Infant During the First 6 Months of Life*. Geneva, Switzerland: World Health Organization. Retrieved from: https://apps.who.int/iris/handle/10665/42519 (accessed on 11 July 2024).

12. Carletti, C., Pani, P., Monasta, L., Knowles, A., & Cattaneo, A. (2017). Introduction of complementary foods in a cohort of infants in northeast Italy: Do parents comply with WHO recommendations? *Nutrients, 9*(1), 34. https://doi.org/10.3390/nu9010034.

13. Clayton, H. B., Li, R., Perrine, C. G., & Scanlon, K. S. (2013). Prevalence and reasons for introducing infants early to solid foods: Variations by milk feeding type. *Pediatrics, 131*(4), e1108–e1114. https://doi.org/10.1542/peds.2012-2265.

14. Domellöf, M., Braegger, C., Campoy, C., Colomb, V., Decsi, T., Fewtrell, M., Hojsak, I., Mihatsch, W., Molgaard, C., Shamir, R., et al. (2014). Iron requirements of infants and toddlers. *Journal of Pediatric Gastroenterology and Nutrition, 58*(1), 119–129. https://doi.org/10.1097/MPG.0000000000000206.

15. European Food Safety Authority (EFSA). EFSA Panel on Dietetic Products, N., & A. (NDA). (2009). Scientific opinion on the appropriate age for introduction of complementary feeding of infants. *EFSA Journal, 7*(3), 1423. https://doi.org/10.2903/j.efsa.2009.1423.

16. Fewtrell, M. S., Lucas, A., & Morgan, J. B. (2003). Factors associated with weaning in full term and preterm infants. *Archives of Disease in Childhood–Fetal and Neonatal Edition, 88*(4), F296–F301. https://doi.org/10.1136/fn.88.4.F296.

17. Fewtrell, M., Bronsky, J., Campoy, C., Domellöf, M., Embleton, N., Fidler Mis, N., Hojsak, I., Hulst, J. M., Indrio, F., Lapillonne, A., et al. (2017). Complementary feeding: A position paper by the European Society for Paediatric Gastroenterology, Hepatology, and Nutrition (ESPGHAN) Committee on Nutrition. *Journal of Pediatric Gastroenterology and Nutrition, 64*(1), 119–132. https://doi.org/10.1097/MPG.0000000000001454.

18. Giannì, M., Bezze, E., Colombo, L., Rossetti, C., Pesenti, N., Roggero, P., Sannino, P., Muscolo, S., Plevani, L., & Mosca, F. (2018). Complementary feeding practices in a cohort of Italian late preterm infants. *Nutrients, 10*(12), 1861. https://doi.org/10.3390/nu10121861.

19. Griffiths, L. J., Tate, A. R., Dezateux, C., Bartington, S., Bedford, H., Cole, T., Hawkins, S. S., Law, C., Peckham, C., Samad, L., et al. (2007). Do early infant feeding practices vary by

maternal ethnic group? *Public Health Nutrition, 10*(9), 957–964. https://doi.org/10.1017/S1368980007247828.

20. Gupta, S., Agarwal, R., Aggarwal, K. C., Chellani, H., Duggal, A., Arya, S., Bhatia, S., Sankar, M. J., Sreenivas, V., Jain, V., et al. (2017). Complementary feeding at 4 versus 6 months of age for preterm infants born at less than 34 weeks of gestation: A randomized, open-label, multicenter trial. *Lancet Global Health, 5*(5), e501–e511. https://doi.org/10.1016/S2214-109X(17)30074-X.
21. Helle, C., Hillesund, E. R., & Overby, N. C. (2018). Timing of complementary feeding and associations with maternal and infant characteristics: A Norwegian cross-sectional study. *PLOS ONE, 13*(6), e0199455. https://doi.org/10.1371/journal.pone.0199455.
22. Kronborg, H., Foverskov, E., & Væth, M. (2015). Breastfeeding and introduction of complementary food in Danish infants. *Scandinavian Journal of Public Health, 43*(2), 138–145. https://doi.org/10.1177/1403494814560844.
23. Newby, R. M., & Davies, P. S. W. (2016). Why do women stop breast-feeding: Results from a contemporary perspective study in a cohort of Australian women. *European Journal of Clinical Nutrition, 70*(12), 1428–1432. https://doi.org/10.1038/ejcn.2016.126.
24. Papoutsou, S., Savva, S. C., Hunsberger, M., Jilani, H., Michels, N., Ahrens, W., Tornaritis, M., Veidebaum, T., Molnár, D., Siani, A., et al. (2018). Timing of solid food introduction and association with later childhood overweight and obesity: The IDEFICS study. *Maternal & Child Nutrition, 14*(1), e12471. https://doi.org/10.1111/mcn.12471.
25. Rebhan, B., Kohlhuber, M., Schwegler, U., Koletzko, B. V., & Fromme, H. (2009). Infant feeding practices and associated factors through the first 9 months of life in Bavaria, Germany. *Journal of Pediatric Gastroenterology and Nutrition, 49*(4), 467–473. https://doi.org/10.1097/MPG.0b013e31818d3602.
26. Schiess, S., Grote, V., Scaglioni, S., Luque, V., Martin, F., Stolarczyk, A., Vecchi, F., Koletzko, B., & European Childhood Obesity Project. (2010). Introduction of complementary feeding in 5 European countries. *Journal of Pediatric Gastroenterology and Nutrition, 50*(1), 92–98. https://doi.org/10.1097/MPG.0b013e3181b0f82a.
27. Scott, J. A., Binns, C. W., Graham, K. I., & Oddy, W. H. (2009). Predictors of the early introduction of solid foods in infants: Results of a cohort study. *BMC Pediatrics, 9*, 60. https://doi.org/10.1186/1471-2431-9-60.
28. Statistics Poland. (2018). *Information Society in Poland. Results of Statistical Surveys in the Years 2014–2018*. Warsaw, Poland: Statistics Poland.
29. Szajewska, H., Horvath, A., Rybak, A., & Socha, P. (2016). Karmienie piersią. Stanowisko Polskiego towarzystwa gastroenterologii, hepatologii i żywienia dzieci. *Standardy Medyczne Pediatria, 13*, 9–24.
30. Szajewska, H., Socha, P., Horvath, A., Rybak, A., Dobrzańska, A., Borszewska-Kornacka, M. K., Chybicka, A., Czerwionka-Szaflarska, M., Gajewska, D., Helwich, E., et al. (2014). Zasady żywienia zdrowych niemowląt. Zalecenia Polskiego towarzystwa gastroenterologii, hepatologii i żywienia dzieci. *Standardy Medyczne Pediatria, 11*, 321–338.
31. Tromp, I. I. M., Briedé, S., Kiefte-de Jong, J. C., Renders, C. M., Jaddoe, V. W. V., Franco, O. H., Hofman, A., Raat, H., & Moll, H. A. (2013). Factors associated with the timing of introduction

of complementary feeding: The Generation R study. *European Journal of Clinical Nutrition, 67*(6), 625–630. https://doi.org/10.1038/ejcn.2013.60.

32. Victora, C. G., Bahl, R., Barros, A. J. D., França, G. V. A., Horton, S., Krasevec, J., Murch, S., Sankar, M. J., Walker, N., & Rollins, N. C. (2016). Breastfeeding in the 21st century: Epidemiology, mechanisms, and lifelong effect. *The Lancet, 387*(10017), 475–490. https://doi.org/10.1016/S0140-6736(15)01024-7.
33. Villar, J., Ismail, L. C., Victora, C. G., Ohuma, E. O., Bertino, E., Altman, D. G., Lambert, A., Papageorghiou, A. T., Carvalho, M., Jaffer, Y. A., et al. (2014). International standards for newborn weight, length, and head circumference by gestational age and sex: The newborn cross-sectional study of the INTERGROWTH-21st Project. *The Lancet, 384*(9946), 857–868. https://doi.org/10.1016/S0140-6736(14)60932-6.
34. Wang, J., Wu, Y., Xiong, G., Chao, T., Jin, Q., Liu, R., Hao, L., Wei, S., Yang, N., & Yang, X. (2016). Introduction of complementary feeding before 4 months of age increases the risk of childhood overweight or obesity: A meta-analysis of prospective cohort studies. *Nutrition Research, 36*(8), 759–770. https://doi.org/10.1016/j.nutres.2016.03.003.
35. Wang, L., van Grieken, A., van der Velde, L. A., Vlasblom, E., Beltman, M., L'Hoir, M. P., Boere-Boonekamp, M. M., & Raat, H. (2019). Factors associated with early introduction of complementary feeding and consumption of non-recommended foods among Dutch infants: The BeeBOFT study. *BMC Public Health, 19*(1), 388. https://doi.org/10.1186/s12889-019-6704-5.
36. Were, F. N., & Lifschitz, C. (2018). Complementary feeding: Beyond nutrition. *Annals of Nutrition and Metabolism, 73*(1), 20–25. https://doi.org/10.1159/000490298.
37. White, J. M., Bégin, F., Kumapley, R., Murray, C., & Krasevec, J. (2017). Complementary feeding practices: Current global and regional estimates. *Maternal & Child Nutrition, 13*(S2), e12505. https://doi.org/10.1111/mcn.12505.
38. World Health Organization (WHO). (2019). *Commercial Foods for Infants and Young Children in the WHO European Region. A Study of the Availability, Composition and Marketing of Baby Foods in Four European Countries*. Geneva, Switzerland: WHO.
39. World Health Organization. (2006). *WHO Child Growth Standards: Length/Height-For-Age, Weight-For-Age, Weight-For-Length, Weight-For-Height and Body Mass Index-For-Age: Methods and Development*. Geneva, Switzerland: WHO.
40. World Health Organization. (2019). *Ending Inappropriate Promotion of Commercially Available Complementary Foods for Infants and Young Children Between 6 and 36 Months in Europe; A Discussion Paper Outlining the First Steps in Developing a Nutrient Profile Model to Drive Changes to Product Composition and Labelling and Promotion Practices in the WHO European Region*. Geneva, Switzerland: WHO.

Chapter 8

COMMUNITY HEALTH POLICIES AND PROGRAMS

Contents

Introduction

Malnutrition, in its different manifestations, is a significant contributing factor to almost 50% of all worldwide deaths. It has a direct and indirect impact on a range of perinatal, infectious, and chronic illnesses. The widespread influence of malnutrition highlights the immediate requirement for focused nutrition interventions incorporated into national development agendas and poverty eradication strategies. When interventions are carried out accurately and following recommended practices, they can greatly reduce the occurrence of malnutrition. This is demonstrated by the impressive accomplishments of countries such as Brazil and China, which have successfully decreased child malnutrition rates by more than 50% in under 20 years. Nevertheless, the issue of malnutrition has worsened in recent years due to worldwide food and fuel crises, coupled with economic downturns, resulting in an unparalleled rise in the number of individuals experiencing hunger in 2009. This concerning pattern emphasizes the need for a thorough analysis of the obstacles to advancement, such as the increasing inequalities within and between countries, and to learn from those nations that have made substantial progress in addressing malnutrition.

The development and execution of policies and programs demonstrate a concrete expression of a nation's determination to address malnutrition and advance community health and nutrition. However, the mere presence of these policies does not ensure the achievement of their objectives. Difficulties frequently arise due to the vagueness and imprecision of policy objectives, making it more complicated to convert them into practical plans. Moreover, even clearly established policies may struggle in the absence of sufficient resources or the ability to enforce them efficiently. The purpose of this chapter is to provide readers with fundamental knowledge about the complexities of community health and nutrition policies and programs. This document provides insight into the present patterns and difficulties in the field of community health and nutrition, highlighting the crucial importance of consistent and well-backed policies in combating malnutrition and promoting a healthier global population. The chapter aims to enhance the ongoing discussion on enhancing nutritional outcomes and community health globally by comprehensively grasping these dynamics.

Orientation and Directional Terms

Term	Definition	
Health Policy	A set of decisions and actions undertaken by governments or organizations aimed at improving health outcomes, ensuring equitable access to health services, and addressing health issues within a community or population.	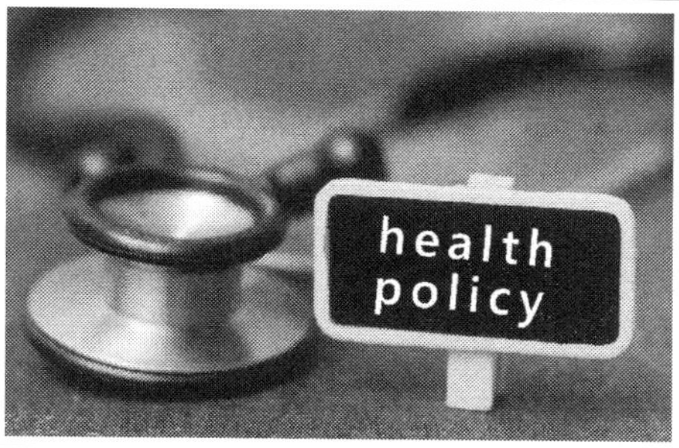
ICDS Scheme	The Integrated Child Development Services (ICDS) scheme is an Indian program designed to improve the nutritional and health status of children under six years, pregnant women, and lactating mothers through a network of Anganwadi centers.	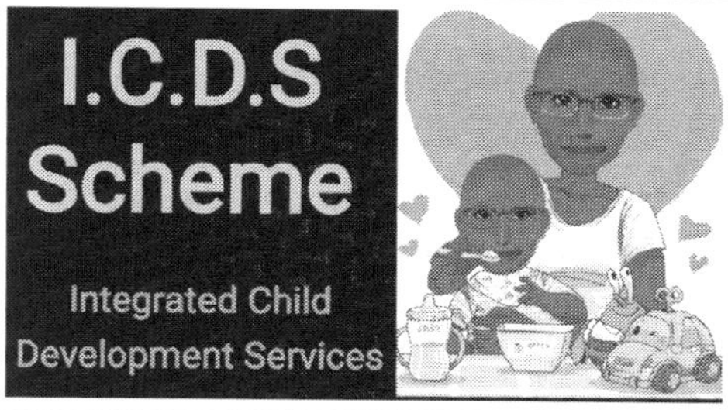
Mid-Day Meals	A government program providing free meals to school children during midday in order to improve their nutritional intake, support educational participation, and enhance learning outcomes.	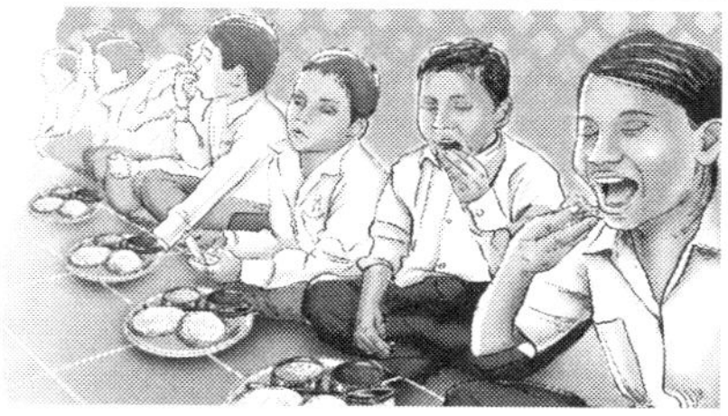
Adolescence	Adolescence is the phase of life between childhood and adulthood, from ages 10 to 19. It is a unique stage of human development and an important time for laying the foundations of good health.	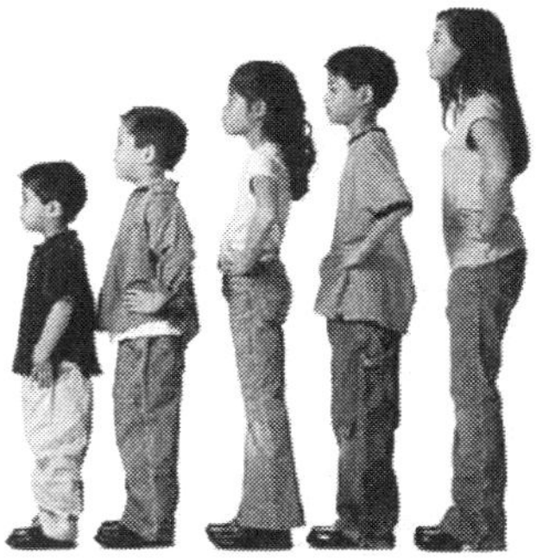

8.1. What Is Community Health Policy?

When it comes to the overall health and safety of a population, community health policy is an absolute necessity. Community health policy establishes clear goals and solutions toward total health by taking into account the needs of a community and determining how to best meet those needs.

The laws, regulations, actions, and decisions that are implemented within society to promote wellness and ensure that particular health goals are met are what are referred to as a community health policy.

Policies pertaining to community health can take many forms, ranging from formal legislation to community outreach initiatives. Community health policy plays a role in multiple sectors, including: health care, insurance, education, agriculture, business, etc.

An unambiguous definition of community health policy can be challenging to pin down due to the fact that it encompasses multiple disciplines. On the other hand, a singular mission toward health is at the center of every single effort to improve community health.

The World Health Organization, the Centers for Disease Control and Prevention, the Food and Drug Administration, and a variety of other governmental and non-governmental organizations all play a significant part in the formulation of community health policy. These organizations conduct research and put into action educational and health initiatives for a population. They also create laws and policies that ensure the society has access to health care, clean water to drink, nutritious food to eat, and vaccines for those who are sick (Figure 8.1).

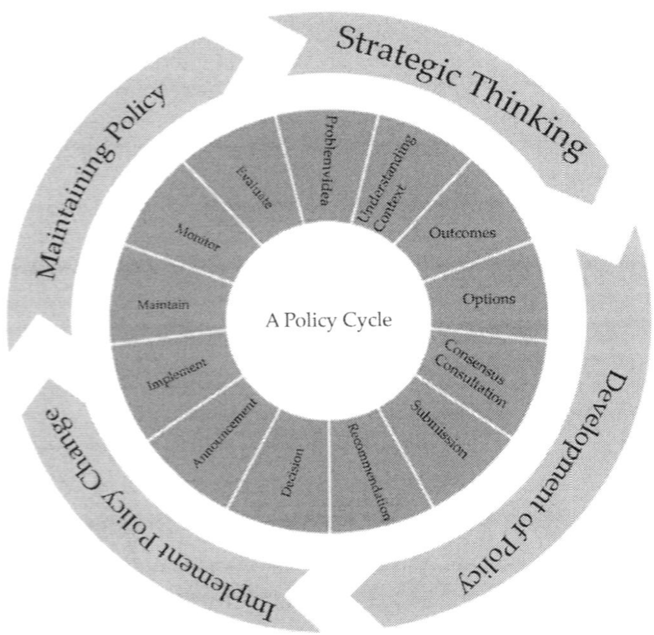
Strategic Thinking
Development of Policy
Implement Policy Change
Maintaining Policy
A Policy Cycle
Problem/idea
Understanding Context
Outcomes
Options
Consensus Consultation
Submission
Recommendation
Decision
Announcement
Implement
Maintain
Monitor
Evaluate

Figure 8.1. *An illustration of public health policy.*

Source: By Anthony F. Camilleri – Own work, CC BY-SA 4.0, https://commons.wikimedia.org/w/index.php?curid=78147458.

8.1.1. The Importance of Community Health Policy

Since it brings the theory and research of community health into the real world, community health policy is an extremely important aspect of community health. Policymakers in the field of community health take action based on research and search for widespread solutions to problems that have been identified in the past.

As an official in charge of community health policy, it is your duty to initiate strategies and policies concerning health intervention as well as health prevention. It is necessary to address not only the physical health of your target population, but also their mental health, social well-being, and economic well-being to maximize their potential for success.

8.1.1.1. Exemplifications of Community Health Policies

Policymakers and officials will conduct extensive research before the implementation of community health policies. The purpose of this research is to identify the community health issues that require attention and to devise the most effective solutions for addressing those issues. The following is a list of some of the most fundamental community health policies that have become an integral part of modern society:

1. **Food Safety Policy:** Policies that ensure food safety are of utmost significance to the overall health of individuals as well as the health of society as a whole. Food-related illnesses are a major cause for concern, and it is the responsibility of community health officials to devise policies that will guarantee that the public will only have access to food that is entirely risk-free for consumption.
2. **Tobacco Use:** To lessen the likelihood of deaths and illnesses brought on by tobacco use and smoking, several community health officials have implemented several preventative measures. To shield non-smokers from the adverse effects of secondhand smoke, some of these policies include raising the price of tobacco and establishing tobacco-free zones within communities.
3. **HIV:** When it comes to educating the general public about HIV prevention, how to live with the virus, treatment options, and preventing stigma, community health policy plays a significant role. There has been a significant reduction in the impact and spread of the virus in several communities because of the implementation of community health policies. These policies include increased access to testing, birth control, and medicine.
4. **Alcohol:** Abuse of alcohol is one of the leading causes of a variety of negative outcomes, including but not limited to health complications, sexual assault, and vehicular accidents. In the fight to reduce the negative effects of alcohol on users and to reduce the prevalence of alcohol dependence, community health policies are of the utmost importance. Policy regarding alcohol varies from community to community, but the most common example is the imposition of age restrictions on the consumption and purchase of alcoholic beverages within the community (Pappas, 2011; Rahman et al., 2011).

8.2. Food and Nutrition Plans and Policies

Food and nutrition policy encompasses the collective efforts of the government and other stakeholders to influence the decision-making environment of food producers, food consumers, and food marketing agents to improve the nutritional status of the population. This is done specifically with the goal of enhancing the nutritional status of the population (Figure 8.2).

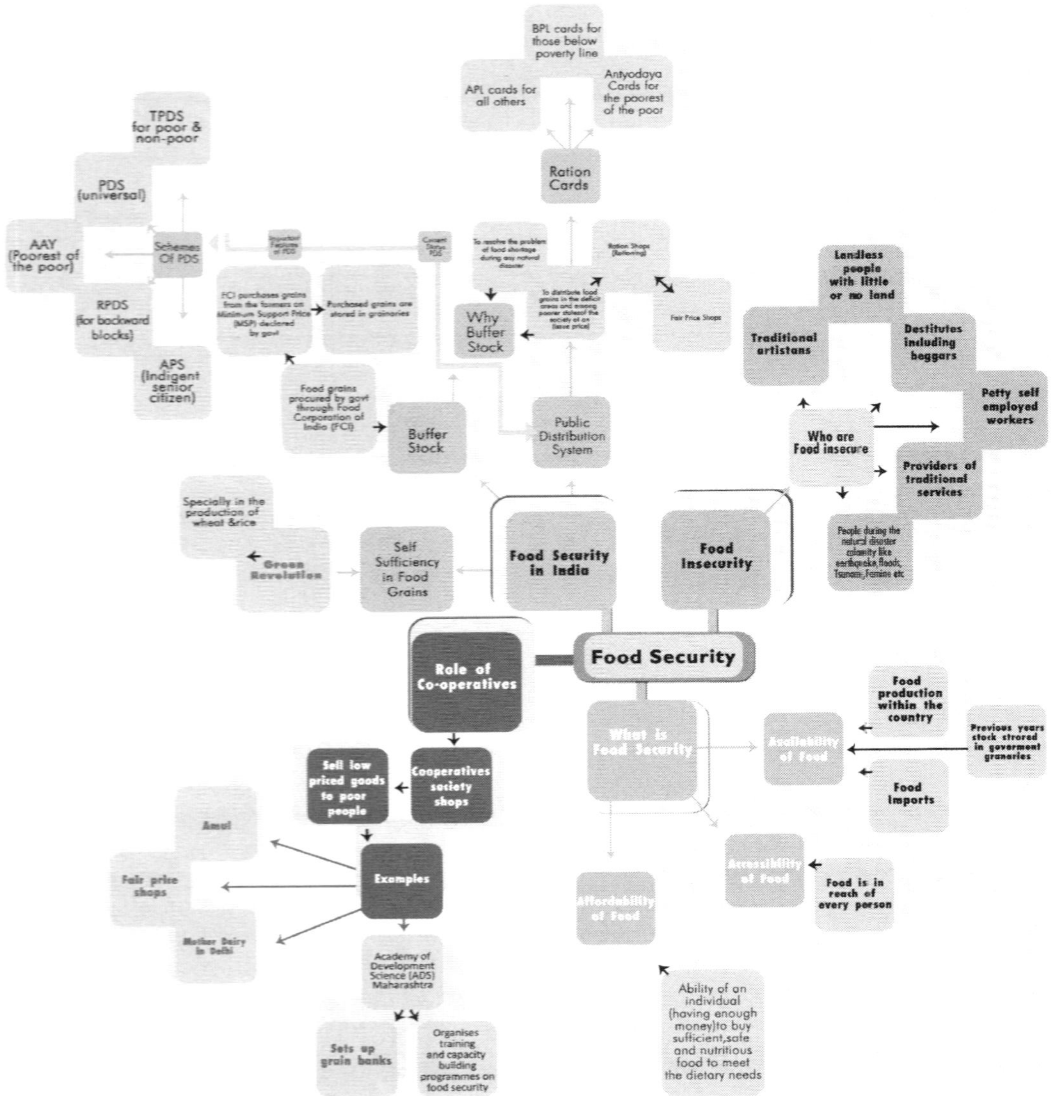

Figure 8.2. *Food and nutrition policy.*

Source: By ciet.ncert – http://nroer.in/static/img/ciet.ncert/2_copy_copy.JPG, CC BY-SA 3.0, https://commons.wikimedia.org/w/index.php?curid=27713253.

Key elements for developing the food and nutrition policy:

- Sustainable food production, processing, distribution and consumption;
- Ensure optimal food quality and safety;
- Collective/multi-sectorial efforts for sustainable food and nutrition security; and
- Achieve and maintain nutrition well-being and healthy lifestyle of the population.

Key stakeholders for developing food and nutrition policy:

- Government;
- UN agencies;
- International organizations;
- Nongovernmental organizations (national and international);
- Industry;
- Professional bodies;
- Academia/researchers;
- Consumers; and
- Mass Media.

Steps involved in developing the food and nutrition policy:

- Understanding the need for a policy;
- Review the current food and nutrition status of the population;
- Review the existing the policies (if any) and identify the lacunae;
- Develop appropriate food and nutrition policy using:
- Direct policy instruments; and
- Indirect policy instruments;
- Develop plans of action for implementation;
- Evolve an effective and strong monitoring and evaluation mechanism; and
- Establish a nutrition surveillance system to facilitate program appraisal and follow-up action.

Each country representative made a presentation of his/her country's nutrition policies/ national plans of action highlighting the following aspects:

- Status of the plan (adopted, not adopted, revised/not revised);
- Whether there is any specific timeframe;
- Coordination between various sectors (as an advantage as well as a barrier) and how it is envisaged in the plan or policy; and
- Linking goals, commitments, strategies and policies.

8.2.1. ICDS Scheme

Under the Integrated Child Development Services (ICDS) scheme, the government is working to ensure that children under the age of six receive comprehensive development in all aspects of their lives, including education, nutrition, and health. In addition to providing pre-school education, its primary objective is to lower the rates of infant mortality and child malnutrition. To ensure that mothers and children, particularly those who come from socially excluded groups, have access to these services in a manner that is not discriminatory, PACS has continued its efforts (Figure 8.3).

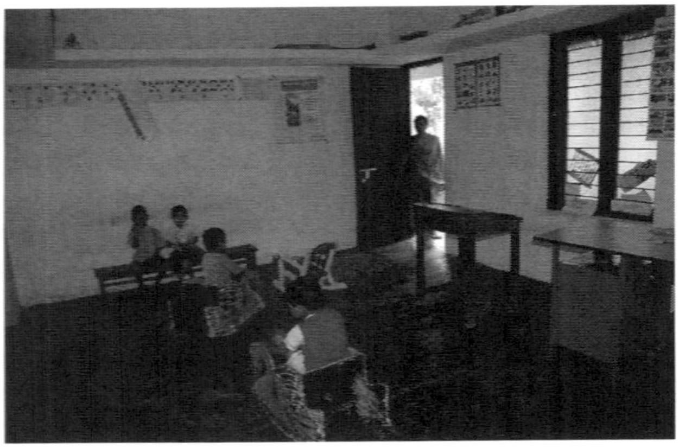

Figure 8.3. *An Anganwadi in India.*

Source: By Jaisuvyas – Own work, CC BY-SA 4.0, https://commons.wikimedia.org/w/index.php?curid=94007923.

8.2.1.1. What Is the Integrated Child Development Services Scheme?

The International Child Development Services (ICDS) program is currently one of the most extensive and distinctive early childhood development programs in the world. The purpose of this program is to reduce the number of deaths, cases of malnutrition, and cases of students dropping out of school by providing pre-school education, healthcare, and nutritional support to children under the age of six, as well as to mothers who are pregnant or breastfeeding themselves. Children under the age of six and mothers who are either pregnant or breastfeeding are eligible to receive the following four primary services through the ICDS program:

- **Supplementary Nutrition:** For mothers and children who are exhibiting symptoms of malnutrition, there are vitamin A tablets, food grains and rice, and food packages that have been fortified with additional nutrients available. All children younger than six years old should have their weight recorded on growth cards that are proportional to their age. Children younger than three years old should be weighed once a month, and children between the ages of three and six should be weighed every three months.
- **Immunizations:** Vaccinations against poliomyelitis, diphtheria, pertussis, tetanus, tuberculosis, and measles should be administered to children in their entirety. These diseases are preventable for the most part. To reduce the risk of maternal and neonatal mortality, pregnant women should receive a vaccination against tetanus.
- **Health Check-Ups:** It is important to provide children with a variety of health services, such as the treatment of diarrhea, the distribution of simple medicines, and the deworming of intestinal parasites (in addition to monitoring their weight and height and administering immunizations). The provision of prenatal and postnatal checkups is something that should be made available to pregnant women and new mothers.
- **Referral Services:** Children and mothers who, following a health checkup, are found to be in need of medical attention should be referred to either the Primary Health Centre or a sub-center by the attending physician. It is recommended that children who are severely malnourished be referred to Nutrition Rehabilitation Centers (NRCs), and that young children who have disabilities be referred to specialists.

Additionally, under the ICDS, children between the ages of three and six should be able to participate in pre-school non-formal education. It should also be possible for women and adolescent girls (between the ages of 15 and 45) to have access to nutrition and health education. This would enable them to receive guidance and assistance in meeting their own health, nutrition, and development requirements, as well as those of their children and families.

PACS has been working on the issue of ICDS to:

- Increase community awareness
- Increase the representation of socially excluded groups (especially women) in health committees
- Support local health committees

PACS's work on the Integrated Child Development Services (ICDS) has been primarily focused on ensuring that children under the age of two are receiving supplementary nutrition through the Supplementary Nutrition Program (SNP), that ICDS centers are located in places that are convenient for socially excluded groups to access, and that ICDS scheme services are provided without discrimination. This is even though the overarching goal of the program has been to increase the access of women and children to their rights under this scheme.

As the importance of proper nutrition to one's health became more widely recognized in the latter half of the 19th century, the first hospitals became places of employment for dietitians and nutritionists. The United States Community Health Service began incorporating dietitians into the staff of PHS Hospitals in 1919, following World War I, to assist in the monitoring and improvement of the health of World War I veterans. Subsequently, dietitians became increasingly involved in the healthcare system of the nation and beyond, even entering the private sector.

8.2.2. Mid-Day Meals

The midday meal scheme is one of the primary schemes that aims to improve the nutritional status of students while simultaneously increasing enrollment, retention, and attendance rates. When children are required to sit in class with an empty stomach, they are unable to concentrate on learning, which is the philosophy that led to the establishment of the MDM Scheme. In addition to meeting the nutritional requirements of children from economically disadvantaged sections, the establishment of a midday meal program has proven to be an efficient method for reducing the high dropout rates of these children.

They are the citizens of the future, and they are the children of today. The National Program of National Support to Primary Education (NPNSPE), which is more commonly referred to as the "Mid-Day Meal Scheme" (MDMS) for the children, is an element that contributes to the overall design of the school to make it appealing to the children and encourage them to consider it their second home. In the beginning, the provision of Midday Meal was considered to be a form of charitable giving; however, as time went on, it evolved into a component of child welfare. Nevertheless, it was not until much later that it was recognized as a component of the child development program. Subsequently, the nutritional improvement approach started to receive more attention from plans. The Nutrition Support to Primary Education program, also known as the midday meal program (MDM), is being considered as a potential method for enhancing enrollment, school attendance, and student retention. Through the provision of a hot, freshly cooked meal, the MDM program aims to fulfill approximately one-third of the daily nutrient requirement for each and every school-aged child. Some people believe that when it comes to children who come from low-income families, the school meal may end up being more of a replacement for the meal that they eat at home than it is a necessary supplement. In addition to the long-term effects that the school meal has on the nutritional status of the students, it is also important to note that the short-term effects of the school meal on improved attention, memory, and learning are significantly more significant. The school meal has been shown to have positive short-term effects on students' ability to learn, according to several reports that have been published and are based on studies that have been carried out effectively. There is a lack of concentration in the saying, "A hungry child is a poor learner." An important tool for preventing hunger in the classroom and fostering improved learning is the provision of a meal in the middle of the day. Because some families do not make eating a nutritious breakfast in the early morning a regular part of their routine, many children arrive at school with an empty stomach. Taking into consideration these conditions, it is essential to recognize the short-term effects that MDM has on the learning process. As a result, MDM has the potential to not only increase the number of students enrolling in schools but also improve the quality of education. A result children from different communities and castes eating together also plays a significant role in fostering better social integration. MDM has the potential to serve the important purpose of increasing school enrollment and attendance, particularly among girls, which would contribute to the advancement of gender empowerment. Both parents and teachers will find it simpler to convince their children to attend school with the help of MDM. This will also make it simpler for teachers to keep their students in the classroom. Additionally, MDM has the potential to contribute to gender equality by lowering the gender gap in education and increasing the number of female students who attend school. Particularly important is the fact that MDM has the potential to initiate comprehensive development of the entire educational system, which would result in improved infrastructures in schools, teaching facilities, School Health Service, and community involvement.

8.2.2.1. Importance of the Mid-Day Meal Program

One of the most common ways that people express their affection is through feeding. When it comes to fostering friendship and affection, not even the most eloquent religious sermon can compare to the power of giving and sharing food. The provision of a cooked midday meal in secondary schools makes the atmosphere of the school less hostile for the child. There is a high incidence of verbal humiliation and physical brutality in the school environment, and children rarely receive expressions of appreciation or encouragement from their teachers. The school environment is frequently suffocating and unfriendly. In a situation like this, the Midday Meal has the potential to play a significant part in boosting the morale of the students who are attending school. In addition to enhancing the health status of children, the parent, the local community, and the local self-governing body, both official and voluntary, have taken the initiative to organize the Mid-Day Meal Program (MDMP). The purpose of this program is to improve children's participation in school education, to increase their overall enrollment, retention, attendance, and achievement statistics. Not only does the Midday Meal provide children with nutritional education, but it also helps to reduce the gender gap in education, protect children from hunger in the classroom, and foster a sense of social equality throughout the community. As a result of widespread poverty, illiteracy, and a lack of awakening, as well as the demand for formal school education, the midday meal for school children has been assuming a certain level of symbolic significance.

8.2.2.2. Mid-Day Meal Motivates Schoolchildren

The children's midday meal program (MDMP) was initially considered to be an "act of charity" by those who participated in it. After a certain amount of time had passed, it was eventually regarded as an "item of child welfare." After some time had passed, it was considered "a component of child development," which led to the introduction of the nutritional approach. It was not until much later that it was considered to be a component of "a movement to make the school attractive" for the child and "to enhance the environment for learning in the school." The parents, the local community, the local self-governing body in the form of municipality or corporation, the state and union government, and international organizations (official and voluntary) have come forward to initiate or support Mid-Day Meal Programs for not only improving children's health but also increasing their school participation in terms of enrollment, regularity in attendance and performance leading to certain levels of achievement of objectives of school education. To achieve the goal of universalizing elementary education (UEE) and primary education (UPE) as a matter of priority, the directive principles of state policy of the constitution, the reports of the education commission and committee, and the policy, plan, and program documents have recommended several incentive programs. These programs include MDM, free textbooks and stationery, free uniforms, and attendance scholarships, among others. During the planning phase, we are required to analyze this incentive program in terms of its cost-effectiveness and cost-benefit for the population that will be receiving services. It is the responsibility of educational researchers and planners to propose methods that will maximize the returns on public investment in basic education. If the returns on particular programs are not satisfactory, they should propose alternative strategies to achieve the national aspirations and goals in this regard.

8.2.2.3. Objective of the Program

The main objectives of the program are:

i. To increase enrollment, and retention and to tone up the learning abilities of the beneficiaries, especially of children belonging to poor and downtrodden sections of the society;

ii. To provide nutritious meals to the school-going children to achieve the goal of a healthy mind in a healthy body;

iii. To promote friendship and feelings of common brotherhood among the children belonging to different castes, colors and creeds by providing meals to them together and also to increase their retention in schools. Also, the mid-day meal scheme is viewed as an opportunity to inculcate hygiene and sanitation practices among children.

iv. Encouraging poor children, belonging to disadvantaged sections, to attend school more regularly and help them concentrate on classroom activities.

v. Providing nutritional support to children of the primary stage in drought-affected areas during summer vacation.

8.2.2.4. Causes of the MDM Program

- **Promoting School Participation:** The midday meal has a significant impact on school participation, not only in terms of increasing the number of children who are enrolling in the registers, but also in terms of the regular attendance of students daily.
- **Preventing Classroom Hunger:** Many children reach school with an empty stomach. Even children who have a meal before they leave for school get hungry by the afternoon and are not able to concentrate – especially children from families who cannot give them a lunch box or are staying a long distance away from the school. Mid-day meals can help to overcome this problem by preventing "classroom hunger."
- **Facilitating the Healthy Growth of Children:** Mid-day meals can also act as a regular source of "supplementary nutrition" for children, and facilitate their healthy growth.
- **Intrinsic Educational Value:** A well-organized mid-day meal can be used as an opportunity to impart various good habits to children (such as washing one's hands before and after eating), and to educate them about the importance of clean water, good hygiene and other related matters.
- **Fostering Social Equality:** the midday meal can contribute to the dissemination of egalitarian values, as it teaches children from different social backgrounds to sit together and share a meal together. Among schoolchildren, the midday meal in particular has the potential to assist in breaking down barriers of caste and class.
- **Enhancing Gender Equity:** As a result of the Mid-Day Meal Scheme, the gender gap in school participation tends to narrow. This is because the scheme helps to erode the barriers that restrict girls from attending school. In addition to being a valuable source of employment for women, the Midday Meal Scheme also helps to relieve working women of the burden of having to prepare meals at home during the day. In addition to these and other ways, they have a special stake in the Midday Meal Scheme, which is for women and girl children.
- **Psychological Benefits:** Low self-esteem, which in turn leads to feelings of insecurity, anxiety, and stress, is a consequence of physiological deprivation. By addressing this issue and fostering cognitive, emotional, and social development, the Midday Meal Scheme can be of assistance.

8.3. Health Promotion and Education for Women and Children

When taking into consideration the factors that determine health, it is essential to be aware that poor physical circumstances are not the only factors that are detrimental to one's health to consider. For instance, a lack of education can potentially result in a diminished capacity to locate, comprehend, and make use of health information. Education is therefore a significant factor in determining health status in both the developed world and the developing world.

There is no denying the fact that investing in the education of women yields high returns in terms of health. High levels of self-reported health and physical functioning, as well as low levels of morbidity, mortality, and disability, are indicators that individuals with higher levels of education have better health than those with lower levels of education. There is a correlation between low educational attainment and high rates of infectious diseases, many chronic diseases that are not infectious, self-reported poor health, shorter survival times when sick, and a shorter life expectancy.

8.3.1. Women and Health Promotion in the Family

Although the precise mechanism by which education influences health is unknown, it has been hypothesized that the education of women modifies the conventional power dynamic within the family, which in turn causes alterations in the way decisions are made and resources are distributed within the household. Accordingly, mothers who have received an education are more likely to take advantage of modern medicine and adhere to the treatments that are recommended than mothers who have not received an education (Figure 8.4).

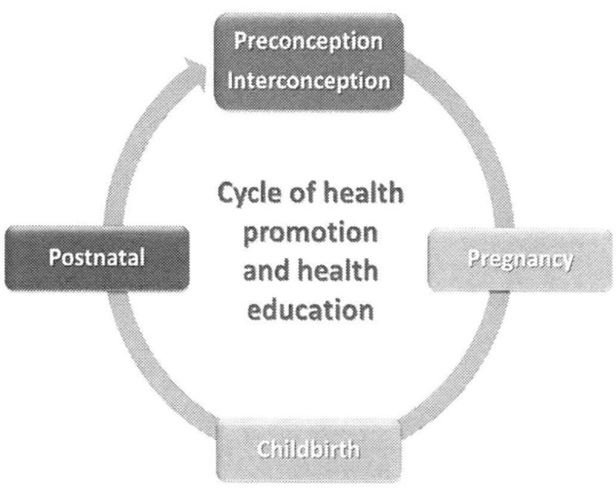

Figure 8.4. *Effective health promotion and health education.*

Source: Bergh A-M, Glob. libr. women's med., ISSN: 1756–2228; doi 10.3843/GLOWM.414253.

In addition, education has the potential to alter the amount of knowledge and perception that mothers have regarding the significance of modern medicine in the care of their children. For instance, children of mothers with higher levels of education benefited more from access to healthcare services than children of mothers with lower levels of education, according to the findings of a study on child nutrition in the Philippines. This finding suggested that mothers with higher levels of education were more likely to make use of the community health services that were available.

Take, for instance, the findings of numerous studies of infant and child mortality carried out in developing countries over the course of the past decade. These studies have shown that there is a nearly universally positive association between maternal education and child survival. Education has the potential to alter women's beliefs regarding the causes of disease, which in turn has an impact on the practices of childcare as well as the utilization of contemporary medical services. Considering these facts, women play a significant role in promoting health education and practices within the home, and the advantages of their education extend to their children as well as to other people.

8.3.2. Teachers and Health Promotion

Teachers serve as role models and have the potential to play a valuable role in the promotion of health in the classroom, just as mothers are important providers of health information about their children in the home. It is necessary for educators to have a "health literacy" for them to be able to encourage healthy behaviors. Health literacy for educators can be characterized as "the capacity of teachers to obtain, interpret, and understand basic health information and services, with the competence to use such information and services in ways that enhance the learning of health concepts and skills by school students."

Even though there have been significant advancements in community health promotion to address traditional early childhood diseases, there are still incredible obstacles to overcome to improve the health status of children and adolescents who are of school age.

The issues of health illiteracy, low self-esteem, and risk-taking behavior among young people are becoming more visible in the community and public schools in the United States of America, for instance. The alarmingly rising rates of health problems in young people are a direct result of risky behaviors and social morbidities. Educating students who may not be health literate and who have significant health needs is a challenge that schools in both developed and developing countries must face. These students have significant health needs. For teachers to promote health practices, they must be "health literate." Teacher health literacy may be defined as "the capacity of teachers to obtain, interpret, and understand basic health information and services, with the competence to use such information and services in ways that enhance the learning of health concepts and skills by school students."

While significant advances occurred in community health promotion to address traditional early childhood diseases, tremendous challenges remain in improving the health status of school-aged children and adolescents.

For example, in America, the problems of health illiteracy, low self-esteem, and youth risk-taking behavior are becoming more visible in the community and public schools. Risk behaviors and social morbidities have produced alarmingly rising rates of health problems in youth. Schools in the developed and developing world face the challenge of addressing the needs of students who may not be health literate and who have significant health needs.

8.3.3. Health Education Strategies

Many different approaches can be taken to teach students about health in the classroom, with varying degrees of emphasis placed on biological, behavioral, and pedagogical concepts. Educators and other professionals working in the health field must be well-equipped to deal with the intricate social, developmental, and health-related issues that young people bring into the classroom. To maximize the learning of important concepts and issues pertaining to the health of children and adolescents, one should continue to make efforts.

School teachers in developed countries receive training in health education that focuses on several different topics, including the following:

The first step is to teach health pedagogy skills. The second step is to provide health information from the ten traditional health content areas, which are community health, consumer health, environmental health, family health, mental health, injury prevention/safety, nutrition, personal health, diseases, and substance abuse. The third step is to investigate the six categories of risk behaviors that adolescents exhibit, as identified by the Centers for Disease Control and Prevention. Finally, the fourth step is to describe the eight components of a coordinated school health program.

It is necessary to conduct additional research to determine the health education strategies that are known to be the most effective for both students and mothers. To give one example, innovative approaches have the potential to improve upon conventional educational models. The best strategies will promote the four fundamental skills that are inherent in individuals who are health-literate. These skills are as follows:

1. the ability to think critically and solve problems;
2. the ability to be responsible and productive citizens
3. the ability to learn on their own initiative; and
4. the ability to communicate effectively.

8.4. Programs for the Welfare of Adolescent Girls and Women

The period of time known as adolescence is an important one in the life of a woman. At this point in time, she is on the verge of entering adult responsibilities. Not only is this stage the most eventful for mental, emotional, and psychological well-being, but it also serves as an intermediary between childhood and womanhood. However, if adolescent girls are not included in the developmental programs that are geared toward human resource development, the life-cycle approach to holistic child development will not be addressed.

A window of opportunity for the improvement of nutritional status and the correction of poor nutritional practices begins during the adolescent years, which are the transitional periods between childhood and adulthood. This is roughly the same period that marks the beginning of puberty, which typically occurs between the ages of 10 and 13 years old in females. There is a period known as the growth spurt that occurs during adolescence. This is a time when growth is extremely rapid. Changes in one's lifestyle may have an impact on one's eating habits and the foods that one chooses to consume during this period. Physical changes have an impact on the nutritional requirements of the body. To support the body's physical growth and to prevent future health problems, it is therefore essential for adolescents to consume properly. Therefore, it is imperative that every parent pays special attention to the necessities of their adolescents in terms of nutrition.

8.4.1. Nutrition Is Essential for Adolescent Girls

Any nutritional deficiency experienced during this critical period of life can influence the future health of the individual and their offspring. For example, failure to consume an adequate diet at this time can result in delayed sexual maturation and delayed or retarded physical growth. The rapid physical changes of adolescence have a direct influence on a person's nutritional needs. Increased demands for energy and nutrients are brought about by the growth spurt that occurs during adolescence, which is second only to the growth spurt that occurs during the first year of life. Therefore, optimal nutrition is a requirement for reaching one's full growth potential. This is because nutritional status and physical growth are dependent on one another.

Even though the nutrition of the adolescent girl is of utmost importance, under-nutrition, which can be defined as either an insufficient amount of food or food that is deficient in essential nutrients, is frequently overlooked by the families of adolescents or by the young people themselves. Preparing for the nutritional demands of pregnancy and lactation, which may be experienced by girls later in life, is something that should be done during the adolescent years.

Undernutrition has a negative impact on adolescent girls in several ways, including the following: it hinders their capacity to learn and work at their highest level of productivity; it raises the likelihood of unfavorable obstetric outcomes for teenage mothers; it impedes the healthy development of future children; it hinders sexual maturation and growth; and it negatively affects their ability to learn and work.

If a young person does not consume an adequate amount of calcium, it stops them from developing healthy teeth and preventing them from reaching normal bone strength.

The fact that children born to women who are short and thin have a higher likelihood of being stunted and underweight (low weight for age) themselves is another well-established fact. The fact that the adverse effects of malnutrition in adolescents continue to carry over into a woman's reproductive years is a more concerning aspect of the situation.

8.4.1.1. Energy

The level of activity, the basal metabolic rate, and the increased requirements to support pubertal growth and development all have an impact on the amount of energy that adolescents require. Teenagers require additional energy to continue their growth and activities. Girls in their teenage years require approximately 2,200 calories daily. Compared to the requirements for children, this represents a significant increase. To fulfill these calorie requirements, adolescents should select a wide range of nutritious foods, including lean protein sources, dairy products with a low-fat content, whole grains, fruits, and vegetables. Advertisements that are unhealthy, aggressive, and coercive can be a source of temptation for adolescents who are trying to satisfy their energy requirements. Therefore, it is necessary for them to have a solid understanding of the selection of nutritious foods both at home and at school.

8.4.1.2. Fats and Oils

Dietary fat continues to play important roles throughout the adolescent years, including serving as a source of energy, a significant component of cell structure, a precursor to biological agents that perform metabolic functions, and a powerful regulator of gene expression. 25% of total energy should come from fat, according to the dietary guidelines for children and adolescents. For children aged 15 and older, the percentage of energy that comes from saturated fat should be less than 10%. When determining the effects of dietary fat on one's health, the type of fat it contains is more important than the quantity of fat it contains. This is because research has demonstrated that following a diet low in fat for a period of eight years did not prevent cardiovascular disease, breast cancer, or colon cancer, and it did not have a significant impact on weight loss either. The consumption of skim milk and the selection of only lean meat options are two effective strategies for lowering the amount of fat that children consume. An adolescent population has shown that there is a positive association between the amount of saturated fats in the diet and the total cholesterol level. However, it is possible that dietary factors are more significant in girls.

8.4.1.3. Protein

Protein requirements of adolescents are based on the quantity of protein that is necessary for the preservation of the lean body mass that is already present as well as the development of additional lean body mass during the growth spurt that occurs during the adolescent years. When it comes to the development and preservation of muscle, protein is an essential component. The recommended daily intake of protein for adolescents is between 45 and 60 grams. Considering the amount of beef, chicken, eggs, and dairy products that most adolescents consume, this requirement is easily satisfied. Tofu and other soy-based foods, beans, and nuts are all plant-based sources of protein. Other vegetable sources of protein include nuts and beans. It is especially important for vegetarians to incorporate these foods into their diets. There can be a reduction in linear growth, a delay in sexual maturation, and a reduction in the accumulation of lean body mass when protein intakes are consistently inadequate.

8.4.1.4. Calcium

It is estimated that 45% of peak bone mass is achieved during adolescence, it is essential to consume an adequate amount of calcium to facilitate the development of dense bone mass and the reduction of the risk of fractures and osteoporosis throughout one's lifetime. Furthermore, due to the increased demand for skeletal growth, the calcium requirements during adolescence are higher than they are during either childhood or adulthood. Children and adults have lower calcium requirements. Enough calcium consumption is also necessary for the development of strong and dense bones during the growth spurt that occurs during adolescence. Osteoporosis is a condition that can develop later in life if an individual does not consume an adequate amount of calcium during their teenage years and early adulthood. It is recommended that adolescents consume three to four servings of foods that are high in calcium daily to accomplish the daily calcium intake requirement of 1,200 milligrams. Cheese, ice cream, and frozen yogurt are the next most calcium-rich foods that adolescents consume, after milk, which is the source of the most calcium in their diets.

As a result of their preoccupation with body shape, young women may find themselves in a difficult position when it comes to incorporating calcium-rich dairy foods into their diets. According to the findings of the National Nutrition Survey that was conducted in 1995, 56% of young girls between the ages of 9 and 13 did not consume the amount of calcium that is recommended for them to consume.

A recent study that was carried out in Canada discovered that there was no significant difference in the percentage of body fat that changed over a period of two years between girls who consumed different amounts of calcium from food. This suggests that the fear of gaining weight because of consuming dairy products is premature and may therefore not be a significant factor in the development of obesity-related conditions. Actually, it is more important to keep an eye on the kind of fat we consume than it is on the amount of fat we consume.

There is empirical evidence that suggests that unhealthy fats, specifically saturated and trans fats, are associated with an increased risk for certain diseases, whereas healthy fats, specifically monounsaturated and polyunsaturated fats, are associated with a decreased risk. One of the most fundamental ideas concerning the prevention of diseases that are associated with the consumption of fat is to replace unhealthy fats with healthy fats.

8.4.1.5. Iron

Iron plays a critical role in the transportation of oxygen throughout the bloodstream. Iron deficiency is the root cause of anemia, which in turn causes symptoms such as fatigue, confusion, and weakness. Because of the rapid growth that occurs during adolescence, as well as the expansion of blood volume and muscle mass, the requirement for iron rises. This is a direct consequence of their rapid growth. As adolescents increase their muscle mass, they require a greater quantity of iron to assist their newly formed muscle cells in obtaining oxygen for energy. In girls, the onset of menstruation brings about an increase in their requirements for iron.

8.4.1.6. Zinc

Because of its role in both growth and sexual maturation, zinc is an essential nutrient during the adolescent years. As a result of the rapid growth and hormonal changes that take place during adolescence, it is common knowledge that serum zinc levels decrease. There was a range of 18% to 33% of female adolescents who had serum zinc levels that were indicative of a mild zinc deficiency.

The recommended daily allowance (RDA) for zinc for males and females between the ages of 9 and 13 is 8 milligrams (about the weight of a grain of table salt) per day. RDA 9 mg (about the weight of a grain of table salt) per day for females between the ages of 14 and 18. Red meats, shellfish, and whole grains are known to contain a high concentration of zinc. A significant number of breakfast cereals also contain zinc as an added ingredient.

There is a competition between zinc and iron for absorption, which means that increased intakes of one can reduce the absorption of the other. If the intake of iron is more than twice as high as the intake of zinc, then adolescents who take iron supplements may be at an increased risk of developing a mild zinc deficiency.

8.4.1.7. Folate

In the process of synthesizing DNA, RNA, and proteins, folate is an essential component. As a result, the amounts of folate that adolescents require during puberty are significantly higher. Certain foods, such as ready-to-eat cereal, orange juice, bread, milk, and dried beans or lentils, are among the dietary folate sources that adolescents consume in large quantities. Adolescents who have developed the habit of skipping breakfast or who do not include orange juice and ready-to-eat cereals in their meals may be at a greater risk of having a low folate intake.

8.4.2. Potential nutrition-Related Problems for Adolescent Children

The development of poor eating habits during the formative years of adolescence can have both immediate and long-term effects on a person's health, including the development of obesity, osteoporosis, and delays in sexual maturation. Several health problems, including obesity, chronic diseases related to obesity, and eating disorders, are associated with adolescents.

8.4.2.1. Obesity

Overweight and obesity among adolescents is on the rise all over the world. According to reports, the prevalence of overweight and obesity among children and adolescents is on the rise, which suggests that there may be a problem with energy imbalance. There is a correlation between obesity and an increased risk of diseases that are associated with obesity, such as diabetes and heart disease. This rise in obesity has been linked by experts to a lack of physical activity as well as an increase in the amount of fast food and "junk food" that is available to adolescents. Adolescents can maintain a healthy weight by engaging in physical activity and avoiding foods and beverages that are high in fat and sugar.

8.4.2.2. Eating Disorders

It is possible for eating disorders, excessive eating, and undereating to have a negative impact on one's health. Self-image refers to the fact that adolescents are typically very self-conscious about their appearances and may experience feelings of pressure to be thin or to look a certain way. Eating habits that are excessively restrictive may be the result of a fear of becoming obese. Sometimes, to maintain control of their weight, adolescents will even resort to self-induced vomiting to achieve their goals.

8.4.3. High-Risk Adolescent Group

Certain groups of adolescents may be at a greater risk for nutritional deficiencies than others, even though adolescents in general are vulnerable in terms of their nutritional status.

This category of adolescents includes the following:

- **Pregnant Adolescents:** When an adolescent becomes pregnant, she has a greater requirement for nutrients than her coworker who is not pregnant. This is because she needs to provide support for her baby as well as her own continued growth and physical development. If her nutritional requirements are not satisfied, her child may be born with inadequate fetal growth, which may result in a low birth weight or other health issues.
- **Athletes:** Adolescents involved in athletics may feel pressure to be at a particular weight or to perform at a certain level. Some young athletes may be tempted to adopt unhealthy behaviors such as crash dieting, taking supplements to improve performance, or eating unhealthy foods to fulfill their hearty appetites. A balanced nutritional outlook is important for good health and athletic performance.
- **Vegetarians:** Many people believe that a vegetarian diet is the healthiest option. Nevertheless, adolescents who adhere to a vegetarian diet, whether for religious or personal reasons, are required to carefully plan their consumption to ensure that they obtain the necessary amounts of protein and minerals. Individuals who adhere to a strict vegetarian diet, also known as vegans, and who do not consume any eggs or dairy products may require nutritional supplements to fulfill their requirements for calcium, vitamin B12, and iron (UN HABITAT, 2006, 2007).

A Closer Look

Food Safety Policy

Food safety policy is a critical framework designed to protect public health by ensuring that food consumed is safe, wholesome, and free from contaminants. At the core of food safety policy are regulations and standards that govern the entire food supply chain, from farm to table. These policies are crafted to prevent foodborne illnesses, which can have severe health consequences and economic impacts. Key components include hygiene standards, proper handling and storage procedures, and the use of safe agricultural practices.

Governments play a pivotal role in enforcing food safety policies through regulatory bodies such as the Food and Drug Administration (FDA) in the United States or the European Food Safety Authority (EFSA) in the European Union. These agencies are responsible for conducting inspections, issuing guidelines, and taking corrective actions when necessary. They also work closely with international organizations like the World Health Organization (WHO) and the Food and Agriculture Organization (FAO) to harmonize food safety standards globally.

Traceability is another critical aspect of food safety policy, allowing for the tracking of food products through all stages of production, processing, and distribution. This is essential for quickly identifying and responding to food safety incidents, such as contamination or outbreaks of foodborne diseases. Advanced technologies, including blockchain and RFID, are increasingly being integrated into food safety systems to enhance traceability and transparency.

Public awareness and education are also vital components of food safety policy. Consumers must be informed about safe food handling practices and the importance of food safety to reduce risks at the household level. Educational campaigns and clear labeling on food products help in achieving this goal.

Summary

The purpose of this chapter is to investigate the significant part that nutrition plays in community health as well as the numerous approaches, programs, and policies that have been developed to address nutritional challenges in communities all over the world. It discusses the significance of nutritional assessments in determining the deficiencies and excesses that are present in the diets of the population, which can result in the development of chronic diseases and outcomes that are detrimental to health. The text highlights successful community health initiatives and interventions, such as fortification, supplementation, and educational campaigns, to reduce the prevalence of malnutrition, obesity, and other non-communicable diseases to improve dietary habits and reduce the prevalence of these diseases. In addition to this, it investigates the policy frameworks that have been established and the collaborative efforts that have been made by governments, non-governmental organizations, and the private sector to develop healthier food environments and improve access to nutritious foods. To effectively improve community health, the chapter emphasizes the importance of utilizing evidence-based approaches, cultural sensitivity, and sustainable practices in the process of designing and implementing nutrition programs and policies.

References

1. African Population and Health Research Center. (2002). *Population and Health Dynamics in Nairobi's Informal Settlements: Report of the Nairobi Cross-Sectional Slums Survey*. Nairobi, Kenya: African Population and Health Research Center.
2. Bell, D. M., Weisfuse, I. B., Hernandez-Avila, M., Rio, C., Bustamante, X., & Rodier, G. (2009). Pandemic influenza as 21st Century urban public health crisis. *Emerging Infectious Diseases, 15*(12), 1963–1969. https://doi.org/10.3201/eid1512.091232.
3. Burra, S. (2005). Towards a pro-poor framework for slum upgrading in Mumbai, India. *Environment and Urbanization, 17*(1), 67–88. https://doi.org/10.1177/095624780501700105.
4. Burris, S., Hancock, T., Lin, V., & Herzog, A. (2007). Emerging strategies for healthy urban governance. *Journal of Urban Health, 84*(3), 154–163. https://doi.org/10.1007/s11524-007-9163-7.
5. Diaz, C. (2012). Preventing dengue at the local level in Havana City. *Eco Health Research and Practice, 1*(2), 163–171. https://doi.org/10.1007/s10393-012-0764-7.
6. Ezzati, M., Vander Hoorn, S., Lawes, C. M. M., Leach, R., James, W. P. T., Lopez, A. D., Rodgers, A., & Murray, C. J. L. (2005). Rethinking the 'Diseases of Affluence' paradigm: Global patterns of nutritional risks in relation to economic development. *PLoS Medicine, 2*(5), e133. https://doi.org/10.1371/journal.pmed.0020133.
7. Fidler, D. (2007). Architecture amidst anarchy: Global health's quest for governance. *Global Health Governance, 1*(1), 1–17.
8. Galea, S., Freudenberg, N., & Vlahov, D. (2005). Cities and population health. *Social Science & Medicine, 60*(5), 1017–1033. https://doi.org/10.1016/j.socscimed.2004.06.036.
9. Gostin, L., & Mok, E. (2009). Grand challenges in global health governance. *British Medical Bulletin, 90*(1), 7–18. https://doi.org/10.1093/bmb/ldp014.
10. Grimond, J. (2007). The world goes to town: A special report on cities. *The Economist, 383*(8531), 3–18.

11. Gruebner, O., Staffeld, R., Khan, M. M. H., Burkart, K., Krämer, A., & Hostert, P. (2011). Urban health in megacities extending the framework for developing countries. *International Human Dimensions Programme on Global Environmental Change: Update, 1*(1), 42–49.

12. Katz, R., Kornblet, S., Arnold, G., Lief, E., & Fischer, J. (2011). Global health diplomacy: Changing demands in the era of globalization. *The Milbank Quarterly, 89*(3), 503–523. https://doi.org/10.1111/j.1468-0009.2011.00638.x.

13. Khan, M. M., Khan, A., Kraemer, A., & Mori, M. (2009). Prevalence and correlates of smoking among urban adult men in Bangladesh: Slum versus non-slum comparison. *BMC Public Health, 9*(1), 149. https://doi.org/10.1186/1471-2458-9-149.

14. Kirton, J., & Mannell, J. (2005). *The G8 and Global Health Governance*. Presented at the global health governance: Past practice: Future innovation conference, Ottawa and waterloo, Canada. Retrieved from: http://www.g7.utoronto.ca/scholar/kirton2005/kirton_waterloo2005.pdf (accessed on 11 July 2024).

15. Krämer, A., Khan, M. H., & Jahn, H. (2011). Public health in megacities and urban areas: A conceptual framework. In A. Krämer, M. H. Khan, & F. Krass (Eds.), *Health in Megacities and Urban Areas* (pp. 3–19). New York, NY: Springer. https://doi.org/10.1007/978-1-4419-9195-9_1.

16. Loewenson, R. (2011). The upcoming Rio conference on social determinants of health. *Health Diplomacy Monitor, 2*(3), 10–12.

17. Lönnroth, K., Jaramillo, E., Williams, B. G., Dye, C., & Raviglione, M. (2009). Drivers of tuberculosis epidemics: The role of risk factors and social determinants. *Social Science & Medicine, 68*(12), 2240–2246. https://doi.org/10.1016/j.socscimed.2009.03.041.

18. Machemedze, R. (2011). Climate change and health: African countries at greater risk of increased disease burden. *Health Diplomacy Monitor, 2*(4), 15–17.

19. McMichael, A. (2010). The urban environment and health in a world of increasing globalization: Issues for developing countries. *Bulletin of the World Health Organization, 78*(9), 1117–1126. https://doi.org/10.2471/blt.10.021010.

20. Miranda, J. J., Kinra, S., Casas, J. P., Davey Smith, G., & Ebrahim, S. (2008). Non-communicable diseases in low- and middle-income countries: Context, determinants and health policy. *Tropical Medicine & International Health, 13*(10), 1225–1234. https://doi.org/10.1111/j.1365-3156.2008.02116.x.

21. Montgomery, M. (2009). Urban poverty and health in developing countries. *Population Bulletin, 64*(2), 1–16.

22. Moore, M., Gould, P., & Keary, B. S. (2003). Global urbanization and impact on health. *International Journal of Hygiene and Environmental Health, 206*(4–5), 269–278. https://doi.org/10.1078/1438-4639-00223.

23. Narayan, V., Ali, M. K., & Koplan, J. (2010). Global noncommunicable diseases—Where worlds meet. *The New England Journal of Medicine, 363*(13), 1196–1198. https://doi.org/10.1056/NEJMp1002024.

24. Ng, N., & Ruger, J. P. (2011). Global health governance at a crossroads. *Global Health Governance, 3*(2), 1–37.

25. Online data set. (2009). HIV/AIDS survey indicators database. Available online: http://www.

measuredhs.com/hivdata/ (accessed on 11 July 2024).

26. Pampel, F. (2008). Tobacco use in sub-Sahara Africa: Estimates from the demographic health surveys. *Social Science & Medicine, 66*(8), 1772–1783. https://doi.org/10.1016/j.socscimed.2007.12.003.
27. Pappas, G. (2011). Conceptual framework: Megacities and public health. In O. Khan (Ed.), *Megacities and Global Health* (pp. 11–33). Washington, DC, USA: American Public Health Association.
28. Rahman, O., Rabbani, K. A., & Tooheen, R. B. (2011). Slums, pollution, and ill health: The case of Dhaka, Bangladesh. In O. Khan (Ed.), *Megacities and Global Health* (pp. 51–76). Washington, DC, USA: Public Health Association.
29. Roy, A. (2002). *Power Politics* (2nd ed.). Cambridge, MA, USA: South End Press.
30. Satterthwaite, D. (2004). The under-estimation of urban poverty in low and middle-income nations. *Human Settlements Working Paper Series Poverty Reduction in Urban Areas; International Institute for Environment and Development*. Retrieved from: http://pubs.iied.org/9322IIED.html (accessed on 11 July 2024).
31. Shetty, P. (2011). Healthcare for urban poor falls through the gap. *Lancet, 377*(9766), 627–628. https://doi.org/10.1016/S0140-6736(11)60222-3.
32. Shiffman, J. (2006). Donor funding priorities for communicable disease control in the developing world. *Health Policy and Planning, 21*(6), 411–420. https://doi.org/10.1093/heapol/czl029.
33. Stephens, C. (2007). Charting a new course of urban public health. In *State of the World 2007: Our Urban Future* (Chapter 7). Washington, DC, USA: Worldwatch Institute.
34. Tana, S., Abeyewickreme, W., Arunachalam, N., Espino, F., Kittayapong, P., Wai, K. T., Horstick, O., & Sommerfeld, J. (2012). Eco-bio-social research on dengue in Asia: General principles and a case study from Indonesia. *Ecohealth Research and Practice, 1*(2), 173–184. https://doi.org/10.1007/s10393-012-0772-7.
35. Taylor, A. (2004). Governing the globalization of public health. *Journal of Law, Medicine & Ethics, 32*(3), 500–508. https://doi.org/10.1111/j.1748-720X.2004.tb00166.x.
36. UN HABITAT. (2002). *Global Campaign on Urban Governance: Concept Paper* (2nd revised ed.). Nairobi, Kenya: UN HABITAT. Retrieved from: www.unhabitat.org/downloads/docs/2099_24326_concept_paper.doc (accessed on 11 July 2024).
37. UN HABITAT. (2006). *State of the World Cities Report 2006/7*. London, UK: Earthscan.
38. UN HABITAT. (2007). *Situation Analysis of Informal Settlements in Addis Ababa*. In *Cities Without Slums: Sub-Regional Program for Eastern and Southern Africa*. Nairobi, Kenya: United Nations Human Settlements Programme.
39. Unger, A., & Riley, L. (2007). Slum health: From understanding to action. *PLoS Medicine, 4*(10), e295. https://doi.org/10.1371/journal.pmed.0040295.
40. United Nations Population Fund. (2007). *Linking Population, Poverty, and Development: Urbanization: A Majority in Cities*. New York, NY, USA: United Nations Population Fund. Retrieved from: http://www.unfpa.org/pds/urbanization.htm (accessed on 11 July 2024).
41. United Nations Population Fund. (2011). *As the World Passes 7 billion Milestone, UN Urges Action to Meet Key Challenges*. New York, NY, USA: United Nations Population Fund. Retrieved

from: http://www.un.org/apps/news/story.asp?NewsID=40257 (accessed on 11 July 2024).

42. Vlahov, D. (2007). Urban as a determinant of health. *Journal of Urban Health, 84*(1), 16–26. https://doi.org/10.1007/s11524-007-9169-1.

43. Vlahov, D. (2011). Urban health in the context of twenty-first-century megatrends. In O. Khan (Ed.), *Megacities and Global Health* (pp. 35–50). Washington, DC, USA: American Public Health Association.

44. Vlahov, D., & Galea, S. (2002). Urbanization, urbanicity, and health. *Journal of Urban Health, 79*(S1), S1–S12. https://doi.org/10.1093/jurban/79.suppl_1.S1.

45. Wilder-Smith, A., & Gubler, D. J. (2008). Geographic expansion of dengue: The impact of international travel. *Medical Clinics of North America, 92*(6), 1377–1390. https://doi.org/10.1016/j.mcna.2008.07.002.

46. Williams, O. D., & Rushton, S. (2011). Are the 'good times' over? Looking to the future of global health governance. *Global Health Governance, 5*(1), 1–16.

47. World Health Organization. (2003). *Severe Acute Respiratory Syndrome (SARS): Status of the Outbreak and Lessons for the Immediate Future—Unmasking a New Disease*. Geneva, Switzerland: WHO. Retrieved from: https://www.who.int/health-topics/severe-acute-respiratory-syndrome#tab=tab_1 (accessed on 11 July 2024).

48. World Health Organization. (2009). *Dengue: Guidelines for Diagnosis, Treatment, Prevention and Control—New Edition*. Geneva, Switzerland: WHO. Retrieved from: https://www.who.int/publications/i/item/9789241547871 (accessed on 11 July 2022).

49. World Health Organization. (2011). *Global Tuberculosis Control: WHO Report 2011*. Geneva, Switzerland: WHO. Retrieved from: https://www.who.int/publications/i/item/9789241564380 (accessed on 11 July 2022).

50. World Health Organization. (2011). *WHO Framework Convention on Tobacco Control: Overview*. Geneva, Switzerland: WHO. Retrieved from: https://fctc.who.int/who-fctc/overview (accessed on 11 July 2024).

51. Worobey, M., Gemmel, M., Teuwen, D. E., Haselkorn, T., Kunstman, K., Bunche, M., Muyembe, J., Kabongo, J. M., Kalengayi, R. M., Van Marck, E., et al. (2008). Direct evidence of extensive diversity of HIV-1 in Kinshasa by 1960. https://doi.org/10.1038/nature07390.

INDEX

T

U

V

W

FSC
www.fsc.org
MIX
Papier | Fördert gute Waldnutzung
FSC® C083411

Kolibri 360 GmbH
Ferdinand-Jühlke-Straße 7
99095 Erfurt, Deutschland
produktsicherheit@kolibri360.de